Second Edition: Updated & Expanded

REVERSING TYPE 2 DIABETES KIDNEY DISEASE & HEART DISEASE

EXPOSING LONGEVITY & OLD AGE SECRETS TO LIVING INTO YOUR 90s

2 Books in 1
By Author Who Did It

VELTISEZAR BAUTISTA

IN HIS 90s

Library of Congress Control Number: 2023908019

Publisher's Cataloging-in-Publication

(Provided by Cassidy Cataloguing Services, Inc.)

Names: Bautista, Veltisezar B., 1933- author.

Title: Reversing Type 2 diabetes, kidney disease, & heart disease : exposing longevity & old age secrets to living into your 90s : 2 books in 1 / by someone who did it, Veltisezar Bautista, age 90.

Description: Second edition, updated & expanded. | Sterling Heights, Michigan U.S.A. : LibroCasa LLC.

[2023] | "Previously published as 'Unmasking Type 2 diabetes, kidney disease, and heart disease' (2021 and 2022)." | Includes bibliographical references and index

Identifiers ISBN: 978-1-7358579-1-6 (paperback) / 978-1-7358579-8-5 (hardcover) | 978-1-7358579-4-7 (ebook) | LCCN: 2023908019

Subjects:LCSH: Type 2 diabetes-- Alternative treatment. | Diabetes-- Alternative treatment. | Kidneys

-- Diseases -- Alternative treatment. | Heart-- Diseases -- Alternative treatment. | Self- care,

Health -- Popular works. | Aging-- Prevention-- Popular works. | Longevity-- Popular works. |

Diet therapy-- Popular works. | Exercise therapy-- Popular works.

Classification:LCC: RC661.A47 B382 2023 | DDC: 616.4/6206--dc23

Disclaimer: This book is for informational purposes and is not a substitute for medical professionals' evaluation, diagnosis, and treatment. Please consult with your doctor or a qualified health care practitioner if you have medical problems or concerns.

https://www.librocasa.com

Email: info@librocasa.com

DEDICATION

I dedicate this book to the light of my life,
the late Genoveva Abes-Bautista;
to my children,
Hubert, Lester, Melvin, Ronald, and Janet;
to my daughters-in-law,
Maria Cecilia Asi-Bautista (Lester's wife),
Faith Gonzales-Bautista (Melvin's wife),
and Reccie Borja-Bautista (Ronald's wife),
and to all patients throughout the world
who have prediabetes, Type 2 Diabetes,
Kidney Disease, and Heart Disease

Amazon Customer Reviews

Reversing Type 2 Diabetes, Kidney Disease and Heart: Exposing Longevity & Old Age Secrets to Living into Your 90s By Veltisezar Bautista

Top reviews from the United States

Rene Korpolinski

5.0 out of 5 stars

Timely, amazing and inspiring book!

Reviewed in the United States on October 28, 2023

Verified Purchase

A talented, seasoned writer presents his personal journey reversing type two diabetes, kidney disease, and heart disease. This book is well researched and a first hand depiction of longevity approaches many of which mirror blue zone research findings and principles. Happy 90th birthday Mr. Bautista!

PhotoPen

5.0 out of 5 stars Lots of information

Reviewed in the United States on December 1, 2023

Verified Purchase

The book was an easy read and lots of information from the author's experience. My spouse has type 2 and this was a very helpful book for us on what to change in our diet and lifestyle. Definitely highly recommended. Thank you for publishing this book.

Lolinda Takahashi

5.0 out of 5 stars Great read and very informative

Reviewed in the United States on November 22, 2023

Verified Purchase

The author did tremendous research on several diseases, and applied everything to reverse his type 2 diabetes, kidney disease, and heart disease.

I admired his knowledge, preserverance, and self discipline to reach his goal in life... Longevity!

-Lolinda Takahashi

Preface

Maybe you already have read a book or several books on diabetes, kidney disease, or heart disease, and secrets to healthy aging and longevity. But I think that after just browsing this book, titled *Reversing Type 2 Diabetes, Kidney Disease, Heart Disease: Exposing Longevity & Old Age Secrets to Living into Your 90s, 2 Books in 1,* By Author Who Did It, Veltisezar Bautista, you'll notice that the book is easy to read and understand, well-organized, and has countless vital facts and statistics.

In other words, the book is a new—thorough approach to reversing and putting type 2 diabetes and kidney disease into remission and reversing heart disease severity and stabilizing it into a better shape.

Many subjects in this ultimate guide are not discussed or mentioned in other books on diabetes, renal disease, cardiac disease, healthy living, and longevity. It's because it covers a wide range of subjects, compiled into 2 books in 1 volume. Yes, you can find a lot of diabetes information and longevity online. But there's no better way of gaining enough knowledge about these diseases and secrets to living in the 90s, in a shorter time, with a little effort, than reading this comprehensive and interesting book.

That means you don't need to read many books and spend long hours researching health matters and healthy aging online. This author compiled many tips and strategies in this book, based on his hands-on experience and thorough research. In a good reference book, such as this, you'll find a goldmine of information about these body disorders that you can read in the comfort of your home office or bedroom while resting.

In most chapters, the author inserted information on his successful disease journey.

Different from Other Books

I'm sure, in reading it, you'll find this book to be different from other disease books. I think it's the only one of its kind--extensive and chock-full of information and resources.

The book can be your reference guide, now and for years to come. My treatment system works!

The tips and strategies in this book are practical, and I also believe that you'll learn many things about how to treat these chronic diseases with the guidance of your doctor or doctors.

My Journey: Documented Proofs of Reversal of Type 2 Diabetes, Kidney Disease, and Heart Disease and other Conditions.

I have presented laboratory blood test results and procedures in this book to prove that I have reversed and put my type 2 diabetes and kidney disease into remission and reversed my heart failure severity, and stabilized it into a better condition. I got the documents from *My Charts* at my hospital on its website. (The original documents are with the records department of the hospital.)

I also got rid of my tinnitus (ringing in the ears), improved my incontinence, cured my peripheral neurophaty, and stopped my having falls, due to my exercises, techniques and strategies.

How Can This Book Help You?

In this book, a comprehensive guide chock-full of information and resources, *you'll discove*r

- The author's exercise regimen that decreases blood sugar by 30 to 60 points in just a 20-minute exercise, as part of three 20-minute exercise sessions daily
- Steps to reduce HbA1c, increase EGFR or GFR, and jump-start the weak heart
- A new flexible semi-plant-based diet style for people with diabetes, kidney disease, and heart disease
- The liquid that dissolves blood sugar, creatinine, and urea blood nitrogen (BUN), reducing their levels in the blood
- 4 effective vitamins for the treatment of peripheral neuropathy
- The mystery and benefits of the low glycemic index (GI) and glycemic load (GL) value of foods

- The amazing device that works like a robot to energize the heart and increase its ejection fraction
- 60 photos that make the pages alive and book interesting

And much, much more.

Flashback of Events

On that day in 1996, I thought it was the year of the end of my life. When I was having chest pain, an ambulance rushed me to a hospital in the state of Michigan, U.S.A. After being hooked on several machines, the doctor told me that I had a heart attack, and had undergone a medical procedure called angioplasty.

It was a massive heart attack, meaning the cardiac event affected and damaged a large portion of the heart muscles.

But I didn't die. My age then was 63; now, I am in my 90s and look forward to my being 95-100. What a joy to think of it!

Then followed my other disease: kidney disease caused by diabetes. (Details in Chapter 7.)

Angioplasty: Medical Procedure

Then the doctor told me he did an angioplasty. This procedure involves putting a coronary stent, a tiny, expanded metal mesh coil, into the artery's newly opened area. Purpose: To help keep the artery from narrowing and closing again. Then the tissue will start to coat the stent.

After the procedure, the attending doctor told me a blockage of the main artery supplying blood to the heart's left ventricle caused the heart attack.

The Heart Chambers

The heart has four chambers: two atriums and two ventricles.

- **Right atrium: It** receives deoxygenated blood (blood with no oxygen) and sends it to the right ventricle.
- **Right ventricle**: It pumps the blood to the lungs to oxygenate; thus, it becomes oxygenated. The blood is pumped back to the

heart's left side by the pulmonary (lung) artery connected to the left atrium.

- **Left atrium**: It receives the blood with oxygen from the lungs and pumps it to the left ventricle.
- **Left ventricle**: The left ventricle pumps the blood to the aorta, the main artery that carries blood away from the heart to the rest of the body.

Kidney Disease

In 2011, my primary physician diagnosed me with having a third-stage kidney disease as a complication of diabetes.

(I got my heart failure condition during my heart attack in 1996.)

Writing the Book

Based on my studies, research, and experiments, I compiled information, writing it in simple, easily to understand, and well-organized book, containing major diseases and conditions, with causes, symptoms, and treatments, all nutrients, including minerals, and vitamins needed for healthy living to achieve longevity, as the author did.

Through my extensive knowledge of these diseases and experiments, I have become somewhat an authority on the subject, making me a human guinea pig. I am not a doctor, but once, an emergency physician mistook me for a doctor based on how I conversed with him. "*How did you know all these things?*" he asked me.

Ideas From My Brain and the Brains of Medical Experts

As a veteran author (I have written other nonfiction books), I have put a lot of work into this guide, using also the brains of medical experts. Well, writing is my passion and publishing is my business.

When I talk to you about tips and strategies, they can either come from my brain or the brains of medical doctors, dietitians, and other health experts, including well-known medical practitioners, and famous institutions mentioned in this book. That means, sometimes, they are the ones talking to you, not me.

Read the Book and Digest It

I wrote this book because I wanted to share my journey and research information on type 2 diabetes, kidney disease, heart disease, healthy aging, and other diseases and conditions and of course, my longevity.

If you have loved this book, and enjoyed it or have hated it, you may post a review on amazon.com website, expressing your views about your experience in reading and using the ideas and strategists in this guide. Thank you so much.

The Joys of Life!

And finally, two of my last significant dreams in America, to reverse my diseases and put them into remission or a better condition, and to have a long life, which some people say are difficult to accomplish--have been realized. Now I can face the world and proudly say, "These, I have done!" --Veltisezar Bautista

Table of Contents

Chapter 1

The Secrets to My Kicking & Alive at Age 90 Plus

Brief Subject Summary

- My Medical Record and Life Journey
- America, Here I Come!
- Heart Attack
- What Happened?
- Heart Failure After Heart Attack?
- Open Heart Surgery
- Diabetes Diagnosis in 2006
- Diagnosis of Kidney Disease in 2011
- Implantation of ICD (Implantable Cardioverter Device) in 2011
- Implantation of CRT-D (Cardiac Resynchronization Therapy with Defibrillator) in 2018
- Reversal of kidney disease in 2020, when the GFR level increased from 35% in 2016 to 73% in 2020, putting the condition into remission
- An increase of ejection fraction from 15% in 2016 to 47% in 2020, reversing severity of heart failure from Class 3 (Stage 3) to Class 1 (Stage 1)

Hello, World!

I thought I was going to die.

On that day, 27 years ago, while hooked to several machines in a hospital in Michigan, U.S.A, the doctor told me I had a massive heart attack that caused extensive bleeding; I was devastated.

It was a shocker! Why? What happened? I asked myself.

But I didn't die.

God kept me alive. I was then 63; I am now in my 90s and looking forward to being 95-100.

Yes, my medical story began in 1996 when I had a heart attack that led to heart failure, nearly costing my life. But up to this day, I can do moderate-intensity walking, covering a distance of 3.3 miles to 3.5 miles every day.

In 2006, I had a double vision problem. It was similar to being crossed-eyed; my two eyes saw different things or two overlapping views. Also, I could not walk without closing one of my eyes because they were pointed in two different directions.

I had a blood test. The result was I had very high blood sugar, revealing I had type 2 diabetes.

And then, in 2003, I had quadruple open-heart bypass surgery.

Not only that, in 2011, my primary physician diagnosed me with having third-stage kidney disease.

Complications

My doctors attributed my diseases: heart disease and kidney disease to complications of diabetes. I had a heart attack due to the accumulation of plaques and blood sugar that clogged my arteries. Diabetes blood sugar obstructing the small eye veins brought on my blurred vision. It went away after three months.

Summary of Author's Medical History and Life Journey

- Age: 90
- Education: in The Philippines
- Occupation: Retired U.S. federal employee and a multi-award-winning author
- Diet: Semi-Plant-Based Diet
- Immigration to the U.S.A: March 13, 1976
- Back to U.S. After 13 Years Living in the Philippines: Dec 2016

Medical Records

- Heart attack: February, 1996
- Implantation of 1st Implantable Cardiac Device (ICD/Pacemaker: 2011
- The author has slowed, reversed, stabilized, and put his type 2 diabetes and kidney disease into prolonged remission

- Kidney Disease: Diagnosed with G3-B (Third-B Stage) Kidney Disease: 2011
- Reversing and Putting His Type 2 Diabetes in 2015
- Kidney Disease: GFR 35% in 2016 increased to 73% (normal function) in the later part of 2020, the year that he put his kidney disease into remission. The GFR this year was also 73%.
- 2020: The year that he improved his ejection fraction from 15% in 2016 to 47% in 2020, reversing the severity of his heart failure from 3rd-B to Class 1 (Stage 1).

America, Here We Come!

My wife, Dr. Genoveva Abes-Bautista, (deceased), and I, landed as immigrants (aboard a Pan Am plane) in Hawaii on March 13, 1976, during which I said: "America here we come!"

And later, we flew to California to settle there for our American dream. Later, we moved to Michigan to live and work here for 30 years. I'm back here in Michigan after retiring for 13 years in the Philippines, during which I lived there with my wife until she died in 2016.

The Beginning of My Medical Adventure

My journey goes back to 1996 when I had a massive heart attack. But I am a survivor. And now, after 26 years, at the age of 89, I can still walk at moderate intensity, walking 3.3 miles to 3.5 miles every day, week after week, month after month.

I: Heart Attack

As already mentioned, I had my first and only heart attack in 1996, which was one of the most frightening and devastating events in my life.

John Hopkins Medicine describes heart attack as follows:

"When a plaque breaks (ruptures), a blood clot quickly forms. The blood clot is the actual cause of the heart attack. If the blood and oxygen supply is cut off, muscle cells of the heart begin to suffer damage and start to die. Irreversible damage begins within 30 minutes of blockage."

What Happened?

God kept me alive. I became a living testimony on how to recover from a massive heart attack and tell the story of what it's like to be a diabetic and afflicted with kidney disease and heart disease.

Heart Failure Immediately After Heart Attack?

My cardiologist and primary doctors say that I have heart failure. But neither one of them can determine when my heart failure started.

My present doctor, who has been my cardiologist for the past 20 years, can not determine when I suffered heart failure. I am not surprised because he was not the one who attended to me when I had a cardiac event.

WebMD says, "Sometimes, heart failure comes on suddenly after a heart attack."

I agree with WebMD's statement: My congestive heart failure occurred after I had the heart attack. No doubt about that.

My Heart Attack

My primary doctor says that I might have had heart failure when my heart weakened. Therefore, because of this reasoning, I have had heart failure since my heart attack.

The heart attack severely damaged 40% of my heart. And that cardiac event was the beginning of my heart failure, as I have said.

I had my open heart surgery at a hospital in Royal Oak, Michigan, U.S.A., because several arteries had suffered artery blockages. The surgeon did two procedures on my heart in the early part of 2003.

Removal of Dead tissues from My Heart (Dor Procedure)

Besides the quadruple open heart bypass, the surgeon also did a procedure called Dor Procedure, slashing away the damaged tissues of my heart to prevent the occurrence of aortic aneurysm. The process makes the heart lighter but stronger to pump blood throughout the body.

The Texas Heart Institute says, "An aneurysm is a balloon-like bulge in the wall of a weakened blood vessel. If the bulging stretches the vessel wall too far, the vessel may burst."

Background

It was in 1996 when I had a massive heart attack. After it happened, my ejection fraction was only 27%. With medicines and rehabilitation, I was able to increase my ejection fraction to 36%.

Cleveland Clinic says, "Ejection fraction (EF) refers to how well your left ventricle (or right ventricle) pumps blood with each heartbeat." It adds, "Most times, EF refers to the amount of blood being pumped out of the left ventricle each time it contracts. The left ventricle is the heart's main pumping chamber. Your EF is expressed as a percentage."

Pacemaker Replacement

On September 7, 2018, an electrophysiologist implanted a cardiac resynchronization therapy (CRT-D) device with a defibrillator in my left chest to replace the old implanted cardioverter device (ICD) that ran out of battery.

There are two types of cardiac resynchronization therapy (CRT) devices: the CRT-P and the CRT-D. In other words, each of them is a two-in-one device. The CRT-P has a pacemaker, and the CRT-D has a pacemaker and a defibrillator. (See Chapter 8.)

What's the Purpose of CRT-D?

The purpose of the CRT-D is to resynchronize the pumping by the left and right ventricles so that they can do their actions simultaneously. The device can make the heart stronger, increasing the heart's ejection fraction to supply enough blood to the whole body.

Back to Almost Normal Ejection Fraction

Wow! My ejection fraction rose from 15% in 2016 to 47% in 2020, recorded on August 15, 2020, by an echocardiogram test. That meant I had reversed the severity of heart failure.

According to the American Heart Association, the normal ejection fraction is 50% to 75%. A borderline ejection fraction can range between 41% and 50%.

As a result, I improved my heart failure from Class 3 (Stage 3) to Class 1 (Stage 1). The condition has been based on the New York Heart Association (NYHA) guidelines established in 2005 for managing congestive heart failure (CHF). CHF identifies four stages of heart failure: Class 1 Class 2. Class 3. and Class 4.

Borderline Ejection Fraction

An ejection fraction (EF) from 41% to 49% may be considered "borderline." It does not always indicate that a person has developed or is developing heart failure. Instead, it may indicate damage, perhaps from a previous heart attack.

Physicians mostly use these NYHA guidelines to gauge the stages of their heart failure patients.

Reversal and Stabilization of Heart Failure into Almost Normal Condition

Now, as I have said, I have reversed the severity of my heart failure and stabilized it into a better condition.

The NYHA (New York Heart Association) guidelines define class 1 (Stage 1) HF as patients with structural heart disease but no current or prior HF symptoms. As of now, I have no signs of heart failure.

II. Type 2 Diabetes Diagnosis in 2006

Doctors diagnosed me with type 2 diabetes in 2006 while retiring in the Philippines. I had a double vision as if I were crossed-eyed and could not walk without closing one of my eyes.

But after several years, with my complete treatment system, I halted, reversed, stabilized, and put my diabetes into remission without taking any diabetes medicines.

III. Kidney Disease

My previous primary doctor diagnosed me with having 3rd stage kidney disease in 2011.

With my treatment system, my estimated glomerular filtration rate (eGFR or simply GFR) that measures kidney function increased from 35% in 2016 to 73% in 2020, reversing the severity of my kidney disease from 3rd-B stage to 2nd stage.

It simply means that I have reversed and put my kidney disease into remission, according to guidelines on an estimation of GFR function percentage.

IV. What Is Heart Failure?

The American Heart Association says, “Heart failure is a chronic, progressive condition in which the heart muscle is unable to pump enough blood to meet the body’s needs for blood and oxygen. The heart can’t keep up with its workload.”

For full details on congestive heart failure, read it on page 155 in Chapter 8.)

Why I’m Still Alive and Kicking at Age 90 Plus

You may ask me, “How did you do it?”. It was just a simple answer: I have been following mytreatment system, lifestyle changes, adopting a semi-plant-based diet, and doing my regiment of exercise every day! Enjoy reading!

Veltisezar Bautista, Author

Chapter 2

The Enigma of Insulin Resistance

Brief Subject Summary

- What Is Insulin Resistance?
- Risk Factors for Developing Insulin Resistance, Prediabetes, and Type 2 Diabetes
- What Is Metabolic Syndrome?
- How Does Insulin Resistance Develop?
- How Does Insulin Resistance Become Prediabetes?
- How Does Prediabetes Turn into Type 2 Diabetes?
- Insulin Resistance vs. Sensitivity
- Can You Prevent or Avoid Insulin Resistance?
- Can Vitamins or Minerals Decrease Insulin Resistance?

Have you been wondering and asking these questions: What is insulin? Is it a plain substance, a complex chemical, or just a simple matter? How does it work in the body?

What Is Insulin?

"Insulin is a hormone made by the pancreas that helps glucose in your blood enter our muscle, fat, and liver, where it's used for energy," says the National Institute of Diabetes and Digestive and Kidney Diseases (NIDDK).

"The liver," it adds, "also makes glucose in times of need, such as when you're fasting." Furthermore, it says, "When blood glucose, also called blood sugar, levels rise after you eat, your pancreas releases insulin into the blood."

Yes, it's a fact. Insulin, when appropriately used, lowers blood sugar to keep it in the normal range.

As described by the Centers for Diabetes Control and Prevention (CDC), this is the normal process of digesting the food after you eat:

- The food you eat breaks down into glucose.
- Then the glucose enters the bloodstream.
- The liver reserves some insulin to use when another need arises.
- When insulin is already in the cells, glucose levels in the blood decrease, so insulin lowers, too.
- When insulin decreases, the liver is alerted to give stored glucose so that energy can be available anytime, even if you don't eat a meal or a snack for a certain period.

What Is Insulin Resistance?

"Insulin resistance occurs when excess glucose in the blood reduces the ability of the cells to absorb and use blood glucose for energy," according to *Medical News Today*.

In simple words, the pancreas makes insulin to help the glucose enter the body cells.

But over time, because of its hard work, the pancreas loses its ability to make and release insulin. Then follows the build-up of too much sugar in the bloodstream.

Risk Factors for Developing Insulin Resistance, Prediabetes, and Type 2 Diabetes

- **Race**: A family history of diabetes (especially if you are a Pacific Islander, Asian-American, African-American, Mexican American, or Native American)
- **Age**: (the older you are, the more your risk increases)
- **Health problem:** Examples such as being alcoholic with fatty liver disease and polycystic ovary syndrome
- **Hormonal issues:** Example of conditions such as Cushing's syndrome and acromegaly (abnormal growth of the hands, feet, and face)
- **Some medications**: Avoiding certain drugs, such as steroids and antipsychotics

- **Smoking:** Quitting smoking if you're smoking
- **Sedentary lifestyle:** Going out and doing some activities such as moderate-intensity walking (not jogging or running), swimming
- **Lack of Sleep:** Getting enough sleep, especially for those with sleep apnea

What Is Metabolic Syndrome?

A metabolic syndrome is a group of conditions that occur together, increasing your risk of type 2 diabetes, heart disease, and stroke.

They are:

- **Obesity**, or excess fat around the middle and upper parts of the body
- **High triglycerides** with levels of 150 or higher, or taking medication to treat high levels of these blood fats
- **Low-density lipoprotein (HDL) levels** of 40 and below
- **High fasting blood sugar** with levels of 100-125 mg/dl (the prediabetes range) or over 125 (type 2 diabetes)
- **High fasting blood sugar (**or you may be taking medicine to treat high blood sugar)

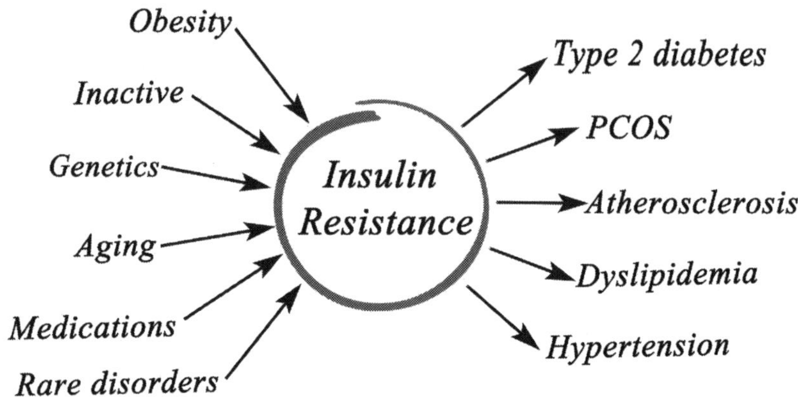

Causes of Insulin Resistance

Illustration Credit: Shutterstock

How Does Insulin Resistance Develop?

"While genetics, aging, and ethnicity play roles in developing insulin sensitivity, the driving forces behind insulin resistance include excess body weight, too much belly fat, a lack of exercise, smoking, and even skimping on sleep," says *WebMD.*

As insulin resistance worsens, the body fights back by producing more insulin.

Over time, the beta cells in the pancreas, trying to make more insulin, get worn out. Thus, they won't keep pace with the demand for more insulin.

As a result, after the insulin has been silent for years, your blood sugar begins to rise. Then later, you may learn that you already have prediabetes or type 2 diabetes.

How does Insulin Resistance Become Prediabetes?

What does prediabetes mean? It merely means that the blood sugar levels are higher than normal but not high enough to be diagnosed as type 2 diabetes.

In simple words, there's an assigned boundary between prediabetes and type 2 diabetes (so-called full-blown diabetes). The border is 125 mg/dL That is, up to 125 mg/dL, it is called prediabetes, and when the blood sugar is above 125 mg/dL and beyond, that's called type 2 diabetes.

In terms of A1c, the boundary between normal blood sugar and prediabetes is 5.6%. Up to 5.6 A1c is normal, while 5.7% up to 6.4% is prediabetes, and so 6.5% and above is type 2 diabetes (full-flown diabetes).

How Does Prediabetes Turn Into Type 2 Diabetes?

When you have not made any lifestyle changes, you have not done any measures to stop prediabetes in its tracks; the disease will lead to type 2 diabetes.

Resistance Vs. Sensitivity

Says *Healthline:* "Insulin resistance and insulin sensitivity are two sides of the same coin. If you are sensitive to insulin, you have low insulin resistance."

How to Prevent or Avoid Insulin Resistance

- **Overweight:** If you are obese or overweight, you must lose some weight based on your doctor's advice on body mass.
- **Sedentary lifestyle:** If you are inactive, go out and do some activities such as moderate-intensity walking (not jogging or running), swimming, and lower glucose in the bloodstream when muscles get the glucose for energy
- **High triglycerides levels:** If you have high triglycerides with 150 or higher levels, take some medications prescribed by your doctor. My normal triglyceride levels are 60 and below.
- **Low-Density Lipoprotein (LDL):** If you have too much LDL (bad cholesterol), the LDL cholesterol can build up on the walls of your blood vessels. This buildup is called "plaque."
- **High-Density Lipoprotein (HDL):** If you have low levels of HDL (good cholesterol, 40 and below), take steps to increase it.

- **High blood sugar levels:** High fasting blood sugar with levels of 100-125 mg/dl (the pre-diabetes range) or over 125 (type 2 diabetes). Concerning this disease, you can take medicine to lower it. And of course, you have to exercise, doing moderate-intensity walking, for instance, after each meal of the day.
- **Smoking:** If you're smoking, stop it. That's the advice of diabetes experts. For me, I tried to smoke during my college days. But I quit it for the simple reason that I didn't get any good things, and I didn't enjoy it.
- **Lack of sleep:** Yes, get enough sleep, at least 7 to 9 hours per night, to help the body rest and reenergize.
- **Managing stress:** You may try to reduce your stress because stress raises blood pressure and blood sugar, too.
- **Fewer Carbohydrates:** If you have insulin resistance, prediabetes, type 2 diabetes, and type 1 diabetes, cut down on carbs.

Limiting or avoiding trans fats: Scientists' animal studies have provided strong evidence linking high trans fat intake to deficient blood sugar control and insulin resistance. However, experts cannot say that artificial trans fat intake increases insulin resistance in human studies.

- **Reduction of added sugar:** Processed foods have lots of sugar. In some food production processes, these sugars consist of table sugar, known as sucrose, and high-fructose corn syrup. Some studies have shown that a higher intake of these sugars can increase insulin resistance.

Supplements and Minerals

Healthline reports consistent evidence showing that specific vitamins or supplements decrease insulin resistance. Such supplements are magnesium, berberine, chromium, and resveratrol

Magnesium: Magnesium, a mineral, works well with insulin receptors to store blood sugar. Some studies have revealed that low magnesium level has a connection to insulin resistance. So taking magnesium, may reduce insulin resistance.

Berberine: A plant molecule extracted from various herbs, including the plant Berberis; its antioxidants bind to and neutralize molecules called free radicals that cause harmful inflammation in the whole body.

Chromium: A mineral that is involved in carbohydrates and fat metabolism reduces blood sugar. But you have to take chromium picolinate supplements in doses of 1,000 to 2,000 mcg to improve insulin receptor ability to reduce glucose or blood sugar.

Resveratrol: It is an antioxidant and anti-inflammatory properties to protect you from certain diseases, including diabetes, cancer, and cardiovascular diseases.

If you want to take any of these supplements, you may talk to your doctor first because any one of them may interact with any of the medicines you're taking.

Chapter 3

Prediabetes: If You Can't Stop it, You're Bound for Trouble

Brief Subject Summary

- What Is Prediabetes?
- Diagnosis of Prediabetes
- Prediabetes and Type 2 Diabetes Chart
- What Is HbA1cc
- What Is a Normal HbA1c Level?
- Causes of Prediabetes
- Symptoms of Prediabetes
- The Bautista Treatment System
- Medications to treat Prediabetes

What Is Prediabetes?

According to the Centers for Disease Control and Prevention (CDC), "Prediabetes is a serious health condition where blood sugar levels are higher than normal, but not high enough yet to be diagnosed as type 2 diabetes.

"Approximately 88 million American adults, more than 1 in 3, have diabetes. Of those with prediabetes, more than 84% don't know they have it."

Diagnosis of Prediabetes

The American Diabetes Association (ADA) says doctors decide the diagnosis of prediabetes if test results show the following measurements:

- Fasting blood sugar levels of 100–125 mg/dl
- Glucose tolerance levels of 140–199 mg/dl
- An HbA1C test result of 5.7%–6.4%

Prediabetes and Type 2 Diabetes Chart

	Normal	Prediabetes	Type 2 Diabetes
HbA1c	5.6% or less	5.7%-6.4%	6.5% or more
Fasting Glucose	99 mg/dl or less	100-125 mg/dl	126 mg/dl or more
Oral glucose tolerance	140 mg/dl or less	140-199 mg/dl	200 mg/dl or more

What Is HbA1c?

HbA1c refers to the amount of glucose attached to hemoglobin, a protein found in red blood cells. The HbA1c blood test determines the average blood sugar levels over the past three months.

Hence, if your average blood sugar is high, your HbA1c for the past three months will be high, too.

In simple words, if you already have prediabetes or type 2 diabetes, you should have low or normal blood glucose to have a lower A1C. Your development of prediabetes into type 2 diabetes increases if your HbA1c is high.

HbA1c Levels

Normal less than 5.7% (at least 5.6 and below.)
Prediabetes 5.7% to 6.4%
Diabetes 6.5% or higher
Source: American Diabetes Association

What Is a Normal HbA1C Level?

Diabetes associations around the world don't agree on this matter. The American Diabetes Association advises that people with diabetes should keep their HbA1c results below 7.0 percent.

Meanwhile, the American Association of Clinical Endocrinologies recommends that you set the A1C level at 6.5 percent and below.

On the other hand, The International Diabetes Federation (IDF) says people with diabetes should have levels below 6.5 percent.

Blood Sugar Lavels

Result	Fasting Plasma Glucose (FPG)
Normal	less than 100 mg/dl
Prediabetes	100 mg/dl to 125 mg/dl
Diabetes	126 mg/dl or higher

Source: American Diabetes Association

Causes of Prediabetes

The CDC explains, "Insulin is a hormone made by your pancreas that acts like a key to let blood sugar into cells for use as energy. If you have prediabetes, the cells in your body don't respond normally to insulin."

In other words, the pancreas makes more insulin so that the cells can get it. However, later your pancreas won't be able to keep up with its work load. Therefore, your blood sugar in the bloodstream increases.

That will be the occurrence of prediabetes, which can lead to type 2 diabetes, if you can't stop it in its tracks.

The risk factors that increase the probability of developing prediabetes may include:

- Insulin resistance
- Are older, especially over age 45
- Being overweight or obese
- Age (even if prediabetes can develop at any age, the risk of prediabetes usually develops after age 45)
- Family history (having a parent or sibling who has developed type 2 diabetes)
- Race (People of certain ethnic groups, including Hispanics, Asian Americans, African Americans, and Pacific Islanders, are more susceptible to diabetes)
- High carbohydrate foods, sugary juices, and soft drinks
- Frequent eating of red meat and processed meat
- Not much eating of plant-based foods
- Lack of activity or exercise, such as walking

- Smoking
- People with obstructive sleep apnea, a condition that disrupts sleep repeatedly
- High blood pressure
- Low levels of high-density lipoprotein (HDL) cholesterol, "the good" cholesterol
- High levels of triglycerides, a type of fat in your blood
- Hypnea or work changing shifts or night shifts

Symptoms of Prediabetes

As explained by the Mayo Clinic, "Prediabetes doesn't usually have any signs or symptoms in the beginning. But one possible sign of prediabetes is darkened skin on certain parts of the body. Affected areas can include the neck, armpits, elbows, knees, and knuckles."

Yes, there are no clear symptoms of prediabetes; that's why you can have it undetected for a long time. That's what happened to me.

By the time that you may notice some symptoms, your prediabetes has already become type 2 diabetes, or full-blown diabetes, when you have already signs that may include:

- Fatigue
- Numbness in or tingling in feet
- Dry, itchy skin
- Black marks on legs
- Blurry eyesight
- Double vision
- Frequent urination

Furthermore, as determined by ADA, an estimated 10 to 23 percent of people with prediabetes, also called borderline diabetes, will develop type 2 diabetes within five years.

Generally, prediabetes affects adults between the ages of 40 and 60. The condition tends to be silent and rarely causes any noticeable symptoms.

8 Top Ways to Prevent Prediabetes

- **Eat healthy foods** with a plant-based diet or a semi-plant-based diet with low glycemic index (GI) and glycemic load (GL) value foods. You should have low-carbohydrate and higher fiber intake with this diet.
- **Do moderate-intensity walking or slow-intensity walking**: If you are an older adult and not comfortable with moderate-intensity walking, do the low-intensity walk based on your physical fitness. A 20-minute walk one hour after each meal can lower blood sugar by 30 to 60 points, based on my experience. (See Chapter 9.)
- **Check your body mass index (BMI)**: See if you're overweight, underweight, or have a healthy weight. You'll know your BMI number based on height and weight. (See chapter 13.) The BMI indicates whether you have a healthy weight or you're overweight or underweight. Then if you're underweight, eat more calories. If you're overweight, then lose about 5% to 7% of your body weight.

  (Note: To know your BMI without any calculation, you may google "BMI calculator," and you'll see several calculators. You type your height and weight in the spaces provided, and click *Calculate*, and you'll know your BMI number.)

- **Drink enough water**: Drinking about 8 to 10 or more cups of water, based on height and weight, you can lower your blood glucose. Sugar is water-soluble, so water dilutes sugar to get out of the body with the urine.
- **Stop smoking if you're smoking**: Smoking can make your body more resistant to insulin. It can also lead to higher and uncontrolled blood sugar glucose levels that can cause serious complications from diabetes, such as problems with your blood vessels, kidneys, and heart.
- **Limit or avoid drinking alcohol**: A moderate amount of alcohol may cause blood sugar to rise, while excess alcohol drinking can decrease your blood sugar level, causing it to drop into dangerous levels for people with diabetes. Beer and sweet wine contain carbohydrates that can increase blood glucose.

- **Monitor your blood sugar regularly**: When you reach 45 years or over, check your blood glucose levels at least every three months to see if your blood sugar increased. At least you'll know if prediabetes has already hit you; by then, you can act to stop it in its tracks.
- **Take medicines, if needed**: If you discover that your fasting blood sugar is already high, and you can't decrease it totally by a moderate-intensity walk, in three 20-minute sessions of exercise one hour after each meal, then you may take diabetes medicine. For me, I don't take medication; I only do walking exercises.

My Journey: Prediabetes Ignorance

I was one of those 88 million American adults, who didn't know they had already prediabetes.

That's it. I didn't realize that I already had prediabetes because there were no symptoms. The disease caught me off guard; I lost the fight without my resistance. Had I known, I should have taken steps to stop it in its tracks.

That's why my prediabetes led to full-blown type 2 diabetes, without my knowing it. What the heck!

Yes, prediabetes doesn't usually have any signs or symptoms. For many years, I didn't know I had prediabetes, which led to type 2 diabetes. I didn't do any blood sugar monitoring, thinking that I had no family history of diabetes.

As for further clarification, prediabetes also means that your blood glucose rises and accumulates in the bloodstream because you already have insulin resistance.

That indicates that your body resists insulin or doesn't produce enough insulin to be accepted by cells for energy.

The Bautista Treatment System (Including Standard Treatment)

- Adopting effective diets for prediabetes, type 2 diabetes, and type 1 diabetes, such as the Mediterranean diet, Flexitarian (or semi-vegetarian diet), or a plant-based diet. (See chapter 11.)
- Doing moderate-intensity walking 20 minutes after each meal of the day (See chapter 9.)
- Drinking enough water at least 8 to 12 cups or glasses of water (8 ounces, each cup), based on your height and body weight.
- Eating low carbohydrates and more fiber
- Avoiding sugary foods and drinks
- Limiting or avoiding foods with high fructose
- Reducing stress
- Getting enough sleep
- Avoiding eating in restaurants that serve sugary and high carbohydrate foods
- Increasing HDL levels and decreasing triglycerides and LDL (bad cholesterol)
- Eating healthy fats and limiting or avoiding saturated fats and trans fats

Common Medications to Treat Prediabetes

Metformin, approved by the US FDA, is the most common medicine used to treat prediabetes, type 2 diabetes, and Type 1 Diabetes for blood sugar control.

The metformin works by stopping the liver from producing excess glucose. If you successfully make life changes, eat a healthy diet, and exercise to stabilize blood glucose, you may stop taking it.

You should have blood tests to see if you are deficient in vitamins and minerals, such as vitamin D, magnesium, and other supplements.

Other Medications

- **Glucagon-like peptide-1 (GLP-1) receptor antagonists:** They slow digestion and improve blood glucose levels.
- **Sulfonylureas**: They are oral medications that help your body make more insulin.
- **Sodium-glucose cotransporter-2 (SGLT2) inhibitors**: They help prevent the kidneys from reabsorbing glucose into the blood and sending it out in your urine.
- **Meglitinides:** These are fast-acting, short-duration medications that stimulate your pancreas to release more insulin.
- **Thiazolidinediones**: They make your body more sensitive to insulin.
- **Dipeptidyl peptidase-4 inhibitors**.:These are milder medications that help reduce blood glucose levels.

Chapter 4

Type 2 Diabetes & Its Complications

Brief Subject Summary

- A Day to Remember
- What Is Type 2 Diabetes?
- Diabetes: Quick Facts About It
- Causes, Symptoms, and Standard Treatment of Type 2 Diabetes
- Medications for Type 2 Diabetes
- What Is Diabetic Neuropathy?
- Types of Diabetic Neuropathy
- Peripheral Neuropathy: Why It Happens
- Types of Vascular Diseases
- Peripheral Vascular Disease (PVD)
- Peripheral Artery Disease or Peripheral Arterial Disease (PAD)
- Chronic Kidney Disease (CKD)
- Coronary Artery Disease (CAD) or Coronary Heart Disease (CHD)
- Diabetes and the Lungs
- Carotid Artery Disease
- Diabetic Retinopathy

A Day to Remember

One early morning in 2006, when I was already retired in the Philippines from my work in Royal Oak, Michigan, U.S.A, I went into the bathroom to pee after I woke up. But my eyes saw two different things or overlapping visual views in the mirror. Everything was double; that is, double vision.

I got scared! What's happening to me? Am I dreaming? Or is this real? I asked myself. I went back to bed, closed my eyes, and tried to sleep. But I could not sleep.

Eye Problem

Without closing one of my two eyes, I could not walk because I didn't know which way to go. So I had a patch over my left eye and just used the other eye for seeing.

Doctors in a hospital in Cabanatuan City in Nueva Ecija, the Philippines, told me I should have therapy for my eyes in Manila. I didn't do it.

Emergency Flight

After two days, I enplaned back to the United States to seek medical treatment. After seeing a doctor at a hospital in Royal Oak, Michigan, the doctor told me:

"We can not do anything about it right now. In three months, that double vision will disappear. Diabetes caused your double vision."

Yes, after 3 months, the double vision was gone.

What a Life!

Several years back, before my diabetes discovery, I had a massive heart attack. Then the double vision incident. I was sure that diabetes contributed to the damage and blockage of one of my heart's main arteries that resulted in my heart attack. And the cardiac event caused my heart failure; there's no doubt about that.

What Is Type 2 Diabetes?

Type 2 diabetes (T2D) is the most common form of diabetes, which happens when blood glucose levels, also called blood sugar, increase due to problems with the use or production of insulin. It can appear at any age, but it is more likely to occur after 40 years.

When you have type 2 diabetes, the cells in your body cannot respond to insulin as well as they should. Then your blood glucose or sugar levels build up in the bloodstream. The hormone insulin moves the sugar from your blood into your cells. It's there that the body uses it for energy. So if there's not enough insulin, then the process won't work.

What Can Diabetes Do?

Yes, as we can see, diabetes can cause severe complications: you can have heart disease, kidney disease, retinopathy, peripheral neuropathy, and other conditions. So, if not treated, you can be blind or amputated. Or you can have a stroke or heart attack due to heart disease. Or you will require dialysis if you already have kidney failure. What a scary thing to think about it!

Diabetes Quick Facts from the U.S. Centers for Disease Control and Prevention (CDC)

- More than 34 million people in the United States have diabetes, and 1 in 5 persons don't know they have it
- More than 88 million US adults, over one-third, have prediabetes, and more than 80% of them are unaware of it
- Diabetes is the 7th leading cause of death in the United States.
- Type 2 diabetes accounts for approximately 90% to 95% of all diagnosed diabetes cases; type 1 diabetes accounts for about 5%-10%

Causes of Type 2 Diabetes

- Unable to stop prediabetes in its tracks
- Lack of blood sugar monitoring
- Uncontrolled blood glucose
- Uncontrolled blood pressure
- Lack of enough exercise, such as walking
- Unresolved high triglycerides and LDL levels
- Unable to increase the HDL level (the good cholesterol)

Symptoms

Classic signs and symptoms that suggest you've moved from prediabetes to type 2 diabetes include:

- Increased thirst
- Fatigue
- More frequent urination
- Excess hunger
- Erectile dysfunction (ED, impotence)
- Blurry vision
- Double vision

Standard Treatment of Type 2 Diabetes

The management of type 2 diabetes includes:

- Regular exercise
- Weight loss
- Diabetes medication or insulin therapy
- Blood sugar monitoring to make sure that your blood sugar remains within your target range
- More vegetables and fruits
- More foods with fiber
- Fewer foods containing saturated fats
- Less refined carbohydrates and incredibly sweet foods

The Bautista Treatment System (Including Standard Treatment)

- Adopting an effective diet based on low glycemic and low glycemic load foods such as whole grains, fruits, and vegetables
- Doing a moderate-intensity 20-minute walk, one hour after each day meal (See chapter 9.)
- Eating low healthy carbohydrates and more fiber foods
- Losing 5% to 10% of your body weight (as recommended by the Centers for Disease Control and Prevention (CDC); that's less than 20 pounds if you weigh 180 lbs
- Having enough sleep

- Reducing stress
- Stabilizing blood sugar and controlling LDL (bad) cholesterol and triglycerides
- Eating low calories, low carbohydrates, and more fiber, fruits, and vegetables
- Avoiding sugary foods and drink
- Stopping smoking
- Limiting or avoiding alcohol
- Using Truvia and SweetLeaf (Stevia), which both contain the ingredient of stevia, a natural sugar, as alternative sugars, instead of other sugar substitutes
- Drinking more water to dilute blood sugar, except if you have heart failure and eating high protein; but low protein if you have kidney disease

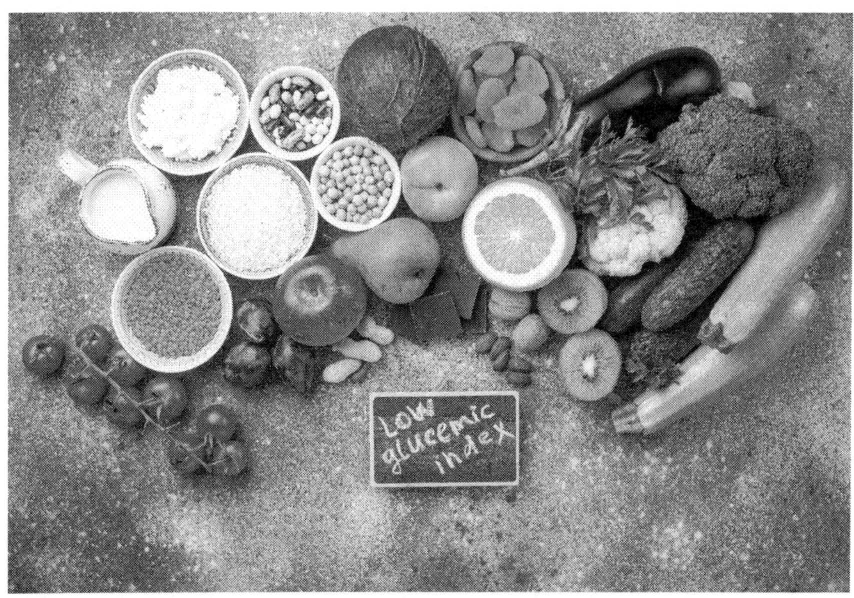

Low Glycemic Index Foods for Diabetes

Photo Credit: Shutterstock

Green Tea and Moringa Tea: Do They Reduce Blood Sugar?

Some studies have shown that several teas, particularly green tea and Moringa oleifera (called *malunggay* in the Philippines), reduce blood sugar levels due to their compounds and antioxidant properties.

Toby Smithson, RDN, CDE, author of *Diabetes Meal Planning and Nutrition for Dummies*, says that the catechins, an antioxidant in green tea, help reduce the effects of insulin resistance by decreasing the digestion and absorption of carbohydrates. (See information about green tea and Moringa tea in Chapter 17.)

Natural vs. Refined Sugars

Natural sugars occur in nature. For instance, fruits have fructose, and dairy products contain lactose. Natural sugars are paired with fiber. Why? Because fiber aids in slowing down the speed at which the sugar may affect your blood sugar levels.

When manufacturers produce refined sugar, a natural ingredient is processed. They extract sugar from the source, such as sugar cane.

Manufacturers remove some nutrients. In addition, they separate the sugar from the fiber.

Also, sugar can be manufactured chemically. Sucrose is the end product when the sugar is chemically processed and refined. The body can easily break down the sucrose, increasing blood sugar and insulin levels.

Added Sugar Recommended Limit Per Day

The American Heart Association (AHA) recommends limiting added sugars to no more than 6 percent of calories each day.

That means, for men, there should be a limit of no more than 150 calories per day, or about 9 teaspoons or 36 grams. On the other hand, there should be no more than 100 calories per day or about 6 teaspoons or 25 grams of sugar for most women.

What Are the Added Sugars?

Added sugar may include:

- Table sugar
- Sucrose

- Honey
- Dextrose
- Brown sugar
- Concentrated fruit or vegetable syrups
- Corn syrups
- Added sugar in sweetened beverages, desserts, and sweet snacks

Which Foods to Eat for People with Diabetes

You can also look for carbohydrate foods that contain less than 10 grams of sugar and more than 3 grams of fiber per serving. Look at the nutritional label to find these numbers. The more fiber you have in the food you consume, the fewer carbs your body will absorb. That means to say, carbohydrates minus fiber = net carbs.

Medications for Type 2 Diabetes

Metformin, approved by the US FDA, is the most common medicine used to treat prediabetes and type 2 diabetes. It works by stopping the liver from producing excess glucose. If you successfully make life changes, eat a healthy diet, and exercise, you may stop taking it.

Other Medications

Same as that for prediabetes (See them in Chapter 3.)

Major Complications

Based on my experience and extensive research, the most severe consequences of diabetes may include the following:

- High cholesterol
- High blood pressure
- Kidney disease
- Nerve damage
- Heart disease
- Heart attack
- Stroke
- Vision problems
- Lung disease
- Amputations

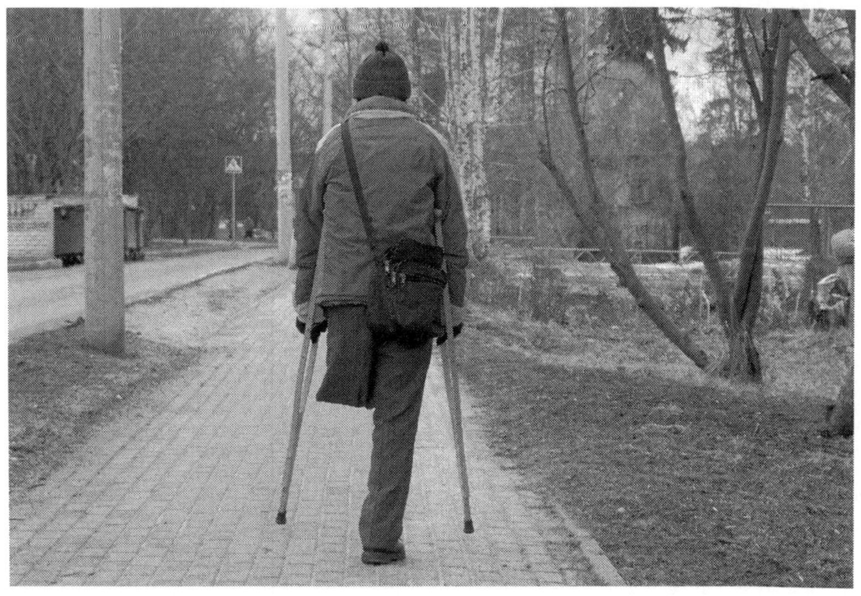

Something to Think About

Photo Credit: \Shutterstock

Type 1 Diabetes Complications

Same as those of Type 2 Diabetes. (See discussions of Type 1 Diabetes in Chapter 6.)

Complications

High blood sugar damages some body organs, such as the heart, nerves, blood vessels, eyes, kidneys,.and the lungs.

I. Peripheral Neuropathy or Diabetic Peripheral Neuropathy

What Is Peripheral Neuropathy?

John Hopkins Medicine describes diabetic neuropathy in this way: "Neuropathy is a complication of diabetes that can lead to problems throughout the body. Diabetes can affect nerves that control movement, sensation, and other functions."

Types of Diabetic Peripheral Neuropathy

The types of neuropathy are:

- Autonomic Neuropathy
- Proximal Neuropathy (Diabetic Polyradiculopathy)
- Mononeuropathy (Focal Neuropathy)
- Peripheral Neuropathy (the most common)

1. Autonomic Neuropathy

The autonomic nervous system involves the functions of your lungs, heart, stomach, intestines, bladder, eyes, and sex organs. Thus, diabetes can affect the nerves in these areas, possibly causing:

- Difficulty swallowing
- Bladder problems, including urinary retention, urinary incontinence, and urinary tract infections
- Erectile dysfunction in men
- Slow stomach emptying (gastroparesis), which may cause nausea, vomiting, and loss of appetite
- Increased heart rate

Autonomic neuropathy occurs when the nerves that control involuntary bodily functions are damaged. It can affect blood pressure, temperature control, digestion, bladder function, and even sexual function.

The nerve damage interferes with the messages sent between the brain and other organs and areas of the autonomic nervous system, such as the heart, blood vessels, and sweat glands.

In a nutshell, nerve damage interferes with the messages sent between the brain and other organs and areas of the autonomic nervous system.

2. Proximal Neuropathy (Diabetic Polyradiculopathy)

Like peripheral neuropathy, proximal neuropathy affects nerves situated closer to the body's center, such as nerves in the legs, thighs, hips, and buttocks. Also called diabetic amyotrophy, proximal neuropathy is more common in people with type 2 diabetes and older adults.

Signs and symptoms include:

- Severe pain in the leg, thigh, hip, and buttock
- Difficulty rising from a sitting position
- Shrinking and weakness of the thigh muscles

3. Mononeuropathy (Focal Neuropathy)

Mononeuropathy, also called focal neuropathy, involves damage to specific nerves, such as in the face, torso, or leg.

Symptoms may include:

- Double vision, aching behind one eye, and difficulty in vision focusing
- Pain in your shin, foot, or in front of your thigh
- Carpal tunnel syndrome: Numbness or tingling in the thumb, middle finger, index finger, and ring finger
- Weakness in the hand results in dropping anything by someone holding it. Source: Mayo Clinic

4. Peripheral Neuropathy

"Peripheral neuropathy refers to the many conditions that involve damage to the peripheral nervous system," reports the National Institute of Neurological Disorders and Stroke (NINDS).

The NINDS explains that the peripheral nervous system is a communication network in the body. Its function is to send signals between the central nervous system, the brain, spinal cord, and other parts of your body.

Nerves and blood vessels are branched structures that travel together to supply blood to almost every tissue and muscle with oxygen and nutrients throughout the body.

When nerves malfunction due to damage, the nerves' normal functioning suffers. As a result, they may send pain signals when nothing is causing it.

The nerve malfunctioning may be due to:

- Infections
- Inherited disorders
- Illnesses
- Injuries

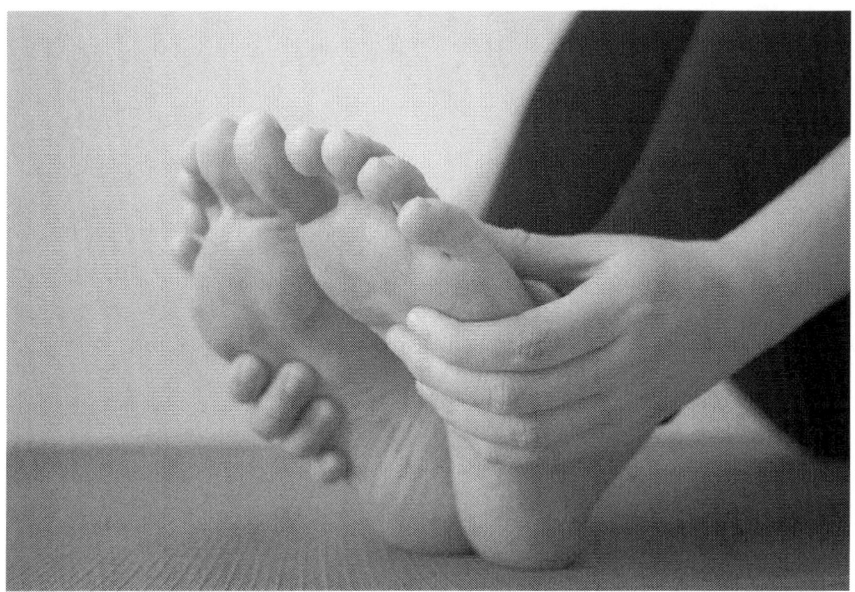

Peripheral Neuropathy

Photo credit: Shuttershock

Types of Peripheral Nerves

There are three types of peripheral nerves:

- Sensory nerves receive sensations, such as pain, temperature, and touch, from the skin.
- Motor nerves control muscle movements.
- Autonomic nerves manage heart rate, blood pressure, bladder, and digestion.

Peripheral Nervous System

The peripheral nervous system connects the nerves from the brain and spinal cord to the rest of the body. They comprise the central nervous system, including the mouth and face, arms and hands, legs and feet, and internal organs.

The nerves deliver signals regarding your physical sensations back to the brain. The nerves monitor food digestion and blood circulation to ensure that they are functioning well.

Epinephrine and Norepinephrine

Epinephrine and norepinephrine are chemicals that belong to a group of compounds called catecholamines. Though they are substances similar in structures, they affect the body differently.

For instance, epinephrine is commonly known as adrenaline. On the other hand, norepinephrine is also known as noradrenaline. These hormones and neurotransmitters play a role in regulating the nervous system. They are part of the automatic nervous system controlling the body's "fight or flight" response.

Causes of Peripheral Neuropathy

Certain conditions can cause peripheral neuropathy. These may include:

- Diabetes
- Autoimmune diseases
- Inflammatory diseases
- Infections
- Bone marrow diseases
- Tumors
- Toxins
- Injuries
- Vitamin B12 deficiency
- Kidney disease
- Liver disease
- Underactive thyroid (hypothyroidism)

Symptoms of Peripheral Neuropathy

The symptoms of peripheral neuropathy may include:

- Numbness
- Muscle cramps
- Muscle twitching
- Muscle weakness
- Paralysis
- Loss of balance
- Loss of bowel control
- Difficulty emptying bladder
- Sexual function problems
- Prickling or tingling sensation
- Abnormal feelings of hot and cold
- Burning or sharp pain

Source: *Healthline*

9 Best Supplements for Peripheral Neuropathy

Here are 8 best supplements for the treatment of peripheral neuropathy and PAD, including:

- Benfortiamine (Vitamin B1, thiamine)
- Curcumin
- Vitamin B6
- Vitamin B12
- Alpha-lipoic acid
- Curcumin
- Acetyl-L-carnitine
- N-Acetyl cysteine
- Omega-3 polyunsaturated fatty acids (PUFAs)

Bentifotiamine: Benfotiamine is a lipid-soluble form of thiamine (B-1.) Japan developed benfotiamine in the early 1960s. The Germans had long been using benfotiamine to treat alcoholic neuritis. Furthermore, it is the most effective metabolic precursor of active thiamine.

Studies have shown that benfotiamine improves neuropathy scores significantly, increasing nerve conduction and reducing pain in the body.

Vitamin B6: Vitamin B6 is known for aiding in maintaining the cover of the body's nerve endings. However, there's a limit to taking it. You should not take more than 200 milligrams because of possible nerve damage and neuropathy systems. Worst, it may cause permanent nerve damage.

Vitamin B12: A mild deficiency may affect the nervous system and the brain's proper functioning. It's because lack of enough B12 damages the so-called myelin sheath around the nerves. In other words, the sheath is the protector of the nerves.

Curcumin: A cooking herb recognized for its anti-inflammatory, antioxidant, and analgesic properties, curcumin helps relieve numbness and tingles in hands and feet.

Alpha-lipoic acid: Alpha-lipoic acid is a vitamin-like chemical called an antioxidant. This acid delays or reverses peripheral diabetic neuropathy due to its multiple antioxidant properties. Treatment with alpha-lipoic acid increases reduced glutathione, an important endogenous antioxidant. In clinical trials, 600 mg alpha-lipoic acid showed improved neuropathic deficits.

Acetyl-L-carnitine: Research has shown that acetyl-L-carnitine helps promote the action of nerve growth factor (NGF). It also stimulates peripheral nerve regeneration and alleviates pain for patients with this condition.

N-Acetyl cysteine: This vitamin reduces the peripheral neuropathy associated with liver cirrhosis. In other words, it improves peripheral liver neuropathy.

Omega-3 fatty acids: Fish oil, such as the omega-3-Acid Ethyl Esters Capsules, is the first fish oil containing omega-3 fatty acids approved by the FDA as a medication. The acids reduce pain and increase functional improvement for neuropathic disorder patients.

II: Types of Vascular Diseases

Vascular diseases include:

- Abdominal Aortic Aneurysm
- Atherosclerosis
- Carotid Artery Disease (Carotid Artery Stenosis)
- Intermittent Claudication
- Deep Vein Thrombosis
- Peripheral Vascular Disease
- Pulmonary Embolism
- Retinopathy
- Reynaud's Phenomenon
- Renal Vascular Disease
- Thoracic Aortic Aneurysm
- Varicose Veins

Source: Stanford Care

Vascular System

The vascular system is a network of blood vessels that transports blood, nutrients, and hormones throughout the body. The blood contains red blood, which carries oxygen to other organs. It is pumped from the left side of the heart to the rest of the body.

The system is divided into two main groups:

- **Arteries** carry oxygenated blood away from the heart.
- **Veins** carry the oxygen-depleted blood back to the heart to be recirculated.

Descriptions of Several Vascular Diseases

Atherosclerosis: The Johns Hopkins Medicines defines atherosclerosis: "Atherosclerosis is thickening or hardening of the arteries caused by a buildup of plaque in the inner lining of an artery.

Risk factors may include high cholesterol and triglyceride levels, high blood pressure, smoking, diabetes, obesity, physical activity, and eating saturated fats."

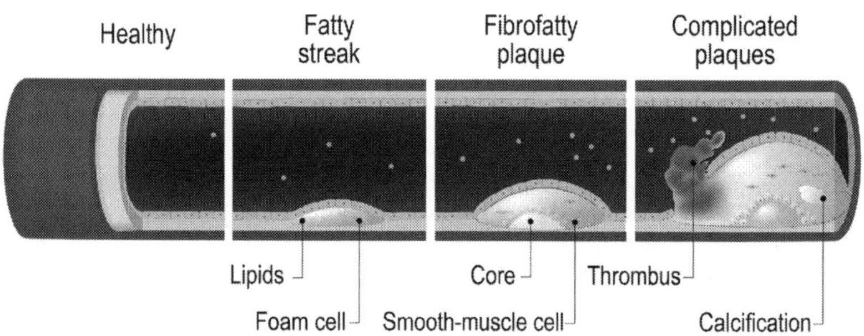

Photo Source: Shutterstock

Pulmonary embolism (PE): The American Lung Association says, "Pulmonary embolism (PE) is when one of the arteries in the lungs gets blocked by a blood clot. In most cases, the clot travels from the leg or another part of the body (called deep vein thrombosis) and blocks blood flow to the lung, making it life-threatening."

Deep vein thrombosis (DVT): Deep vein thrombosis, or DVT, occurs when a blood clot forms in one of the deep veins of your legs. If the blood clot breaks off, it travels through your bloodstream, blocking blood flow in your lungs. Doctors call that blockage a pulmonary embolism which can be fatal.

Chronic venous insufficiency (CVI): Your leg veins have one-way valves that won't close to keep blood from flowing backward instead of going back to the heart. If you have chronic venous insufficiency, the valves won't work as they should. As a result, some of the blood may go back down your legs.

Pelvic congestion syndrome (PCS): This results from the pooling or accumulation of blood in the pelvis due to insufficient outflow. In some women, veins in the lower abdomen sometimes stop working properly. When this happens, the pelvis can get bigger, like varicose veins. Then this leads to pain and other symptoms in the pelvic area. This condition occurs mostly in women of childbearing age, but it may be common to women who have given birth to more than one child.

Renal vascular disease: Renal vascular disease involves a variety of complications affecting the arteries and veins of the kidneys. The condition damages the kidney, leading to kidney failure if a patient doesn't take proper actions. It also causes high blood pressure, which is dangerous.

Thoracic aortic aneurysm: A thoracic aortic aneurysm is a bulge in the aorta in the chest. A bulge is a rounded swelling or lump in the blood vessel that occurs due to an injury to the chest, infection, or hardening of arteries.

If the bulge occurs in a weak spot in the blood vessel, it may burst under stress. If this happens, bleeding may occur that may lead to death.

Abdominal aortic aneurysm (AAA): Dr. Michael J. Singh, in an article published online by the Society for Vascular Surgery, explains: "When the wall of a blood vessel weakens, a balloon-like dilation called an aneurysm sometimes develops.

This occurs most often in the abdominal aorta, an essential blood vessel that supplies blood to your legs."

Diabetes: Its Link to Vascular Diseases

Diabetes is linked to several vascular conditions, especially to the following diseases.

- Atherosclerosis (hardening of the arteries in peripheral vascular disease (PVD), peripheral artery disease (PAD)
- Nephropathy (a kidney disease)
- Coronary artery disease (CAD) or coronary heart disease (CHD)
- Carotid Artery Disease (damage to arteries leading to the brain)
- Retinopathy (an eye disease)

These conditions arise from hyperglycemia, having a high level of glucose (blood sugar) in the bloodstream.

How Does Diabetes Damage Your Blood Vessels?

The Society for Vascular Surgery says, "Both Type 1 and Type 2 diabetes cause high blood sugar. The sugar, also called glucose, damages the inner linings of both big and small arteries. The arteries respond by layering on the plaque, a substance that fills the arteries so that oxygen-rich blood has a hard time getting through to the eyes, kidneys, legs, and feet."

III. Peripheral Vascular Disease (PVD) and Peripheral Artery Disease (PAD)

What Is PVD?

Peripheral vascular disease (PVD) is an umbrella term for many diseases that affect blood vessels outside the heart and brain, most often in the lower extremities. The diseases result from circulatory dysfunction caused by plaque on artery and vein walls. PVD also involves lymph vessels that transport lymphatic fluid to the body.

To clarify, conditions that involve blocking blood flow through a vessel, whether an artery or a vein, are classified as PVD. The body's network of blood vessels comprises the arteries, veins, and capillaries that carry blood with oxygen to and from the heart.

Among the most known PVD are:

- Peripheral artery disease (PAD)
- Chronic venous insufficiency (CVI)
- Deep vein thrombosis (DVT)

All the diseases involve atherosclerosis, the build-up of plaque, consisting of fatty deposits, cholesterol, calcium, and other substances in the artery walls and veins.

Affected by the accumulation of plaques include:

- Heart
- Kidneys
- Brain
- Pelvis
- Legs, feet, or arms

Causes of PVD

The most common causes of PVD may include:

- Diabetes
- Stress
- Drugs
- Injury
- High cholesterol levels
- High blood pressure
- Cold temperature
- Infection
- Blood vessel inflammation
- Muscle or ligament abnormal structures

People with coronary artery disease (CAD) more often suffer from PVD.

PVD Symptoms

Symptoms of peripheral vascular disease may include:

- Claudication: Pain in legs, thigh, calf, or buttocks during exercise or any activity, which may disappear at rest
- Sexual dysfunction
- Loss of hair on legs
- Slow toenail growth
- Weak leg pulses
- Paleness when legs are elevated

Treatments

To prevent or to treat PVD, take some steps, which may include:

- Quitting smoking
- Changing diet to semi-plant-based or plant-based diet, including reducing intake of saturated and unsaturated foods and eating an increased amount of grains, vegetables, fruits, and healthy fats
- Treating high cholesterol and triglycerides, and high blood pressure with medicine
- Taking some vitamins and minerals
- Reducing weight
- Limiting or avoiding alcohol intake
- Doing moderate-intensity walking as a form of exercise every day
- Controlling diabetes

What Is PAD?

Peripheral artery disease or peripheral arterial disease (PAD) affects only the arteries, primarily in the legs or the lower extremities. In other words, it only refers to one of the diseases that fall under the category peripheral vascular disease (PVD).

PAD signifies that fatty deposits and calcium build up in the artery walls (atherosclerosis). The substances interfere with the distribution of blood throughout the body. PAD primarily causes atherosclerosis, which means it's a type of PVD.

How Is PAD Related to PVD?

Arteries bring oxygenated blood from the heart to the rest of the body, while veins carry oxygen-depleted blood from the rest of the body to the heart.

For patients with PAD, the damaged arteries prevent blood flow. For this reason, the extremities suffer from decreased blood supply that may result in the development of chronic or non-healing wounds.

Causes of PAD

The causes of PAD include:

- Diabetes
- Smoking
- High blood pressure
- Elevated cholesterol level
- Infection
- Blood vessel inflammation
- Abnormal structures of muscles or ligaments

Symptoms of PAD

The PAD affects your feet and legs first, followed by your arms and hands occasionally.

With it, your limbs, typically your legs, don't get enough blood. It usually occurs because of the damaged arteries and nerves that narrowed. Your legs may feel weak or numb when you walk.

The symptoms include:

- Restless legs
- Losing your balance more often
- Leg pain that doesn't go away when you stop exercising
- Foot or toe wounds that won't heal or heal very slowly
- The decreased temperature in your lower legs or feet
- Loss of reflex response
- Impotence
- Swollen legs and feet (and sometimes arms)

Generally, the most common lower-extremity peripheral artery disease symptoms include painful muscle cramping. They may be in the hips, thighs, or calves. Muscle cramping occurs while walking, exercising, and climbing stairs.

Treatments of PAD

The treatments for PAD may include:

- Elevating your legs or arms above the level of your heart a few times a day or while sleeping at night, if you have swollen legs, ankles, or feet
- Quitting smoking if you smoke
- Managing diabetes
- Lowering blood pressure
- Following a healthy diet, adopting a plant-based or semi-plant-based diet consisting of grains, vegetables, fruits, and healthy fats
- Limiting or avoiding the use of saturated and unsaturated fat
- Avoiding certain cold medications (Advil Cold & Sinus and Aleve-D Sinus & Cold)

How Does PAD Cause Swollen Legs and Feet?

Here's a clear explanation from LAM Vascular & Associates on how legs and feet become swollen: "Venous or vascular insufficiency can cause peripheral edema in the ankles and feet; this occurs when the veins have trouble transporting enough blood back to the heart.

Thus, fluid gathers in the legs. Then it is forced out of the blood vessels into the surrounding tissue (ankles and feet)."

The Cleveland Clinic describes edema as "a swelling caused by fluid trapped in your body's tissues. Causes include diseases, medications, and allergies. Treatment involves lifestyle changes, including diet and exercise."

Differences Between Peripheral Neuropathy and Peripheral Artery Disease (PAD)

Although peripheral neuropathy and PAD share some of the symptoms of the conditions, they are different from each other. They are two distinct but related conditions.

Peripheral neuropathy involves nerve damage caused by diabetes. The condition causes tingling, burning, and weakness in the legs, feet, and hands.

The PAD involves narrowing the arteries found in the lower region of the body, including the legs, calves, thighs, hips, or buttocks, which causes symptoms and complications.

My Journey: Peripheral Neuropathy

Because of my peripheral neuropathy and peripheral artery or arterial disease (PAD), discussed in this chapter, I must confess that a while back, the pain, muscle spasms, and other symptoms occurred at night while I was trying to sleep. While asleep, the stabbing pain and tingles in my legs and feet woke me up, and sometimes it was hard for me, to go back to sleep.

Peripheral neuropathy and PAD share some of the symptoms. So if you have these conditions, you'll be experiencing some symptoms that can be symptoms for one or both of them.

Last year, I decreased my treadmill's speed and my moderate-intensity walking outdoor because my feet were hurting. Later, I was not able to continue my exercise outside anymore. I tried putting self-sticking salonpas patches around my left leg at night to lessen the pain, but the patch didn't work. Salonpas, which has a variety of topical medications for treating inflammation, is an adhesive patch approved by the FDA to relieve mild to moderate pain caused by arthritis and other conditions.

But now, I have no more symptoms of the conditions, excruciating pain, restless legs, and muscle spasms caused by peripheral neuropathy and PAD because I found solutions to the problem.

Those pain, tingling, and feeling like pins and needles that gave me sleepless nights and discomfort are gone. What a relief! What a joy!

List of My Supplements I take (Self-Prescribed)

- Benfotiamine, 600 mg per day
- Vitamin B-6 tablet, 25 mg per day
- Alpha-lipoic acid, 600 mg per day
- Vitamin B-12 tab, 1,000 mcg per day
- Omega-3-Acid Ethyl Esters (Lovaza) capsules, 4,000 mg or 4 grams (Available only by prescription.)

Due to the above supplements, I had been back (since late last year) to moderate-intensity walking outside or on the treadmill. If you have peripheral neuropathy and PAD and want to take these vitamins, you may first ask your doctor if you can take them because they may interact with your medications.

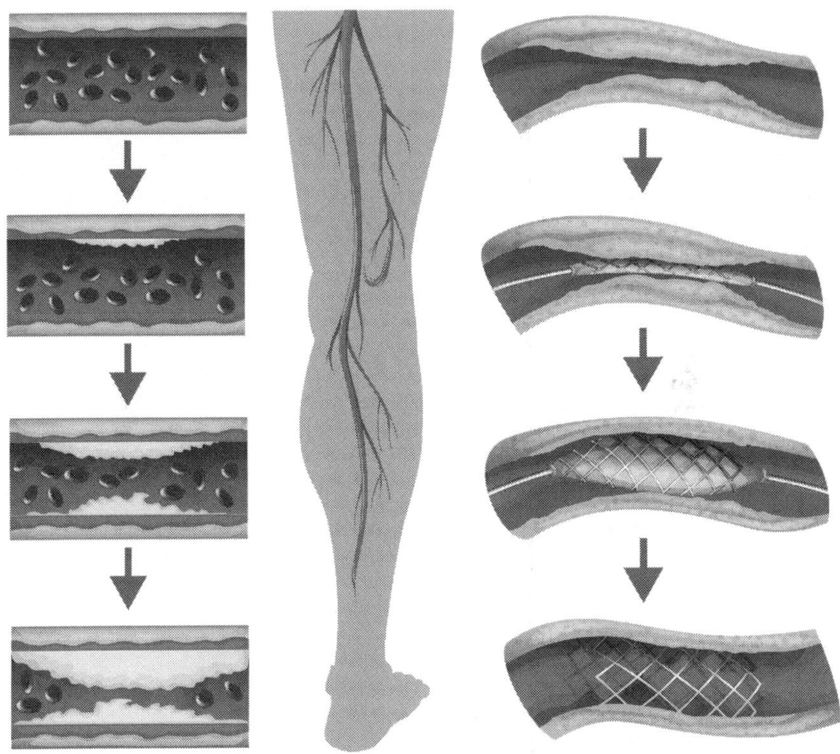

Treatment of Peripheral Artery Disease

Photo Source: Shutterstock

IV. Chronic Kidney Disease (CKD)

What Is Chronic Kidney Disease?

Chronic kidney disease, also called chronic kidney failure, involves a gradual loss of kidney function: filtering waste and excess fluids from your blood, which are then removed from the body through the urine you excrete.

Advanced chronic kidney disease can cause dangerous levels of fluids, electrolytes, and toxins to build up in your body.

You might have few signs or symptoms in the early stages of chronic kidney disease.You might not realize that you have kidney disease until the condition becomes advanced.

One million people are at risk for CKD. Meanwhile, according to the CDC, it is the 9th leading cause of death in the U.S., killing more people than breast cancer or prostate cancer.

The National Kidney Foundation (NKF) estimates that one of every three adults – some 80 million people – is at risk for chronic kidney disease (CKD).

Treatment for chronic kidney disease focuses on slowing the progression of kidney damage, usually by controlling the cause. Without artificial filtering (dialysis) or a kidney transplant, chronic kidney disease can progress to end-stage kidney failure.

IV. Coronary Heart Disease (CHD) or Coronary Artery Disease (CAD)

What Is Coronary Heart Disease?

Coronary heart disease (CHD) is the most common type of heart disease in the United States. That's why it's no wonder that it's the leading cause of death for men and women in the U.S.

(For details see Chapter 8.)

CHD, also called coronary artery disease (CAD), develops when plaques buildup in the body. Next comes the hardening of arteries that carry blood and oxygen to your heart and other body parts.

As a result, blockages may occur in one or more arteries resulting in the insufficiency of flowing blood to the heart, ending in a heart attack or stroke. (For details about this disease, see Chapter 8.)

Diabetes affects much of all body systems and some of the long-term implications of Type I and Type 2 Diabetes.

Type I diabetes is often caused by genetics alone, while genetic and environmental factors cause type 2 diabetes.

A recent study published by *Diabetes Care* of the American Diabetes Association found that people with diabetes are:

- 8% more likely to have asthma
- 22% more likely to have a chronic obstructive pulmonary disease (COPD)
- 4% more likely to have pulmonary fibrosis and nearly twice to be hospitalized for pneumonia

As a result, patients suffering from chronic lung diseases, like asthma or COPD are more likely to have a further decline in lung function with the onset of diabetes. Also, diabetes and chronic lung disease combine to raise lung inflammation, worsening the condition.

V. Carotid Artery Disease (CAD)

What Is Carotid Artery Disease?

The National Institute of Health describes carotid artery disease as "a disease in which a waxy substance called plaque builds up inside the carotid arteries. You have two common carotid arteries, one on each side of your neck."

They are called internal and external arteries. The internal carotid arteries provide oxygen to your brain, while the external arteries supply oxygen-rich blood to your scalp, face, and neck.

Usually, carotid artery disease does not cause symptoms. However, if you have this condition, you have an increased risk of stroke or transient ischemic attack (TIA, or mini-stroke), which may involve sudden numbness and weakness in the face, arm, or legs, and slurred speech.

A ruptured or blocked narrowed artery reduces oxygen flow to the brain, causing a stroke. As a result, a stroke can cause:

- Lasting symptoms
- Brain damage
- Long-term disability, including vision or speech problems or paralysis, or death

Symptoms

Carotid artery disease may not cause signs or symptoms in the early stages. It can have symptoms only after the carotid arteries are severely narrowed or blocked.

Treatments of Carotid Artery Disease

- Healthy lifestyle changes
- Medicines
- Carotid endarterectomy, a surgery to remove the plaque
- Angioplasty and placement of a stent

Endarterectomy Surgery

When you have an endarterectomy procedure due to a blocked carotid artery, you lie on your back on an operating table. Then, turn to one side, opposite the side which is to be fixed. The surgeon will insert a temporary, flexible tube so that blood can flow around the blocked area as the procedure continues.

The surgeon will make a small cut or incision on the affected part of the carotid artery. After the surgeon removes the plaques, he closes the artery and neck incisions with stitches.

Angioplasty and Stenting

Another option is angioplasty and stenting. The doctor will place a balloon in the artery to open it, inserting a stent in the blood vessel to open it and hold it open.

VI. Diabetic Retinopathy

What Is Diabetic Retinopathy?

Diabetic retinopathy is an eye disease caused by diabetes complications; the condition causes damage to the blood vessels of the light-sensitive tissue at the back of the eye (retina).

Chapter 5

Can Prediabetes & Type 2 Diabetes Be Reversed and Put into Remission?

Brief Subject Summary

- Comments from Different Authoritative Sources
- Diabetes Remission Guidance
- Is Diabetes Remission Permanent?
- Restrictions of Sugar for Diabetics
- How to Stabilize Your Blood Sugar Levels
- My Journey: Putting My Type 2 Diabetes into Remission
- Do Diabetics Need More Water?
- How Much Water Should You Drink?
- Losing Weight and How Much
- Weight Status and BMI (Body Mass Index)

Now, here is the question:

Can prediabetes and type 2 diabetes be stopped, reversed, stabilized, and put into remission?

Yes, you can do it!

Comments from Different Authoritative Sources

Here are some comments from different sources on what reversal and remission are:

In its report on prediabetes, the Centers for Disease Control and Prevention (CDC) says:

"It's real. It's common. And most importantly, it's reversible. You can prevent or delay prediabetes from developing into type 2 diabetes with simple, proven lifestyle changes."

From the *University Health News* comes this report:

"Learning how to reverse diabetes is not difficult, and it can be done. Doctors will insist that once you have type 2 diabetes, it cannot be cured—which is why it is so important not to allow yourself to become prediabetic—but most will acknowledge that diabetes can be sent into remission. Remission is believed to occur when all the symptoms have resolved."

From its website, *UW Health* says, "Diabetes can go into remission. When diabetes is in remission, you have no signs or symptoms of it. But the risk of relapse is higher than normal."

It adds: "Of those people who don't need diabetes medicine, some find that their diabetes does 'reverse' with weight control, diabetes-healthy eating, and exercise."

For its part, WebMD says: "Although there's no cure for type 2 diabetes, studies show it's possible for some people to reverse it. Through diet changes and weight loss, you may be able to reach and hold normal blood sugar levels without medication."

Diabetes.co.UK says, "People with type 2 diabetes that are able to get their HbA1c below 42 mmol/mol (6%) without taking diabetes medication are said to have reversed or resolved their diabetes. This is also known as putting diabetes into remission."

It continues, "With time and dedication, type 2 diabetes can be reversed, and the results can be very rewarding, with less tiredness and better all-round health."

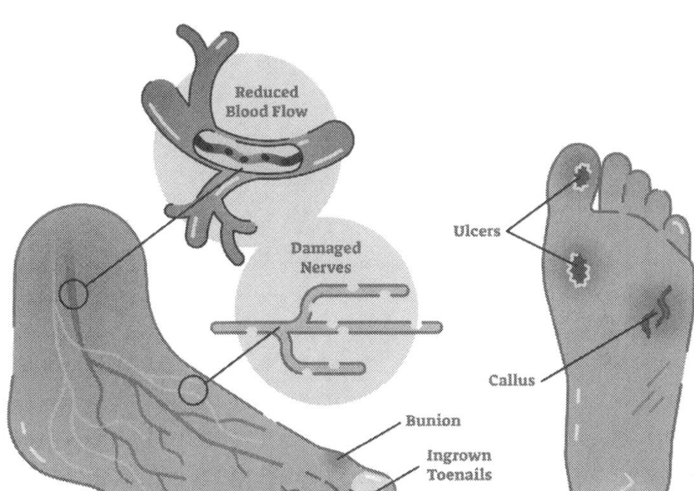

Feet with Common Conditions

Photo Source: Shutterstock

Diabetes Remission Guidance

A panel of international experts from three world diabetes organizations has met in England to define what diabetes remission is. The group members were from the Diabetes UK, the American Diabetes Association, and the European Association for the Study of Diabetes.

The experts agreed on this definition: "Remission is when your HbA1c, a measure of long-term blood glucose levels, remains below 48 mmol/mol or 6.5% for at least six months."

Remission is to be achieved without taking any diabetic medications. It's a fact that reversal can imply a permanent cure, which can't be achieved, so experts decided to use the term "diabetes remission."

So What's the Deal?

In June 2009, a consensus group comprised of experts in the U.S. met to define "cure" or "remission" of prediabetes and type 2 diabetes.

The group consisted of medical professionals, including pediatric and adult endocrinology experts and specialists in diabetes education, metabolism, bariatric and metabolic surgery, and hematology-oncology.

The panel classified remission into three stages: *partial remission, complete remission*, and *prolonged remission.*

(Note: The group's opinions and recommendations are those of the experts and not the official position of the American Diabetes Association.)

The panel's guidelines are as follows:

- *"Partial remission* is having a blood sugar that does not meet the classification for Type 2 diabetes, i.e., either HbA1c <6.5% and/or fasting blood glucose 5.5 - 6.9 mmol/1 (100-125 mg/dl) for at least 1 year while not taking any medications to lower blood sugar.
- *"Complete remission* is the return to normal glucose values, i.e., HbA1c <5.7% and a fasting blood sugar <5.6 mmol/L (100 mg/dl) for at least 1 year while not taking any medications to lower glucose is a return to normal glucose values (i.e. HbA1c <6.0%, and/or fasting blood glucose <5.6 mmol/L (<100 mg/dl) for at least 5 years while not taking any medications to lower blood sugar."
- "*Prolonged remission:* Prolonged remission is complete remission that lasts for more than 5 years and might operationally be considered a cure. The 5-year period was chosen arbitrarily, since there are no actuarial data indicating the likelihood of relapse over various periods of time from the onset of normoglycemia. It is recognized that the risk of relapse likely remains higher for people with diabetes in remission than for age-, sex-, BMI-, and ethnicity-matched individuals who have never had diabetes."

Source: *Diabetes Care*, American Diabetes Association November 2009: https://care.diabetesjournals.org/content/32/11/2133.

Authors of Study: John B. Buse, MD, Ph.D., Sonia Caprio, MD, William T. Cefalu, MD, Antonio Ceriello, MD, Stefano Del Prato, MD, Silvio E. Inzucchi, MD, Sue McLaughlin, BS, RD, CDE, CPT, Gordon L. Phillips II, MD, R. Paul

Robertson, MD, Francesco Rubino, MD, Richard Kahn, Ph.D., and M. Sue Kirkman, MD.

Memorable Day of Type 2 Diabetes Remission

Report on my A1c results at my hospital website follows:

HEMOGLOBIN A1c - Details

Veltisezar B. Bautista

Details

Past Results
Graph of Past Results
Component Results
ComponentYour ValueStandard RangeFlag
Hb A1c 5.7% 4.0 to 6.0% 4.0 - 6.0 %

NOTE: All hemoglobin A1c methods are affected by conditions that decrease or increase red blood cell survival. Falsely high results may be seen with iron deficiency. Falsely normal or low results may be seen with hemolytic anemias, unstable hemoglobins, or following transfusions.

Estimated Average Glucose117 mg/dLmg/dLmg/dL
General Information
Collected on 09/26/2015 7:10 AM
Resulted on 09/27/2015 8:32 AM

On 09/27/2015, I achieved an HhA1c of 5.7%, indicating remission of my type 2 diabetes. To this day, my diabetes stays in remission.

Is Diabetes Remission Permanent?

No. The remission of prediabetes and type 2 diabetes is only temporary. Diabetes symptoms can come back if you resume eating bad foods for diabetes, return to your bad habits, and stop exercising.

However, there were reports that some people have maintained diabetes remission for 15 to 25 years. It all depends on your diet, lifestyle changes, and your exercise

My Journey: Background

Cross-Eyed? It was similar to being crossed-eyed when I had double vision, meaning the two eyes saw different things or overlapping visual views. Without closing one of the two eyes, I could not walk. I didn't know which way to go. The year was 2006.

Prediabetes doesn't usually have any signs or symptoms. I didn't know I had prediabetes for many years, which led to type 2 diabetes. I didn't do any blood sugar monitoring, thinking that I had no family history of diabetes.

So I was diagnosed only with full-blown type 2 after significant complications occurred. First, I had a heart attack in 1996, which doctors attributed to a blockage of the main artery of the left part of the heart, called the left ventricle.

Plaques, a mixture of fat, cholesterol, calcium, and waste from cells, clogged the main left ventricle blood vessel. That's what happened: the blocked artery stopped the blood from reaching the heart, resulting in my heart attack.

It's a fact, too, that diabetes blood sugar had contributed to the damage of the artery walls.

Another Incident: In 2006, my primary physician discovered that I already had full-blown diabetes after a double vision problem.

Restrictions of Sugars for Diabetics

As a general rule, if you have prediabetes, type 2 diabetes, or type 1 diabetes, you should limit or avoid simple carbohydrates such as white rice, white bread, and white pasta to prevent an upsurge of blood sugar after a meal. You should limit or avoid overly-processed products that contain white flour and foods with added sugar

How to Stabilize Your Blood Sugar Levels

There are several ways of stabilizing your blood sugar to treat pre-diabetes, type 2 diabetes, and type 1 diabetes:

The ways include:

- Following a low to moderate carbohydrate diet
- Maintaining a healthy weight
- Doing moderate-intensity walking for 20 minutes after each meal of the day, improving your insulin sensitivity
- Drinking enough water, at least 8 to 10 or more cups or glasses of water (8 ounces) based on your height and weight, to dilute blood sugar
- Maintaining a healthy weight
- Avoiding vigorous-intensity exercise, such as jogging or running that, can result in high blood sugar, not low as you intended to have
- Monitoring blood sugar levels closely
- Consuming more plant-based foods and fewer animal foods
- Increasing dietary fiber intake because fiber reduces carbohydrates level
- Eating low glycemic index and low glycemic load foods
- Having enough sleep, 7 to 9 hours because it promotes good health
- Managing stress
- Limiting or avoiding caffeine, whether it is coming from coffee, tea, or chocolate, because the caffeine in the body increases blood glucose levels
- Eating portion size foods (measured in cups or ounces)
- Choosing whole grains which are slowly digested and don't trigger blood sugar spikes
- Including whole grains in your diet, black rice, brown rice, steel-cut oats, and other foods such as barley, quinoa, tofu, lentils, and chickpeas (See chapter 14: *Rice and Other Grains for Diabetes .)*
- Consuming leafy vegetables, beans, legumes, and selected fruits low in glycemic indexes, such as berries, orange, and grapefruit (if you're not taking Lipitor or any statins)

My Journey: Putting My Type 2 Diabetes into Remission

With my treatment system, including eating more plant foods than animal foods and doing moderate-intensity walking, I have stabilized my blood glucose. In fact, I reduced my high blood sugar to be at always normal level, putting type 2 diabetes into remission.

I have been diabetic for 16 years now. But I have stabilized and put my diabetes into remission, prolonged remission. I have consistently had fasting blood sugar of less than <100 mg/dl and A1c levels ranging from 57% to 59% for the past 7 years. (Years ago, my uppermost fasting blood sugar was 160 mg/dl, and my HbA1c was more than >6.5% A1c.)

Based on diabetes guidelines by a panel of medical experts mentioned earlier, I now have a prolonged remission of my type 2 diabetes with an HbA1c (below < 6% or fasting blood sugar <5.6) mmol/L (<100 mg/dl) for the past 7 years.

Water, Water, Water Everywhere in Our Body

Sixty percent of our body is composed of water, mostly in our brains and muscles; it's like oil to a machine, according to Dr. Roberta Lee in an article in the *Medicine Daily*, published online by *Diabetes Strong*.

Do Diabetics Need More Water?

Yes! And why?

Diabetes.co.UK has this report: "When your blood sugar levels are running high, your body will try to flush excess sugar out of your blood through the urine. As a result, your body will need more fluids to rehydrate itself. Drinking water can help the body with flushing out some of the glucose in the blood."

What Does Water Do to Your Body?

Water nourishes the kidneys and washes away the developing stones. And another benefit? It can lower your BUN and creatinine levels by drinking enough water. With water, you can lessen the effects of bad things on the kidneys. That's a good job of water!

Regarding the importance of water, this can happen to the human body if you have kidney disease: the BUN (blood urea nitrogen) will return to normal with rehydration if the underlying kidney functions are normal.

Quite simply, *Quora* says, "If you have normal BUN and get dehydrated for long enough, the BUN will climb, and then the BUN will fall if you restore normal hydration."

Well, that's a beautiful thing to happen!

Warning: Do not drink water or any fluids in excess. Water can intoxicate you, which may result in death.

Other terms for water intoxication may include hyperhydration, water toxemia, water poisoning, and overhydration.

Water intoxication happens when the amount of salt and other electrolytes in your body becomes too diluted. The condition is called hyponatremia. For this reason, when electrolytes drop too quickly and too low, they can kill you.

Furthermore, the accumulation of fluids in the brain called cerebral edema can affect the brain stem and cause dysfunction of the central nervous system. As a result, the brain can be damaged and cause seizures and even death.

How Much Water Is Enough?

For people with type 2 diabetes, drinking water is a must. Why? Because a little dehydration can significantly impact your blood sugar, rising as high as it can.

So how much water is enough? Well, it may depend on different factors. There is no definitive rule on how much water you should consume, but you can take steps to determine how much you need.

Water is fluid, including other liquids such as soft drinks, coffee or tea, or juices. So in counting water intake of liquids or fluids, you must deduct the volume of such fluids in the form of coffee or tea, from the total amount of water you should drink per day.

Of course, when there's hot weather, you may drink more fluids to stay hydrated. Yes, it is good to drink water, the number 1 drink globally.

According to the Institute of Medicine, men may drink up to about 13 cups (3.08 1 liters) per day, and women may drink about 9 cups (2.13 1 liters).

Drinking-Water Formula

The standard formula for determining daily water intake is a "one size fits all"; that is, eight 8-ounce cups or glasses of water every day. That should not be the case, experts say. Why? Because we have different body sizes and levels of activities.

Determining how much water you should drink per day depends on several factors, including your body size, weight, gender, and levels of exercise or activities.

Simple Formulas

Here's the simple formula available for calculating how much water you drink per day:

Bodyweight divided by 2 = 1/2 (or 50%) of the bodyweight

Now, we should presume 1/2 of the body weight to be in ounces to compute how many ounces of water should be consumed by an individual based on weight.

For instance, If you weigh 150 lbs. you divide it by 2 = 75. In this case, you should drink 75 ounces of water (a little less than 9 measuring cups or glasses of water. A cup contains 8 ounces of liquid.

It's that simple. But in calculating water intake, you should also take cognizance of your walking, exercise, or workout intensity. Also, your water intake may depend on the weather in your area, whether it's cold or hot. Then, if it's hot, you should add some more water.

Example

If I use this formula for me, then the calculation should be like this:

Bodyweight divide by 2 = 1/2 or 50% of body weight
I weigh 125 lbs divided by 2 = 1/2 of body weight
125 lbs. divided by 2 = 62.5 ounces of water

For instance, 62.5 divide by 8 (ounces per cup or glass) = 7.81 cups or make it 8 cups of water.

But I thought that this water volume was insufficient to dilute my blood sugar, blood urea nitrogen (BUN), and creatinine. Blood sugar, blood urea, nitrogen, and creatinine are all water-soluble. Nitrogen gas does not react with water; it does dissolve in water

So I decided to drink 9 to 10 cups of water (including tea), which means 9 x 8 ounces at least 72 ounces of water daily. If I consume 10 cups or glasses of water per day, that equals (10 x 8 ounces) = 80 ounces of fluid.

But I seldom drink 10 glasses of water per day; the average is 9 ½ cups or glasses of water consisting of 3 types of teas: Moringa tea, green tea, and white tea, which some studies showed teas lower blood sugar and boost energy during exercise. I drink 1 cup of tea one hour after each meal before my moderate-intensity walking.

Another Formula

Generally, the computation of how much water to drink is done in two ways: from 1/2 (50%) to 2/3 (67%) of your body weight, which will be calculated as ounces.

With regard to the formula of 2/3 of the body weight, multiply your body weight by 2/3 (or 67%) to determine how much water to drink.

You may want to multiply your weight by 2/3 (or 67%) to determine how much water to drink daily. For example, if you weighed 174 pounds you would multiply that by 2/3 (67%) and learn how you should be drinking about 116.58 ounces of water every day.

Sipping, Gulping, or Chugging Water

Here's an explanation of the words above:

Sipping water (or fluid) means you drink it by taking just a small amount of it at a time; while gulping it, you drink the water quickly by swallowing it in large amounts.

On the other hand, chugging may mean consuming a drink in large gulps without pausing. So it means, too, that chugging is more aggressive drinking.

Some experts say that to be fully hydrated: there is a need to have a slow but steady approach to water consumption. That is, the answer should be you sip your water allocation by dividing the amount of drink at intervals throughout the day.

In sipping, some sources say the water and nutrients go continuously to all body parts, including the cells, for water hydration.

On the other hand, when you gulp or chug water, there will be an overload of water that the kidneys should filter. When the kidneys are overloaded, they naturally respond by flushing out excess water to ensure a correct amount of fluid stays within the body. It's because the kidneys are responsible for balancing fluids in the body.

But for me, I can't do water sipping at all times. It's because if I do that, it will take me a long period sipping water. How about when I'm busy?

So what I do is, sometimes, I do some little gulping of water, and sometimes I do a few sips of water to drink enough water in a certain period. Also, there are days that I bring at least one bottle of water when I go out and sip it little by little.

Yes, it's better to sip water because the body can absorb it slowly. But if you can't do a lot of sipping, you must do some gulps of water, consuming about 8 or more cups of fluid every day, the amount of which depends on your body weight and other factors like age and gender.

Losing Weight and How Much?

According to the CDC, losing weight doesn't mean losing a lot of weight. It says taking off just 5% to 10%—that's 10 to 20 pounds for a 200-pound person—can improve your health and well-being.

If you have diabetes, you may find your blood sugar levels easier to manage with less diabetes medicine after losing weight. Many people who lose weight notice that they have more energy and sleep better.

What Is a Healthy Weight?

Again, here's what CDC reports according to its guidelines:

There are two ways of getting a good idea to see if your weight is healthy or not: Body Mass Index (BMI) and waist circumference.

BMI measures body fat based on weight in kilograms and height in meters. It indicates whether a person has healthy body fat by dividing the body mass by the square of the body height.

BMI Calculation Formula (Metric)

BMI Chart

BMI = Weigh t(kg) / height (m^2)

Weight Status	BMI
Underweight	Less than 18.5
Normal	18.5–24.9
Overweight	25–29.9
Obese	30 or greater

English to metric conversions:

Weight (kilograms): 1 lb / (1 kg / 2.2lbs) = 0.454 kg

Height (meters): 1 ft = 12 inches, 12 inches = 1 ft, 1 ft = 0.3048 m

Sample Calculation

Example: Weight: 125 lbs, Height: 5 ft 5 inches

Weight (kilograms): multiply 125 by 1/2.2 to get lbs converted to kilograms. 125 lbs x (1 kg/2.2 lbs) = 56.81 kgs.

Height (meters): To convert inches to feet, multiply 5 inches by 1/12 then add to 5 ft, 5 inches x (1 ft / 12 inches) = 0.42 ft; 5 ft + 0.42 ft = 5.42 ft;

To convert inches to feet, multiply 5.42 by 0.348/1 = 5.42 ft x (0.3048 m / 1 ft) = 1.652 m

When you have all the conversions calculated, you can determine the BMI by dividing 56.81 kgs by the multiplication of 1.652m to 1.652m = 56.81 kgs / (1.652m) x (1.652m) = 56.81 kgs/2.729 m^2 = 20.82 kgs/m^2

Hence, 20.82 kgs/m^2 is the BMI.

(Note: m^2 means to multiply the number by itself; The symbol / means divide the first number by the second number.

Based on the BMI Category Chart above, the number 20.1 is in the middle range of 18.5-24.9 (normal weight). Therefore, a BMI of 20.82 represents a healthy weight.

Want to Know Your BMI?

Want to do your BMI calculation? If you don't want to do it, you may google: "BMI calculators" and select any BMI calculators, including CDC calculator. You type the height and weight and click Calculate, and you'll get the number instantly.

How Many Grams of Carbs Per Day for Diabetics

The recommendations on how many grams of carbs per day for people with diabetes vary:

- The American Diabetes Association (ADA) says that 150-200 grams per day, or 30-40% of total calories on a 2,000-calorie diet, is a standard low-carb diet. However, the ADA emphasizes that there is no ideal amount of carbohydrates for all people with diabetes. The ADA suggests that you choose healthy carbs or low glycemic index and low glycemic load foods, which are considered healthy carbs.

- The typical American diet is more than 250 grams of carbohydrates per day. But this quota is considered high for most people with diabetes.
- The Recommended Dietary Allowance (RDA) for carbs is 130 grams per day.
- There's no standard definition of a low-carb diet, so medical professionals often consider less than 130 grams per day as a low-carb diet.
- Some dietitians recommend 45 grams to 60 grams of carbs per meal or 135 grams to 180 grams per day

Chapter 6

Pancreas Islets for Type 1 Diabetes; Next, Pig Islets?

Brief Subject Summary

- FDA Panel Endorses Allogeneic Islet Transplant Therapy
- Brittle Diabetes or Labile Diabetes
- Benefits of Treatment
- Who Are Candidates for Islet Transplantation?
- Two Pancreas Procedures
- Allogeneic Islet Transplant
- Process of Transplantation
- Autologous or Auto-Islet Transplant
- Pig Islets for Humans?
- What is Type 1 Diabetes?
- Causes, Symptoms, and Treatment of Type 1 Diabetes
- Complications of Type 1 Diabetes

FDA Panel Endorses Allogeneic Islets Transplant Therapy

A US Food and Drug Administration (FDA) advisory panel has endorsed an allogeneic pancreatic islet transplant therapy to treat people with type 1 diabetes. The product is for type 1 diabetics with severely low blood sugar or hypoglycemia problems.

On April 15, 2021, the FDA's Cellular, Tissue, and Gene Therapies Advisory Committee voted 12 to 4 in favor of the approval of donislecel (Lantidra). There was one abstention.

The therapy, manufactured by CellTrans, is intended for adults with "brittle" type 1 diabetes.

If you have brittle diabetes, you have a condition that's hard to control; both mean "unstable" or "easily changed." Brittle diabetes is also called "labile" diabetes.

When you have this disorder, your blood sugar levels often range from very low (hypoglycemia) to very high (hyperglycemia).

The Pancreas

The pancreas has 2 types of glands:

Exocrine. The exocrine gland secretes digestive enzymes.
Endocrine: The endocrine gland consists of the islets of Langerhans. This gland secretes hormones into the bloodstream.

Insulin and glucagon are the main hormones produced by the endocrine glands. They work together to regulate the glucose levels in the blood.

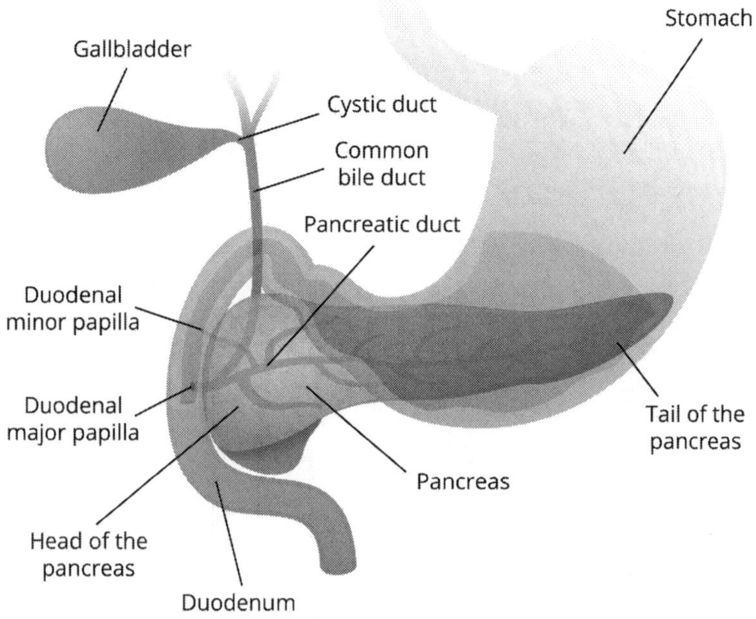

The Human Pancreas

Photo Source: Shutterstock

What Are Islets?

Pancreatic islets, also called islets of Langerhans, are small clusters of beta cells in the pancreas that produce hormones. The islets contain 5 types of cells, one of which is called beta cells that produce insulin groups of beta cells in your pancreas.

As you probably know, insulin helps your body use glucose for energy and controls blood glucose levels.

Because islet transplantation is in its experimental stage, it can only be performed as part of (FDA)-allowed clinical trials.

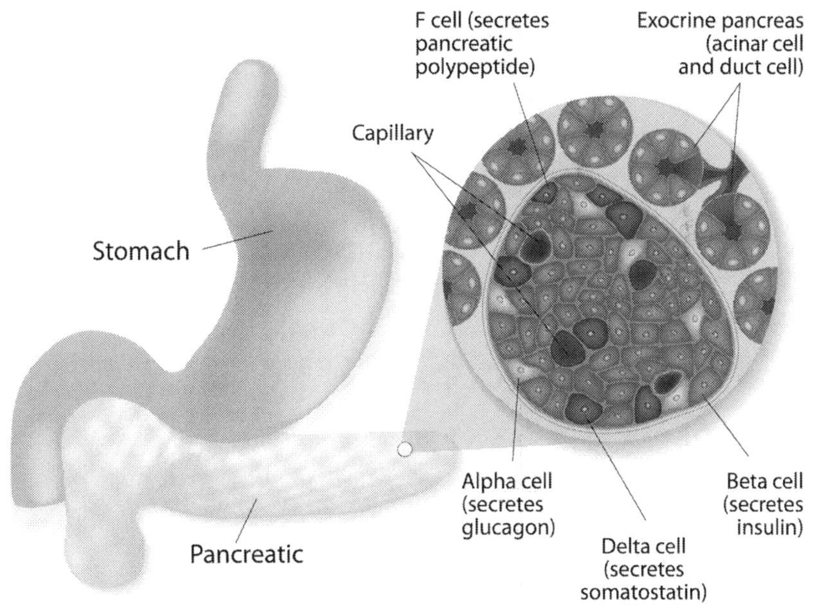

Islets of Langerhans

Photo Source: Shutterstock

Benefits of Treatment

- Potential for insulin independence
- Elimination of severe hypoglycemia

The new product consists of purified allogeneic pancreatic islets of Langerhans taken from deceased donors. The islets are small clusters of cells in the pancreas that secrete several hormones, one of which is insulin produced by the beta cells. A surgeon infuses the islet solution into the portal vein of the recipient's liver. The transplanted islets will then produce insulin in the recipient's liver to manage the body's blood sugar levels.

The potential risks in islet transplant include surgical procedure complications and long-term immunosuppression, taking medicines to prevent the rejection of the product by the recipient's body.

CellTrans manufactures the therapy. According to Jose Oberholzer, MD, the founder of CellTrans, the proposed indication is for adults with "brittle" type 1 diabetes who meet the American Diabetes Association's (ADA's) criteria for whole-organ pancreas-alone transplant (i.e., transplant of the pancreas but not the kidneys).

The allogeneic islet transplantation therapy involves transferring islets from dead persons to people with type 1 diabetes. If the FDA approves the new treatment, the time may come that more people can benefit from this therapy and reverse their type 1 diabetes.

What a great achievement that could be!

Background

So far, the Collaborative Islet Transplantation Registry (CITR) External link has reported that, between 1999 and 2015, 1,086 patients worldwide received islet transplants for type 1 diabetes.

The CITR gets information on pancreas transplants from North America, Europe, Australia, and Asia research centers. The U.S. National Institute of Diabetes and Digestive and Kidney Diseases (NIDDK) established the CITR.

Who Are Candidates for Islet Transplantation?

The ideal candidates for the procedure are those people with type 1 diabetes who have:

- Blood glucose levels that are difficult to manage
- Occurrence of hypoglycemia awareness, a dangerous condition in which a patient can't recognize the symptoms of hypoglycemia
- People who are experiencing severe hypoglycemia
- Type 1 diabetic patients who have had or are planning to have a kidney transplant to treat kidney failure

Two Pancreas Islet Procedures

There are two types of pancreas islet transplantations: the **allogeneic** and the **autologous** or simply **autotransplantation**.

The allogeneic transplant is an experimental procedure rather than a clinical treatment in the United States. However, medical centers in some parts of the world now perform the process.

On the other hand, many universities have been doing pancreas islet autotransplantations in medical facilities approved by the FDA to offer the surgery.

What's the Difference Between the Two Pancreas Procedures?

The allogeneic transplant in pancreas islets taken from a deceased donor to a recipient who has type 1 diabetes. On the other hand, autotransplantation requires a surgeon to remove a patient's pancreas. And infuse the islet solution into the donor and recipient being the same.

I. Allogeneic Islet Transplant

While Americans are still waiting for the approval of the treatment by the FDA, U.S. scientists are still in the third phase of experimental trials on islet transplantations, known as allogeneic pancreas islet transplants. The transplants are for people with type 1 diabetes, endorsed by an FDA panel last year.

Turning Point?

With an FDA panel endorsement of the allogeneic pancreas islet transplant, there's a probability of its approval by the U.S. government agency.

Although it's not automatic for the FDA to approve an endorsed drug or product by a panel, the approval may occur unless documents or other research results are missing.

The allogeneic pancreas islet transplantation is a standard treatment for patients with labile type 1 diabetes worldwide, including in Japan, Australia, the United Kingdom, Canada, and most European countries.

The Process of Pancreas Islet Transplantation

The process involves a surgeon inserting a thin, flexible tube called a catheter through an incision or small cut in the recipient's abdomen.

A radiologist uses ultrasound and x-rays to assist the surgeon in the procedure.

At first, the surgeon injects the islets extracted from a deceased pancreas donor into the vein where the blood flows into the liver of a person with type 1 diabetes.

After that, if the procedure is successful, the beta cells begin to make and release insulin in the recipient's body

Benefits of Islet Transplantation

According to the National Institute of Diabetes and Digestive and Kidney Diseases (NIDDK), the benefits of islet transplantation include:

- Improved blood glucose levels
- Improved awareness of hypoglycemia, which helps prevent episodes of severe hypoglycemia
- Fewer or no episodes of severe hypoglycemia
- May help prevent or slow the development or progression of diabetes complications, such as kidney disease, heart disease, and nerve or eye damage

How About the Risks?

The NIDDK says the risks of islet transplantation may include:

- Bleeding
- Blood clots
- Side effects of anti-rejection medicines, also called immunosuppressants

Side Effects of Immunosuppressants

Immunosuppressants can have serious side effects, which may include:

- Kidney disease
- High glucose levels
- High blood pressure
- High levels of cholesterol and triglycerides in the blood
- Headaches, tremors, and confusion
- Higher chance of getting infections
- Vomiting
- Nausea
- Diarrhea

What's the Success Rate of This Procedure?

Participants in a study sponsored by the National Institute of Health (NIH) included people with type 1 diabetes who had problems managing their blood sugar levels. These issues involve severe hypoglycemia (low blood sugar) and "impaired awareness of hypoglycemia."

The study found out that:

- After one year of islet transplantation, almost 9 out of 10 transplant recipients had an A1c level below 7% (the A1c goal of many people with diabetes).
- Participants did not have any episodes of severe hypoglycemia.
- About 4 out of 10 participants did not need insulin intake.
- Islet transplant recipients experienced significant improvements in their diabetes-related quality of life.

Evolution of Islet Transplantation

According to the U.S. National Institute of Health (NIH), islet cell transplantation started as early as 1893. That happened when Watson-Williams and Harshant transplanted a minced sheep pancreas into the thigh of a young boy with diabetic ketoacidosis. But though the boy's condition improved for 24 hours, the procedure finally failed.

Then in 1980, a patient achieved insulin independence with normal glucose levels at 9 months follow-up. There were reports of less than 10 percent successful insulin independence for one year from that time on.

Somewhere in Switzerland

In 1979, a group from Zurich University led by Largiader, Kolb, and Binswanger reported the first successful transplantation of allogeneic pancreatic fragments.

The procedure was in conjunction with a kidney transplant in a patient with T1D (type 1 diabetes)., resulting in 10 months of exogenous insulin independence until kidney failure occurred. Exogenous insulin is the insulin people inject or infuse via an insulin pump.

Sometime in 1985, the University of Miami in Florida reported promising results of allogeneic islet transplantation. But the research failed, too.

Scientists consider the year 2000 as a milestone in the advancement of islet transplantation. Why? Because the publication of the so-called Edmonton Protocol produced results far more promising than previously reported in Islet Transplant Registry.

The registry had collected data from 267 islet transplants voluntarily reported by several research centers from 1990 to 2001.

What Is the Edmonton Protocol?

The Edmonton protocol is a method of implanting pancreatic islets to treat type 1 diabetes.

Reports indicated more than 1,000 patients worldwide with type 1 diabetes successfully received the treatment. Although up to 80% of the recipients achieved insulin independence for the first year after transplant, many returned to small insulin use over time.

II. Autologous or Auto-Islet Transplant

John Hopkins Medicine describes an auto-islet transplant by saying, "An auto-islet transplant, also known as a total pancreatectomy with auto islet cell transplantation or islet autotransplantation, is an operation where an entire pancreas is removed. The isolated cells are placed in an IV bag with a solution. The solution is then infused into the liver."

An autologous islet cell transplant or an islet cell auto-transplantation is an infusion of a patient's pancreatic islets into his liver portal vein. After that, the islets start making insulin for the patient.

Twenty Programs in the U.S. Offering Auto Islet Transplant

The Johns Hopkins Hospital is one of a few research centers globally to offer autologous (auto) islet cell transplantation.

Twenty medical centers offer this pioneering procedure to restore patients to live without chronic pancreatitis pain or insulin dependence. The FDA has approved these medical facilities to perform this surgery.

In addition, auto islet transplant cures pancreatitis with a lower risk of developing diabetes after the operation. The islet auto-transplant process is a modified islet transplant surgery used to manage severe insulin-dependent type 1 diabetes.

During the transplant, the surgeon gets the islets from a deceased person and infuses them into the recipient's body. On the other hand, in chronic pancreatitis, the patient's islets are used; thus, eliminating the risk of tissue rejection.

In other words, a pancreatectomy, referred to as pancreas removal surgery, relieves severe pain in patients with chronic pancreatitis.

Total Pancreatectomy and Islet Autotransplantation

Who are the candidates for auto-islet transplants? They are those who have acute recurrent and chronic pancreatitis. Usually, these patients have chronic severe abdominal pain and do not respond to conventional treatment.

The procedures involved two parts:

Doctors surgically remove the pancreas in the first part, a procedure known as a total pancreatectomy.

In the second part, the surgeon removes the auto islets (insulin-producing cells) from the pancreas of the dead donor and delivers them to the recipient's liver.

III. Pig Islets for Humans?

Alternative to Human Islets

Insufficient cadaveric islet donors spurred scientists to expand medical research into using pig islets as an alternative to human islets for transplantation for people with type 1 diabetes.

Several years ago, using a $2.5 million, three-year grant from the Juvenile Diabetes Research Foundation (JDRF), Emory University transplant researchers planned to develop pig islets, alternative to human islets for transplant into patients with Type 1 diabetes.

The JDRF, based in New York, NY, is the leading global organization funding type 1 diabetes (T1D) research clinical trials.

Because the pancreas of a patient with Type 1 diabetes cannot produce insulin, the patient must receive sufficient transplanted islets to manufacture adequate insulin.

However, most people require more than one islet infusion to forgo insulin injections. Not only that, the patients must take toxic immunosuppressant drugs to prevent the immune system from attacking the new islets.

Clinical trials continue to see if pig islets will treat people with type 1 diabetes.

Why Use Common Pigs, Not Guinea Pigs?

But why, of all animals, do scientists select pigs to be the donors of pancreas islets?

Here are the reasons:

- The similarity between porcine and human insulin
- The high fecundity (the ability to produce an abundance of offspring or new growth) of pigs
- The availability of efficient and precise techniques for genetic modification
- The possibility of maintaining pigs under designated pathogen-free (DPF) conditions, and
- Less socio-cultural and ethical concerns compared to research involving nonhuman primates (NHPs) or dogs

Sources of porcine islets won't be a problem. There are millions of pigs in the whole world!

Background

As early as 2010, Serena Gorfdin, a reporter, published an article in *HealthDay News* about pancreatic cells from pigs transplanted into humans. Those beta cells called porcine islets have been encapsulated and successfully transplanted into humans without triggering the dreaded immune system attack on the new islets.

And the good thing is the transplanted pig pancreas cells quickly produced insulin in response to high blood glucose levels in the bloodstream.

In some patients, their blood sugar control improved. Two patients stopped their insulin injections for at least a short time. From then on, the search continued.

Now, we'll see what the future holds for this new technology. What a wonderful world!

There are 21 research centers throughout the U.S. participating in this endeavor.

IV. Type 1 Diabetes

What Is Type 1 Diabetes?

Mayo Clinic says: "Type 1 diabetes, once known as juvenile diabetes or insulin-dependent diabetes, is a chronic condition in which the pancreas produces little or no insulin."

"Insulin is a hormone needed to allow sugar (glucose) to enter cells to produce energy," it adds.

Cleveland Clinic says, "Type 1 diabetes occurs when the autoimmune system attacks and destroys cells in the pancreas called beta cells, which produce insulin."

"Insulin is a hormone that helps sugar, or glucose, enter cells to give them energy," it further says.

Yes, when there is not enough insulin entering the cells, too much sugar stays in the bloodstream, which may lead to a life-threatening condition.

However, different factors, like genetics and some viruses, may cause type 1 diabetes.

Also, even if type 1 diabetes typically occurs during childhood or adolescence, it can develop in adults up to 30 years old.

Type 1 diabetes is also different from prediabetes and type 2 diabetes because its immune system destroys the insulin-producing pancreas (called beta cells).

Other Diseases Common to People with Type 1 Diseases

Autoimmune disorders: Medical experts don't know how autoimmune disease occurs. They presume that this disease is caused by genetics, in which the immune system attacks its own body's healthy cells or tissues. And there are no medicines yet to cure this condition.

Thyroid disorders: Kids and teenagers with type 1 diabetes usually become victims of this disorder that affect the thyroid. Thyroid is a part of the endocrine system. And as such, it makes hormones that aid in controlling growth and metabolism.

Celiac disease: Celiac disease is another autoimmune disorder affecting 1 in 20 people with type 1 diabetes. The immune system reacts when foods containing gluten can cause gastrointestinal problems to kids and teens.

Grains such as rye, barley, and wheat have gluten. This disease can cause tiredness, lack of appetite, and weight loss.

Addison's disease: This disorder is a type of adrenal insufficiency that affects the adrenal glands of the endocrine system.

These glands are essential because they make hormones, including cortisol and aldosterone. The glands help control many body functions, including those involved in response to stress.

They are also involved in maintaining body functions, fluid balance, blood pressure, and immune system activities.

Causes of Type 1 Diabetes

Like genetics and some viruses, different factors may cause type 1 diabetes. Also, even if type 1 diabetes typically occurs during childhood or adolescence, it should not be surprising that it can develop in adults up to 30 years old.

There are no known exact causes of type 1 diabetes.

- Thought to be an autoimmune disease
- Exposure to viruses and other environmental factors

Symptoms of Type 1 Diabetes

- Increased thirst
- Unexplained weight loss
- Frequent urination
- Extreme hunger
- Unintended weight loss
- Irritability and other mood changes
- Sores that heal slowly
- Dry and itchy skin
- Weakness and fatigue
- Loss of feeling in feet or having tingles in feet
- Blurry eyesight
- Frequent exhaustion

Treatments of Type 1 Diabetes

To this day, there is no cure yet for type 1 diabetes. Many factors involving genetics and some viruses, as a whole, can cause type 1 diabetes, which can be treated by:

Insulin Therapy

- Pancreas islet transplantation as described in this chapter
- Adopting effective diets for type 1 diabetes, prediabetes, and type 2 diabetes, such as the Mediterranean diet, Flexitarian (or semi-vegetarian diet), or a plant-based diet
- Moderate intensity walking within one hour each meal of the day (See chapter 9)
- Eating low carbohydrates and more fiber
- Avoiding sugary foods and drinks
- Limiting or avoiding foods with high fructose
- Reducing stress
- Getting enough sleep
- Avoiding eating high carbohydrates and sugary foods
- Eating whole grains, such as lentils, quinoa, brown rice, and black rice
- Limiting or avoiding caffeine from coffee, tea, chocolate, and other products, because caffeine affect blood glucose
- Limiting or avoiding salty canned foods, and other well-processed foods such as white rice, white bread, and white pasta

Medicines

Since the launch of Symlin in 2005, it's not unusual that people with type 1 diabetes treat themselves with some supplemental injectable medication besides insulin. Some of them also take oral medicines, known as "type 2 only" drugs.

Symlin (pramlintide) is a manufactured form of a hormone that occurs naturally in the body. Type 1 diabetes and type 2 diabetes patients take pramlintide, together with insulin, to lower blood glucose (of type 1 and type 2 diabetes patients), including the glucose produced by the liver.

Complications of Type 1 Diabetes

If you don't control your blood sugar, you may suffer from the complications, which may include:

- Chronic kidney disease (diabetic kidney nephrology)
- Heart disease
- Stroke
- High blood pressure
- Nerve disease (neuropathy)
- Skin infections
- Foot problems, including ulcers
- Eye disease (retinopathy)

V. Hypoglycemia and Hyperglycemia

1. What Is Hypoglycemia (Low Blood Sugar)?

Hypoglycemia is a condition in which your blood sugar (glucose) level is lower than normal. A fasting blood sugar level of less than 100 mg/dL (<5.6 mmol/L) is normal.

Different people react differently to blood sugar levels. Generally, a fasting blood sugar of 70 milligrams per deciliter (mg/dL), or 3.9 millimoles per liter (mmol/L), or below should serve as a warning for hypoglycemia.

You may ask your doctor how much your numbers indicate an alert for hypoglycemia.

Causes of Hypoglycemia

The causes of hypoglycemia may include:

- Insufficient carbohydrates in the body
- Delaying or skipping meals
- Exercising too much or without eating before doing it
- Drinking alcohol, if you're taking insulin or oral medicines
- Kidney disease insufficiency in clearing insulin from the system
- Body production of too much insulin

- Taking the antimalarial drug Qualaquin (quinine), the antibiotic Zymaxid (gatifloxacin), antiarrhythmic drug cibenzoline, antimicrobial drug Pentam (pentamidine), nonsteroidal anti-inflammatory drug (NSAID), Indocin, and Tivorbex (indomethacin)
- If you have type 1 diabetes, you may not have taken enough insulin.
- If you have type 2 diabetes, your body may have sufficient insulin, but it's not as effective as it should be.
- You have not eaten sufficient carbohydrates, and didn't have enough exercise.
- You may have experienced the so-called down phenomenon, during which the body produces hormones that occur daily around 4 a.m. to 5 a.m.

Symptoms of Hypoglycemia

Causes of symptoms of hypoglycemia may include:

- Fatigue
- Pale skin
- Blurred vision
- Fast or irregular heartbeat
- Headache
- Dizziness
- Heart palpitations
- Mood changes
- Tremor or trembling
- Sweating
- Skin tingling
- Hunger
- Lack of concentration
- Unconsciousness
- Restless sleep
- Frequent urination
- Increased thirst or hunger
- Dry mouth
- Confusion
- High level of sugar in the urine
- Fruity-smelling breath.

Hypoglycemia Emergency Treatment

If you experience hypoglycemia, eat or drink any of the following:

- 1 tablespoon of sugar
- 1 tablespoon of honey
- 2 or 3 pieces of hard candy
- 4 or 5 saltine crackers

Complications

If left untreated, complications may occur, including:

- Damage to eyes, kidneys, and heart
- Damage to the nervous system
- Nerve damage
- Unconsciousness
- Seizures

What Is Hyperglycemia (High Blood Sugar)?

Hyperglycemia is a medical condition characterized by high blood sugar in the bloodstream. Generally, blood glucose may be considered high when it exceeds 11.1 mmol/l or 200 mg/dl.

However, you may not notice it until the value reaches 13.9-16.7 mmol/l or 200 to 300 mg/dl when symptoms occur.

As mentioned in Chapter 3, when you have a fasting glucose level of 100 - 125 mg/dl, you are considered prediabetic; when you have a fasting blood sugar level of more than 125 mg/dl, you are supposed to have type 2 diabetes.

Diabetic Ketoacidosis

If left untreated, hyperglycemia can lead to diabetic ketoacidosis (DKA). DKA is a serious medical condition that leads to diabetic coma or even death. Why?

When your body's cells don't get the glucose they need for energy, they burn fat. The process produces ketones, chemicals that the body makes to break down fat for energy use. It does this because insulin cannot use glucose for energy when it is not sufficient in the body.

As a result, ketones build up in the blood, making it more acidic. When the levels of ketones get too high, it is then that you can develop diabetic ketoacidosis. Usually, this condition happens to people with type 1 diabetes and rarely to people with type 2 diabetes.

Home Treatment of Hyperglycemia

- **Walking**: Moderate-intensity walking, an hour after each meal of the day, is an effective way to lower your high blood sugar caused by eating breakfast, lunch, or dinner. Determine how long you should exercise or how fast you should do it. (See chapter 9, Walking.)
- **Taking your medication as directed**: If you have frequent episodes of hyperglycemia, your doctor may adjust the dosage or timing of your medication.
- **Making your eating plan:** It helps to eat smaller portions and avoid sugary beverages and frequent snacking. If you're having trouble sticking to your meal plan, ask your doctor or dietitian for help.
- **Checking your blood sugar regularly**: Monitor your blood glucose as directed by your doctor. Check more often if you're ill or concerned about severe hypoglycemia or hyperglycemia.
- **Adjusting your insulin doses:** Adjustments to your insulin program or have supplemental short-acting insulin. Insulin can help control hyperglycemia levels. You may ask your doctor how often you need an insulin supplement if you have high blood sugar.

Chapter 7

How to Reverse, Stabilize, & Put Kidney Disease into Remission

Brief Subject Summary

- Chronic Kidney Disease Remission
- How You Can Reverse, Stabilize, and Put Chronic Kidney Disease into Remission
- KDIGO Definition of CKD Remission
- The Kidneys and Types of Kidney Diseases
- Creatine and Creatinine
- Phosphocreatine (PCr) or Creatine Phosphate (CP)
- Creatine Kinase (CK) or Phosphocreatine Kinase (PCK)
- Blood Urea Nitrogen (BUN)
- Estimated Glomerular Filtration Rate (eGFR)

Can chronic kidney disease (CKD) be reversed, stabilized, and put into remission?

Many medical experts say yes; others say no. I have gathered documentation based on several studies, and my personal journey shows that you can reverse and put your kidney disease into remission.

I'm a living testimony of putting kidney disease into remission by doing the steps in my 19 ways of treating this disease.

I. Kidney Disease Remission

How You Can Reverse, Stabilize, and Put Chronic Kidney into Remission

Some experts say that you can reverse CKD and put it into remission. Some say you can slow it down, but you can't reverse kidney disease severity and put it into remission.

I have done it: I have stopped, stabilized, and put my CKD into remission.

KDIGO Definition of CKD Remission

The Kidney Disease Improving Global Outcomes (KDIGO) defines CKD remission as the absence of diagnostic criteria (estimated glomerular filtration rate (eGFR) >60 ml/min/1.73m2 and urine albumin-to-creatinine ratio (uACR) <3 mg/mmol) at any study visit. (A study visit is a short stay for some days or even weeks in a host country for a person or a group understudy.)

In 1995, the National Kidney Foundation (NKF) developed the first broadly accepted clinical practice guidelines in nephrology, known as KDOQI—Kidney Disease Outcomes Quality Initiative.

In 2002, the NFK-KDOQI proposed the definition and classification for chronic kidney disease. The KDOQI endorsed the proposal in 2004.

Based on the NKF-KDOQI guideline, it means that I have reversed and put my kidney disease into remission. My current GFR numbers are from 61% to 73%. I improved my kidney disease GFR from 35% in 2016 to 73% in December 2020, as proven by the results of echocardiogram tests included in this book.

I have a normal albumin value, and I have no albuminuria or elevated protein in the urine (proteinuria).

Large CKD Study Reports Kidney Disease Remission

In a large five-year study by Adam Shardlow et al., published by the National Institute of Health (NIH) in 2016 on its website, the group reports:

- Only 4 (0.2%) developed ESKD (end-stage kidney disease), the last stage of long-term) chronic kidney disease
- 308 participants (17.7%) had CKD progression
- Stable CKD was observed in 593 participants (34.1%)
- 336 (19.3%) met the criteria for remission

The study included 1,741 patients from general practices around the United Kingdom from 2008 to 2010. All the participants met the KDIGO criteria for stage 3 chronic kidney disease and eGFR measurements below 60 mL/min per q1.73 m2 over 90 days.

The mean eGFR was 52.5 mL/min per 1.733 m2. And the mean age at baseline was 73 years old. (Mean age refers to the average ages in a different group of individuals.)

The mean age is used in the statistical entry to compare people with a different age group for various reasons and intentions.

Under the guideline, a participant had to have (at least) 2 eGFR tests <90 mL/min/1.73 m2 at least 90 days apart, in line with the definitions under the guidelines of the Kidney Disease Improving Global Outcomes (KDIGO) classification and the UK National Institute for Health and Care Excellence (NICE).

The cohort (a group of people banded together) included individuals with reduced kidney function (median follow-up 4.9 years, 45% men, 19% with CKD, and 74% with only mildly decreased eGFR of 60–89 mL/min/1.73 m2 at entry or 60%-89%.

The researchers based the above results of the large study on the KDIGO's definition of kidney remission. In this study, the results revealed 336 (19.3%) met the criteria for kidney disease remission.

Indeed, kidney disease is feasible for many people who have this condition, depending on how they implement the correct ways of treatment and based on the stage of their illness, at least third stage CKD or below.

In other words, if caught early in the early stages (1-3), reversing the disease is possible. However, doctors often discover kidney disease when it's already in the third stage because of the non-appearance of symptoms.

You must not have albuminuria or proteinuria in your urine if you want to put your kidney disease into remission. That is, your albumin level should be in the normal range.

Albuminuria is a kind of protein in the urine. Proteinuria indicates the presence of abnormal quantities of protein in the urine, which may show damage to the kidneys.

Reference Range

The reference range for albumin testing is 3.5 to 5.5 g/dL or 35-55 g/liter. This range may vary slightly in different laboratories. Indeed, if you have kidney disease, you can put it into remission, too, depending on what you'll be doing.

New Practice Guideline About Chronic Kidney Disease (CKD)

KDIGO (Kidney Disease: Improving Global Outcomes) has released a new CKD practice guideline, updating the 2002 NKF-KDOQI guideline. (NKF stands for the National Kidney Foundation in the United States, whose national offices are in New York City, NY.)

The KDIGO is a global non-profit organization developing and implementing evidence-based clinical practice guidelines in kidney disease. It is an independent, volunteer-led, self-managed charity incorporated in Ghent, Belgium.

According to KDIGO, "CKD is defined as abnormalities of kidney structure or function, present for >3 months, with implications for health," and requires one of two criteria documented or inferred for >3 months: either GFR <60 ml/min/1.73 m2 or markers of kidney damage, including albuminuria.

To further discuss it, CKD is classified based on cause, GFR category (stages G1-G5), and albuminuria category (A-1 to A-3), abbreviated as CGA.

The new guideline didn't change the definition; hence, the description of CKD is not new. The definition of CKD clarifies that kidney disease may affect patients with a GFR below 60%. The normal GFR numbers are from 90%, and above on the stages of kidney disease,

The presence of abnormal quantities of protein in the urine damages the kidneys. On the other hand, the KDIGO says the numbers of >60% and above may mean that the disease is in remission if there was CKD before.)

As already mentioned, the KDIGO guideline classified CKD based on the cause, GFR, and albuminuria categories (CGA). Previously, CKD was classified into 5 stages (1-5) according to GFR alone

The new classification emphasizes that the indication of causes of kidney disease are a high level of albumin in the urine (albuminuria) or an increased protein in the urine (proteinuria).

II. The Kidneys and Types of Kidney Diseases

What Are the Kidneys?

The National Institute of Diabetes and Digestive and Kidney Diseases (NIDDK) says, "The kidneys are two bean-shaped organs, each about the size of a fist. They are located just below the rib cage, one on each side of your spine. Healthy kidneys filter about a half cup of blood every minute, removing wastes and extra water to make urine."

The kidneys are parts of the urinary tract, including the bladder and ureters. The ureters are two thin tubes of muscles located on each side of the bladder, which stores the urine.

The Nephrons

Your kidneys have millions of tiny blood vessel clusters, called nephrons, that filter waste from your blood. The kidneys, when damaged, will later lose their ability to filter your blood and waste products. When your kidneys become impaired, they can't filter blood toxins and other substances as they should.

As a result, wastes build up in your body. Damage to the kidney can cause other health problems.

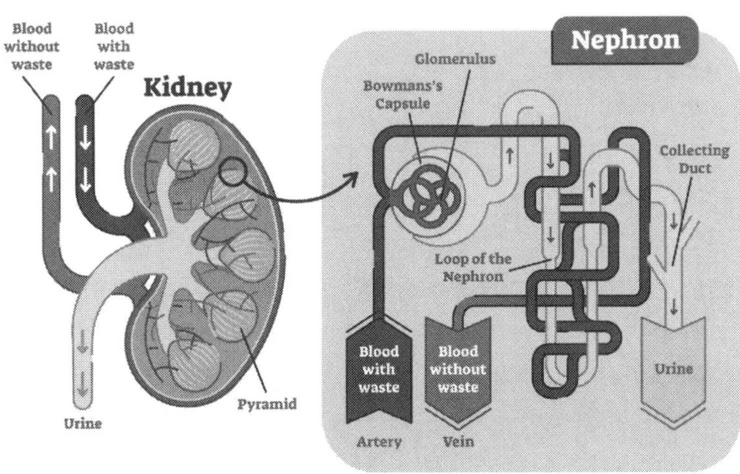

How the Kidneys Work

Photo Source: Shutterstock

Other Functions of the Kidneys

Although the kidneys' main function is filtering wastes and extra liquid out of the blood to make urine, the kidneys also have other tasks.

They include:

- Balancing body fluids
- Taking drugs from the body
- Releasing hormones that regulate blood pressure
- Regulating red blood cell production
  Producing an active form of vitamin D that helps make sturdy and healthy bones

Source: National Kidney Foundation

Types of Kidney Diseases

According to the CDC, one in three people with diabetes also has kidney disease.

Other names for CKD are Diabetic Nephropathy and Diabetic Kidney Disease (DKD).

According to the National Institute of Diabetes and Digestive and Kidney Diseases (NIDDK), "Diabetic kidney disease is a type of kidney disease caused by diabetes."

The NIDDK adds, "Diabetic kidney disease is also called DKD, chronic kidney disease, CKD, kidney disease of diabetes, or diabetic nephropathy.

On the other hand, the National Kidney Foundation (NKF) says, "Chronic kidney disease (CKD) is a condition characterized by a gradual loss of kidney function over time."

Among many kidney diseases, chronic kidney disease (CKD) is the most common.

The National Institute of Diabetes and Digestive and Kidney Diseases (NIDDK) says, "Diabetic kidney disease is a type of kidney disease caused by diabetes."

The NIDDK adds, "Diabetic kidney disease is also called DKD, chronic kidney disease, CKD, kidney disease of diabetes, or diabetic nephropathy.

Other Kidney Conditions

- Acute kidney injury
- Nephrotic syndrome
- Renal stones
- Urinary tract infection

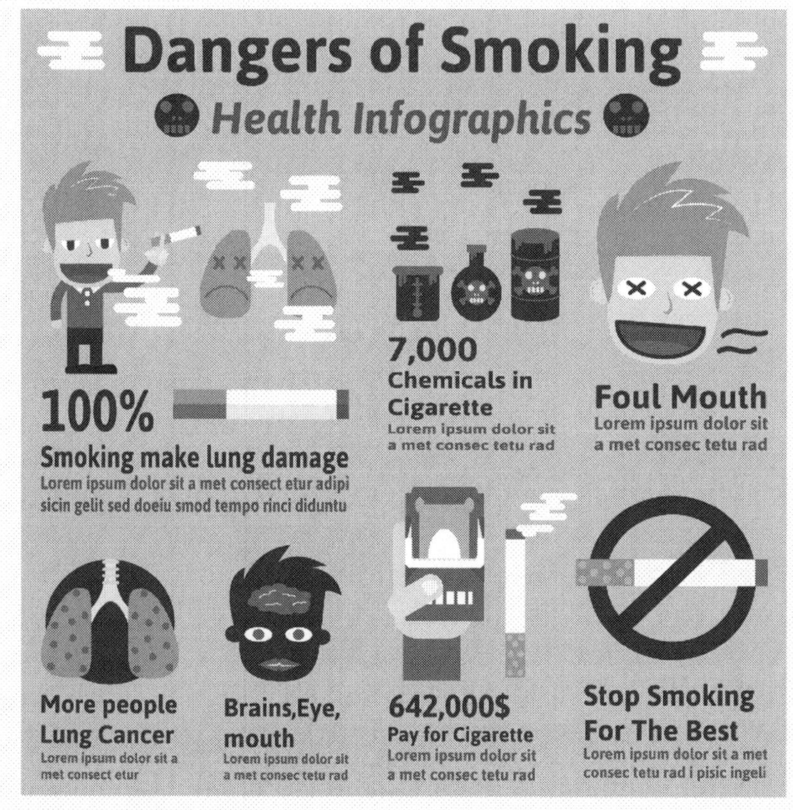

Smoking: Bad for Diabetes, Kidney Disease, and Heart Disease

Photo Source: Shutterstock

Diabetes is the leading cause of chronic kidney disease (CKD). But there are many causes of CKD.

Causes of CKD

- Diabetes
- High blood pressure
- Renal artery stenosis
- Hemolytic uremic syndrome in children
- Drugs that are toxic to the kidneys

- Repeated urinary infections
- Disorders in which the body's immune system attacks its cells and organ
- Rare genetic conditions, such as Alport syndrome
- Glomerulonephritis that is a group of diseases that cause inflammation and damage to the kidney's filtering unit
- Inherited diseases, such as polycystic kidney disease, which causes large cysts to form in the kidneys and damage the surrounding tissues
- Lupus and other diseases that affect the body's immune system
- Disorders caused by problems like kidney stones, tumors, or an enlarged prostate gland in men

Standard Symptoms of CKD

- Frequent urination
- Dry and scaly skin
- Poor appetite
- Sleeping problems
- Lack of concentration
- Swollen feet and ankles
- Puffiness around the eyes
- Muscle cramps
- Foamy urine
- Blood in the urine

Source: National Kidney Foundation

Severe symptoms of CKD

Symptoms that indicate that kidney disease is progressing to end-stage renal disease (ESRD) may include:

- Nausea and vomiting
- Fluid retention
- Occurrence of anemia (a decrease in red blood cells)
- Worsening edema (swollen feet, ankles, and hands)
- Potassium level increase
- Drugs that are toxic to the kidneys

- Repeated urinary infections
- Disorders in which the body's immune system attack the cells and organs
- Malfunctions that occur as a baby develops in its mother's womb
- Lupus and other diseases that affect the body's immune system
- Disorders caused by problems like kidney stones, tumors, or an enlarged prostate gland in men
- Extreme tiredness
- Shortness of breath
- Continuous trouble sleeping

Standard Treatment of CKD

The standard treatment of CKD includes:

- Limiting salt, potassium, and phosphorous (if disease is in third stage)
- Exercising, such as walking, on most days of the week
- Keeping a healthy weight
- Controlling cholesterol levels, decreasing LDL (bad) cholesterol and triglycerides, and increasing HDL (good) cholesterol
- Stabilizing blood pressure at normal level
- Managing your blood sugar if you have diabetes
- Quitting smoking, if you smoke
- Limiting alcoholic drinks

The Bautista Treatment System for CKD and Standard Treatments

My kidney disease is in remission. For years, doctors advised me to control my high creatinine levels and blood urea nitrogen (BUN). I struggled, but later on, I discovered the road to appropriate treatments.

I found out that kidney disease can be reversed, stabilized, and put into remission in different ways, including:

- Drinking enough water (at least 8 to 10 cups or glasses with 8 oz content to dilute creatinine and BUN (blood urea nitrogen), except for those with heart failure and advanced kidney disease stage

- Eating more plant protein than animal proteins because plant foods have no creatine, whose waste product is creatinine, and other factors, such as age, and weight, which are the basis of estimated glomerular filtration rates (eGFR) that measures kidney function
- Reducing intakes of meats high in protein and creatine that becomes creatinine (the waste product) when cooked.
- Limiting or avoiding species of fish that have high levels of protein and creatine, which are bad for the diseased kidneys
- Limiting or avoiding alcohol (I do not even drink beer.)
- Avoiding smoking (I do not smoke.)
- Having enough sleep at night, at least 6 to 8 hours
- Reducing stress, even if there's always bad news
- Exercising (I do moderate-intensity for 20 minutes, 3 sessions of 20 minutes each, totalling one hour a day.)
- Consumption of Omega-3 Polyunsaturated Fatty Acids (PUFAs)

Omega-3 Polyunsaturated Fatty Acids (PUFAs) and Kidney Function in Older Adults

A recent study (published on the website PMC of the U.S. National Library of Medicine, National Institute of Health) showed that PUFA supplementation slowed the rate of loss of renal function in patients with IgA nephropathy, also known as Berger's disease.

IgA neuropathy is a kidney disease that occurs when an antibody called immunoglobulin A (IgA) accumulates in the body. The study was done in Tuscany, Italy, involving older persons.

In particular, the study found that elderly patients with low total plasma PUFA levels had a greater decline in creatinine clearance. The finding suggested that a higher dietary intake of PUFAs may be good protection against the rapid progression of CKD.

Fish Oil

Fish oil containing Omega-3 polyunsaturated fatty acids (PUFAs) comes from oily fish species, such as salmon, tuna, mackerel, cod, and others. They also have high creatine that produces the waste product creatinine. High levels of this waste are bad for diseased kidneys.

Omega-3 acids decrease LDL (bad) cholesterol and increase HDL (good) cholesterol.

In particular, omega-3 fatty acids help prevent inflammation in the body. Health experts recommend kidney patients with IgA and uremic proritus to takeOmega 3 fatty acids. Uremic pruritus, also known as "chronic kidney disease-associated pruritus" (CKD-aP), is chronic itching experienced by patients with advanced or end-stage renal disease.

Omega-3 fatty acids, in general, can be a good supplementation for people with diabetes, kidney disease, and heart disease.

Generic Omega-3-acid Ethyl Esters Capsule, USP, a fatty acid (brand name: Lovaza)) is a prescription medicine for adults called a lipid-regulating medicine.

In other words, Lovaza is made of omega-3 fatty acids. Omega-3 fatty acids, natural substances that your body needs, are found in some plants and the oil of certain fatty fish, such as salmon, cod, tuna, and mackerel.

My Journey

Having these diseases, I have been taking 4 grams (4,000 mg) of Omega-3-Acid Ethyl Esters Capsules, USP 2 capsules twice a day.

Omega-3-Acid Ethyl Esters, considered pure, is the generic of Lovaza, the first fish oil approved by the Food and Drug Administration (FDA) and prescribed only by doctors.

The second fish oil approved by the FDA is vascepa, whose generic name is icosapent ethyl capsules. The FDA has approved the generic version. However, this version is not available yet.

Kidney: Renal Corpuscle (Glomerulus)

The renal corpuscle is the filtration unit of nephrons, functional units of the kidney. It comprises two structures, the glomerulus and the Bowman's capsule.

A glomerulus is a small unit of capillaries containing two cell types: Endothelial cells, large fenestra (a small natural hole or opening), and Mesangial cells. The Mesangial cells are smooth muscle cells that lie between the capillaries.

The nephrons compose the renal corpuscle and the renal tubule that serve as the functional unit of the kidney. The renal corpuscle consists of the Bowman's capsule and the glomerular capillaries that filter plasma.

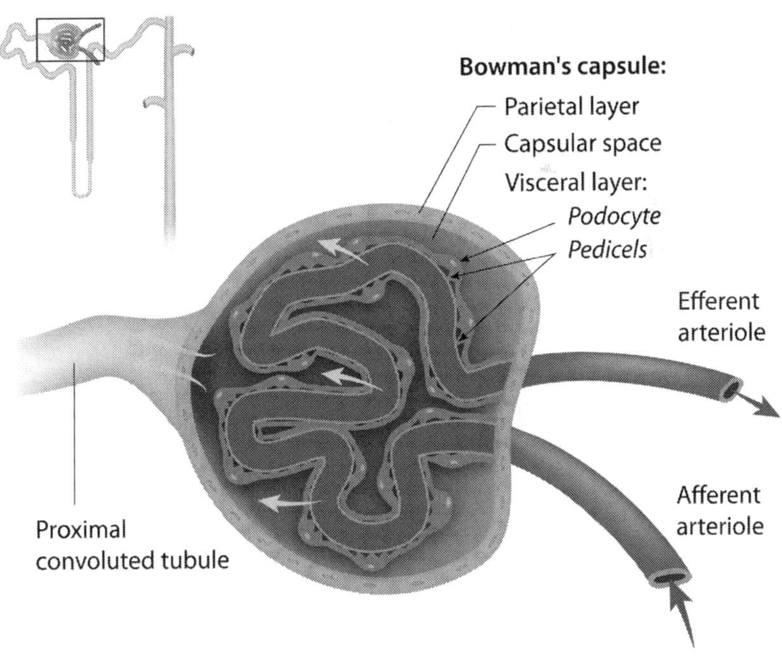

The Renal Corpuscle Structure

Photo Credit: Shutterstock

My Journey

My research shows that water can be a "medicine" for reversing the condition in treating my kidney disease.

What does water do to our bodies? I have already mentioned that creatinine and blood urea are water-soluble. When you drink a lot of water, the more you urinate, whether you like it or not. The more you do this, the more creatinine, BUN, and other toxins come out with the urine from your system.

I do not smoke, and nor do I drink alcohol. That's my advantage over other people who smoke and drink, worsening their kidney disease. That's why I have low creatinine and BUN numbers and a higher GFR number.

How Does Diabetes Damage Kidneys?

The National Kidney Foundation says that diabetes can damage your kidneys in three ways:

Blood vessels in your kidneys: Blood sugar damages the tiny vessels of the kidneys' filtering units. As a result, the blood vessels become narrow, and blood will have difficulty passing through them.

Not having enough blood causes the kidneys to be damaged. The albumin (a type of protein) passes through the filters and ends up in the urine, where it should not be.

Nerves in the body: Diabetes also damages nerves in your body. These nerves act as the carriers of messages throughout the body.

Urinary tract infection: It's terrible if the urine stays longer in your bladder because you may get a urinary tract infection. Thus, the conditions affect the bladder, sometimes spreading to the kidneys. Of course, there are various other complications as a result of diabetes.

Be Aware of These Complications

If you have kidney disease, especially in the early stages of kidney disease, it would be good to start knowing the severe complications you may encounter.

Complications of CKD

- Heart disease
- Heart attack
- Stroke
- High blood pressure
- Weak bones
- Nerve damage (peripheral neuropathy)
- Anemia or low red blood cell count
- Kidney failure (end-stage renal disease or ESRD)

Stages of Chronic Kidney Disease (CKD)

The five stages of CKD are classified as follows:

- Stage 1: Kidney damage with normal or increased GFR (>90 mL/min/1.73 m 2)
- Stage 2: Mild reduction in GFR (60-89 mL/min/1.73 m 2)
- Stage 3a: Moderate reduction in GFR (45-59 mL/min/1.73 m 2)
- Stage 3b: Moderate reduction in GFR (30-44 mL/min/1.73 m 2)
- Stage 4: Severe reduction in GFR (15-29 mL/min/1.73 m 2)
- Stage 5: Kidney failure GFR (< 15 mL/min/1.73 m 2 or dialysis)

End-Stage Renal Diseases (ESRD)

End-stage renal disease, also called end-stage kidney disease (ESKD), is the last stage of the long-term chronic kidney disease during which the kidneys can no longer do their filtering of waste.

5 Stages Of Kidney Disease

Stage 1	Stage 2	Stage 3A	Stage 3B	Stage 4	Stage 5
GFR≧90	89≧GFR≧60	59≧GFR≧40	44≧GFR≧30	29≧GFR≧15	GFR<15
Normal or high function	Mildly decreased function	Mild to moderately decreased function		Severely decreased function	Kidney failure

Photo Credit: Shutterstock

III. Creatine and Creatinine

What Is Creatine?

Creatine, a substance found naturally in muscle cells, is one of the body's natural energy sources for muscle contraction. One-half of the body's supply of creatine comes from meat, and the other half is in the brain, liver, and kidneys. Creatine maintains a continuous supply of energy to working muscles.

About 95% of creatine is in skeletal muscles in the form of phosphocreatine. The other 5% is in the brain, kidneys, and liver.

Creatine consists of three amino acids: L-arginine, glycine, and L-methionine, making up about 1 percent of the total volume of human blood.

Particularly, creatine helps your muscles produce energy for heavy lifting or high-intensity exercise, like running or doing a marathon.

Simply put, it is popular among athletes and bodybuilders to enhance their strength and performance.

Because of this, creatine is often used as a dietary supplement to improve muscle strength and athletic performance. In the U.S., a majority of sports nutrition supplements contain creatine.

Some foods like red meat, chicken, and seafood, in particular, provide creatine that transforms into creatinine when cooked.

When you eat lots of red meat, chicken breast, and some seafood, you eat creatine, creating more creatinine in your bloodstream.

Uses of Creatine

Among others, creatine, which upon cooking, turns into creatinine is needed by the body because it:

- Gives power to the muscles to produce energy especially making intense movement or exercising, whether you're doing slow-intensity or moderate-intensity walking, weight-lifting, and any other activities
- Builds muscles, especially for bodybuilders and athletes, to enhance their strength and performance

- Treats disorders of the so-called creatine metabolism of people with certain conditions whose bodies can't make creatine
- Augments low levels of creatine in the brain, which can cause seizures, autism, and decreased mental function, if not treated
- Improves muscle strength to enhance the upper body and lower body, especially in older adults
- Replaces age-related muscle loss (sarcopenia) in older adults

What Affects the Creatine Content?

Several factors affect the creatine content in your body, involving meat intake, exercise, and amount of muscle mass and hormones, such as testosterone and IGE-1.

The enzyme complex creatine kinase transforms the creatine into phosphocreatine inside the cells. Phosphocreatine breaks down into creatinine, which is then excreted into the urine.

Every day, 1% to 2% of creatine content in the body converts to creatinine as a waste product.

Generally, men have higher creatinine concentrations than women because they have a bigger muscle mass.

Moderate Amount of Protein

Although creatine has many uses, you should not take a high amount of it because it turns into creatinine, the waste product, and substance would be a burden on the diseased kidneys in filtering it.

But it would be best if you did not also have a low level of creatine, either, because the muscles need it to produce energy for the body.

Specifically, you should eat moderate levels of animal protein and creatine and eat more plant protein because plants have no creatine. A high-protein diet is bad for kidney disease.

Remember: foods with high protein also have high creatine.

Creatine in Typical American Diet

According to a 2017 review published by the Journal of the International Society of Sports Nutrition, a typical American diet that includes meat gives 1 gram to 2 grams of creatine per day. The liver, kidneys, and pancreas produce the rest of the creatine you need.

So, to get enough creatine in your diet, it's recommended to aim for 1-2 grams per day of natural food sources if you don't take a supplement.

If you're a man and have no kidney disease, you should take 56 grams of protein; and if you're a woman, you should eat 46 grams of protein.

IV. Creatinine (The Waste Product of Creatine)

What Is Creatinine?

Creatinine is the waste product of creatine that comes from the normal breakdown of muscle tissues. It is filtered through your kidneys and expelled through the urine.

The kidneys' ability to handle creatinine is called the creatinine clearance rate.

If you have kidney disease, you must eat more plant protein than animal protein. Why? Because meat, chicken, and fatty fish provide a high protein, which turns into blood urea nitrogen (BUN), and creatine becomes creatinine.

So these substances accumulate in the bloodstream, which is bad for the diseased kidneys.

As we know, an elevated creatinine in the bloodstream is often an indication of kidney disease. In addition, a high protein diet can bring about a high level of creatinine. In other words, a high protein diet and high creatine foods also pose other health risks besides renal disease.

According to Mayo Clinic, the normal range of creatinine (for an adult) in the blood is typical:

- U.S. units: 0.84 to 1.21 milligrams per deciliter (mg/dL)
- European units: 74.3 to 107 micromoles per liter (umol/L)

Creatinine levels may vary due to several factors such as age, sex, and race. Also, standard reference ranges can be different from laboratory to laboratory.

Other factors that may affect the body's supply of creatine are as follows:

- Amount of meat intake
- Moderate and vigorous exercise or any activity
- Amount of muscle mass
- Cellular processes
- Levels of hormones, such as testosterone
- Hydration

In general, high creatinine levels indicate your kidneys' impairment or that they do not work well.

Creatinine Test

If you have a creatinine level test, a lab technician will draw a blood sample from you as part of the Complete Metabolic Syndrome. Creatine is a chemical that supplies energy, mainly to muscles. The test includes GFR estimation.

Usually, GFR results are reported as mL/min/1.73 m2 but estimated in percentage, such as 73%.

Some laboratories do not collect information on a patient's race when the sample they collect for serum creatinine testing; they may report calculated results for African Americans and non-African Americans.

The lab specialist combines your blood creatinine level with several other factors to estimate your GFR, including some or all of the following:

- Age
- Lean Body Weight
- Race
- Sex

Creatinine Clearance

Creatinine clearance tests your kidneys' function in filtering creatinine out of the bloodstream for excretion into the urine.

Your doctor determines your creatinine clearance within 24 hours.

Lab Report

Lab technicians report creatinine clearance as milliliters of creatinine per minute per body surface area (mL/min/BSA).

The typical range for men, 19 to 75 years old is 77 to 160 mL/min/BSA. The standard content for women 18 to 72 is 78 to 131 mL/min/BSA.

The albumin/creatinine ratio describes how much albumin is relative to the creatinine level in a urine sample. The results are reported as the number of milligrams (mg) of albumin for every creatinine gram (g).

Compare albumin (mcg/L) to creatinine (mg/L) of less than 30. A ratio of 30-300 indicates microalbuminuria, and values above 300 are considered macroalbuminuria.

You must also be aware that a microalbumin creatinine ratio compares the amount of albumin to the amount of creatinine in your urine. If there is any albumin in your urine, the amount can vary greatly throughout the day. But creatinine is released at a steady rate.

Effect of Cooked Meal on Serum Creatinine and GFR

It would be best if you did not have the habit of increasing the ingestion of animal protein. True, if you eat too much-cooked meat, you will increase your total muscle mass. But naturally, it will cause an increase in serum and urinary creatinine. That's bad news, especially for those with renal disease.

A study published by the *Diabetes Care* of the American Diabetes Association (ADA) found that creatine in meat is converted to creatinine during cooking, absorbed by the body, and caused significant increases in serum creatinine.

This fact, of course, impacts the management of the condition, resulting in withdrawing certain medications. Therefore, a fasting serum test on these patients to determine GFR levels is good to reflect the kidney functions better.

If you do vigorous exercise or take certain medications like chemotherapy drugs, creatinine levels also rise temporarily.

How to Lower Creatinine Levels

If your damaged kidneys, in some ways, have lost their ability to filter efficiently waste products through the nephrons, a significant amount of creatinine remains in the blood.

For this reason, you need to take the necessary steps to remove the creatinine from the bloodstream.

Your steps may include

- Drinking enough water at least 8 to 10 cups or glasses (8 ounces each) based on your body weight and kidney and heart condition to dilute the creatinine because it is water-soluble
- Reducing protein intake (especially animal protein like red meat and other protein sources, including dairy products) because they have high creatine content that turns into creatinine when cooked
- Increasing plant-based protein because plants have no creatine to turn into creatinine.
- Reducing or avoiding species of fish that have high protein and creatine content, such as salmon, tuna, and cod.
- Limiting your sodium intake because a diet high in sodium may lead to high blood sugar and fluid retention that might cause increased creatinine levels in your blood
- Avoiding any vigorous or high-intensity exercise or activity such as running or weight-lifting to eliminate blood sugar upsurge and high production of creatinine because of creatine use
- Sleeping well because when you sleep, your body's metabolic rate of body functions decreases; thereby reducing creatinine in the muscles
- Quitting smoking because smoking, in a cardiovascular health study, showed that it is associated with an increase in serum creatinine, resulting in a 0.3 mg/dL rise in creatinine

- Limiting or avoiding alcohol drinking since a 1984 study showed that drinkers of two or fewer drinks per day had higher serum creatinine levels than non-drinkers

Lab Report

Lab technicians report creatinine clearance as milliliters of creatinine per minute per body surface area (mL/min/BSA).

The typical range for men, 19 to 75 years old is 77 to 160 mL/min/BSA. The standard content for women 18 to 72 is 78 to 131 mL/min/BSA.

The albumin/creatinine ratio describes how much albumin is relative to the creatinine level in a urine sample. The results are reported as the number of milligrams (mg) of albumin for every creatinine gram (g).

V. Phosphocreatine (PCr) or Creatine Phosphate (CP)

Two Forms of Creatine

There are two forms of creatine in the body: Phosphocreatine (CPr) or Creatinine phosphate (CP) and free creatine. The high-energy phosphocreatine consists of 60-70% of the total creatine content, while the free creatine is 30-35%.

Creatine consists of three amino acids: L-arginine, glycine, and L-methionine.

What Is Phosphocreatine (Pcr) or Creatine Phosphate (CP)?

Phosphocreatine (PCr)) or Creatine Phosphate (CP) is the phosphorylated form of creatine primarily found in the skeletal muscles of vertebrates. It serves to store phosphates to provide energy for muscular contraction.

It maintains and recycles adenosine triphosphate (ATP) from adenosine diphosphate (ADP) for activities like a contraction.

Simply put, ATP is an organic chemical that provides energy for the cell's intracellular energy transfer. On the other hand, ADP is an organic component for metabolism in the cell.

Recycling chemical compounds is necessary because the human body only produces 250g of ATP daily; hence, ADP converts into ATP because ADP is one of the most numerous in the body.

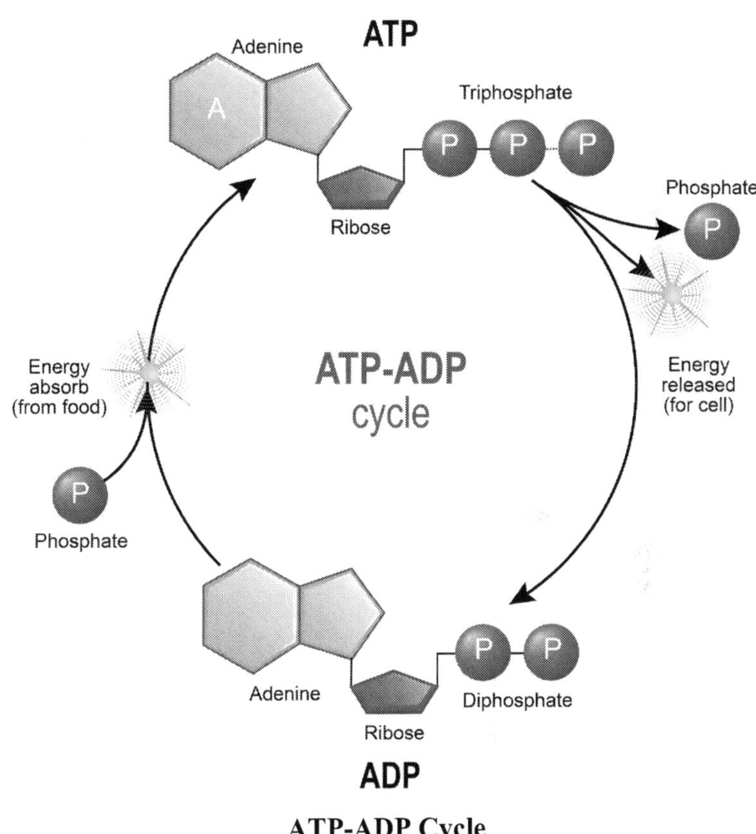

ATP-ADP Cycle

Photo Credit: Shutterstock

VI. Creatine Kinase (CK) or Phosphocreatine Kinase (PCK)

What Is Creatine Kinase (CK)?

MedlinePlus of the (U.S.) National Institute of Health says, "CK is a type of protein, known as an enzyme, mostly found in your skeletal muscles and heart, with lesser amounts in the brain.

Skeletal muscles are the muscles attached to your skeleton. They work with your bones to help you move and give your body power and strength. Heart muscles pump blood in and out of the heart."

Generally, CK forms the core of an energy network known as the phosphocreatine (PCr) circuit. The cytosol isoenzymes combine with glycolysis to produce ATP for muscle activity in this circuit.

CK's function is to add a phosphate group of creatine into the body and turn it into a high-energy molecule known as phosphocreatine. In other words, the substance burns as a source of energy by your cells.

There are three types of CK enzymes:

- CK-MM found mostly in skeletal muscles
- CK-MB found mostly in the heart muscles
- CK-BB found mostly in brain tissues

During muscle degeneration, the muscle cells break open. Therefore, their contents go to the bloodstream. Elevated CK naturally indicates that there has been damage to the muscles, whether in the skeletal muscles, heart muscles, or brain tissues.

Simply put, high KC levels can signal a heart attack that has occurred or is happening. A CK test is very important for medical conditions such as myocardial infarction (heart attack), muscular dystrophy, and cerebral diseases.

What Is a Creatine Kinase Test?

A creatine kinase (CK) or creatine phosphokinase (CPK) test measures CK in the blood. The purposes of the test are to monitor and diagnose damage, injury, and some diseases, including:

- Muscular dystrophy is a rare inherited disease that causes weakness, breakdown, and loss of function of skeletal muscles
- Rhabdomyolysis, a rapid breakdown of muscle tissues
- Damage of muscles caused by eccentric exercises involving running, weight lifting, and other eccentric exercises
- Other disorders

Any small amount of CK normally in the blood comes primarily from skeletal muscles. However, any disorder that causes muscle damage and interferes with muscle energy production and use can cause an increase in CK levels.

For example, strenuous exercise and inflammation of muscles, called myositis, can raise CK, as can muscle diseases (myopathies) such as muscular dystrophy. Significantly elevated levels of CK can cause rhabdomyolysis, an extreme breakdown of skeletal muscle tissues.

A CK activity occurs in muscle (MM isoenzyme), heart tissue (MB isoenzyme), and brain (BB isoenzyme). Serum CK concentrations reflect muscle mass, causing males to have higher concentrations than females.

CK may be measured to evaluate myopathy and monitor rhabdomyolysis patients for acute kidney injury.

What's the Normal Range of Creatine Kinase?

Adult/elderly: (Values are higher after exercise):

Male: 55-170 units/L
Female: 30-135 units/L
Newborn: 68-580 units/L

Isoenzymes:

CK-MM: 100%
CK-MB: 0%
CK-BB: 0%

CK–MB enzymes disappear from the serum more quickly than CK.

Can Eccentric Exercises Raise Creatine Kinase?

According to some small studies, eccentric exercises, such as moderate-intensity and vigorous-intensity walking, running, and weightlifting can raise KC levels in the bloodstream.

However, there is no clear consensus among experts defining CK levels in rhabdomyolysis. Rhabdomyolysis is a condition that results from injury to skeletal muscle and the release of cellular contents into the so-called extracellular fluid and circulation.

No studies have firmly established that a normal range of CK elevation can occur from moderate-intensity exercises, such as moderate-intensity walking or brisk walking.

However, available data support that vigorous-intensity activity does raise CK levels. A study showed that CK level increased for long-distance runners. In this study, triathletes had a 12-fold increase in CK levels as long as 24 hours after the race.

Two Types of Muscle Contraction

Resistance exercises involve two types of movements, concentric and eccentric. You do a concentric exercise when you raise the weight during a biceps curl. The lengthening action would be considered an eccentric contraction as you lower your arm. When the muscle doesn't move at all, it's an isometric status.

Types of Muscle Contractions

Examples of Eccentric Contraction Activities include:

- Vigorous-intensity race walking
- Long-distance running
- Downhill running
- Downward motion of a push-up
- Downward motion of squatting
- Lowering a weight during a shoulder press
- Lowering the body during a crunch

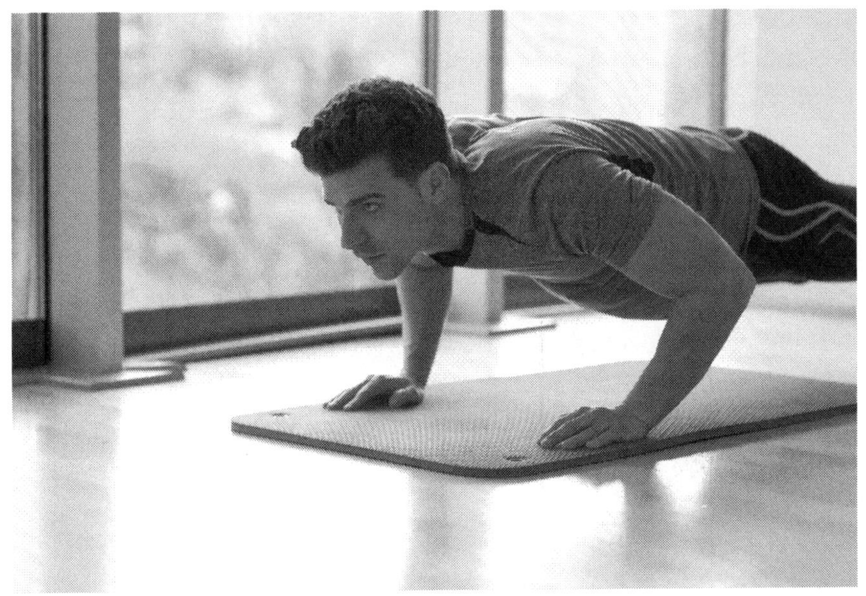

Push-Up: An Example of an Eccentric Exercise

Photo Credit: Shutterstock

VII. Blood Urea Nitrogen (BUN)

The kidneys, lungs, and skin are the body's excretory organs, removing toxic waste products from your body.

They do the following:

- Kidneys get rid of excess salts, water, and urea.
- Lungs remove carbon dioxide.
- The liver breaks down excess amino acids.

How Is BUN Created?

Blood urea nitrogen (BUN) is a normal waste product after the liver breaks down the protein; the urea forms when liver cells transform dietary proteins into amino acids.

After that, the liver breaks down the excess amino acids to produce ammonia, which converts into urea, which is less toxic than ammonia. Urea consists of carbon, oxygen, and nitrogen.

Nitrogen is a component of both urea and ammonia. The liver releases urea into the blood that carries it to the kidneys for filtration. Then the kidneys excrete it into the urine.

If there's something wrong with the kidneys, then a certain amount of urea remains in the blood, and you'll have a high BUN level.

Generally, an elevated BUN level indicates dehydration before the BUN or serum BUN test, included in a routine comprehensive or basic metabolic panel (CMP) laboratory test.

Typically, the panel measures the blood levels of blood urea nitrogen (BUN), creatinine, potassium calcium, carbon dioxide, chloride, glucose, and sodium.

Why Is a BUN Test Needed?

The BUN test is done, together with the creatinine test, to evaluate kidney function. However, while measuring the amount of urea nitrogen in the blood, a BUN test won't necessarily identify the cause of a higher or lower than average urea nitrogen count.

BUN levels naturally increase when the kidneys and liver are damaged. In other words, having too much urea nitrogen in the blood can be a signal that the liver or kidneys may not be functioning well.

An elevation of the BUN level is known as azotemia. A doctor does the BUN test to determine the cause or causes of the elevated BUN level, which may include the following conditions:

- Dehydration
- Impaired kidney function
- Congestive heart failure due to poor renal perfusion
- Acute myocardial infarction (as a result of heart attack)
- Shock or stress
- Excessive protein intake or protein catabolism

Of course, elevated BUN and creatinine levels signify lower GFR, the measure of renal function.

Normal BUN Values

According to Mayo Clinic, around 7 to 20 mg/dL (2.5 to 7.1 mmol/L) is generally considered normal.

How to Decrease BUN Levels

Based on my experience and research, I have found that water is the most effective "medicine" for reducing creatinine and BUN levels to increase GFR numbers and improve kidney function.

The different ways by which you can reduce your creatinine levels in your bloodstream include:

- Drink enough water (at least 8 to 10 cups or glasses of 8 ounces each, to dilute the BUN, like what water does to creatinine. BUN is water-soluble because urea and nitrogen dissolve in water, together with other wastes.
- Avoid taking any protein supplements because overconsumption of proteins is bad for the body. The kidneys have a hard time processing proteins, particularly animal proteins. Don't overwork your kidneys.
- Lessen protein intake, especially red meat and high-protein species of fish.
- Do not over-exercise, like jogging, running, or weight-lifting, because vigorous conditioning also causes elevated BUN levels, as well as creatinine levels.
- Live a balanced, healthy lifestyle, including eating a rounded diet consisting of plant-based foods and little portions of meat, including chicken and fish.
- Exercise moderately, like doing moderate-intensity walking or brisk walking, because it lowers your blood glucose, increases your kidney function, normalizes blood pressure, and raises your heart rate to strengthen your body engine.
- Eliminate persistent stress. You can do this by meditating or doing yoga and doing the things you love to give you calm and positive thoughts.

Waste Products of Protein Metabolism

The waste products of protein metabolism include:

- Urea
- Uric acid
- Creatinine
- Ammonia

Water dilutes the above substances, reducing their levels in the bloodstream. The urine is the main excretory for such wastes. In addition, some wastes are removed away from the body through feces.

.For example, the more you drink water, the more your GFR will increase, and the more creatinine will reduce, which is good for the body.

The University of Waterloo in Ontario, Canada, says, "Ammonia gas is very soluble in water. The relatively high solubility is attributed to the hydrogen bonding between the ammonia and water molecules."

Among the four waste products, the solubility of uric acid, including its alkali metal and alkaline earth salt, is low. And the salts are better dissolved in hot water than cold.

VIII. Estimated Glomerular Filtration Rate (eGFR)

What Is eGFR or GFR?

The National Kidney Foundation describes eGFR or simply GFR as "a measure how well your kidneys filter blood." It is calculated based on your serum creatinine level, age, race, and other factors.

A GFR number tells how much kidney function you have. As chronic kidney disease progresses, your GFR number decreases.

What's the Normal GFR Number?

For adults, 90 or any number above >90 is the normal GFR number. However, GFR declines with age. This occurrence happens too to older adults, even if they are not afflicted with kidney disease.

Normal (or Average) Estimated GFR or eGFR based on Age

Age (Years)/Averaged eGFR
20-29=116 mL/min/1.73 m2 or 116%
30-39=107 mL/min/1.73 m2 or 107%
40-49=99 mL/min/1.73 m2 or 99%
50-59=93 mL/min/1.73 m2 or 93%
70 + =75 mL/min/1.73 m2 or 75%

Source: National Kidney Foundation

On the other hand, The National Institute of Diabetes and Digestive and Kidney Diseases (NIDDK) says that:

- A GFR of 60 or higher is in the normal range.
- A GFR below 60 may mean kidney disease.
- A GFR of 15 or lower may mean kidney failure.

On the Stages of Kidney Disease, the normal values of eGFR, consider 90 or any number above it, are normal GFR.

The NIDDK says, “A GFR of 60 or higher is in the normal range.” On the other hand, under the KDIGO guideline, kidney disease is defined as remission if your GFR is 60 and above. But there must be a CKD before.

Calculating the GFR

Lab technicians use several equations or formulas to calculate the eGFR or GFR number, namely:

- Cockcroft & Gault Equation
- MDRD Formula
- CKD-EZPI Creatinine (2009
- Automatic calculators (available on the internet)

Comprehensive Metabolic Panel (CMP) Test: If you take the Comprehensive Metabolic Panel Test, lab technicians estimate the creatinine level and GFR. based on several factors. You will automatically get the creatine and BUN numbers and GFR.

Automatic Calculators: If you have only the creatine test results, you can use the so-called mechanical calculators on the internet for GFR percentages. You may go to:

https://www.calculator.net/gfr-calculator.html, or

Steps to Increasing GFR

- Eating more plant protein than animal protein because animal protein is hard on the kidneys
- Drinking enough water to dilute the creatinine and blood urea nitrogen (BUN), thereby raising GFR number
- Managing blood sugar levels and lowering blood pressure
- Reducing salt and processed food intake
- Avoiding smoking
- Doing moderate-intensity walking or low-intensity walking, based on your physical condition, at least 1 hour divided into 20-minute each session, 1 hour after each meal
- Limiting or avoiding the so-called NSAIDs (nonsteroidal anti-inflammatory drugs), such as aspirin, Advil, Motrin, Ibuprofen, and Naproxen

Protein Intake for People with Kidney Disease

According to the National Kidney Foundation, here's the way how you should determine your protein needs based on your kidneys' stage or condition and body weight in kilograms.

1. For CKD stages 1 or 2 (GFR of 60% and above), you should eat less protein to slow down the progression of kidney disease. It will help if you get more plant protein than animal protein.

The current protein restriction for stages 1 or 2 is no more than 0.8 grams per kilogram of your body weight.

For example, if you weigh 125 lbs, you should multiply it by 0.8 g/kg. Thus, your weight x 0.8g/kg equals the grams of protein you need. First, you have to convert your weight from pounds to kilograms.

To convert pounds into kilograms, divide the number of pounds by 2.2. (The 2.2 lbs are equal to one kilogram.) If your body weight is 125 lbs or 56.82 kilograms, your protein needs are kg x 0.8 = 45.46 grams per day.

2. For CKD stages 3 to 5 (GFR 59% or lower), people in these stages should lower their protein intake. The protein requirement for these stages should be 0.6 - 0.8 per kilogram of the body weight.

For example, a 65-year-old man is in the CKD stages 3 to 5, and he weighs 140 lbs; the weight should be multiplied by 0.6 - 0.8 per kilogram of his body weight. Thus, his weight divided by 2.2 = 63.64 kg. His protein needs are 63.64 x 0.6 - 0.8 g/kg =37-50 (or 38.18-50.91) grams of protein per day.

For a chart of pounds to kilogram conversion, you may go to: https://www.metric-conversions.org/weight/pounds-to-kilogrtams.htm

Creatine Source

Beef, pork, chicken, tuna, salmon, and cod contain between 1.4 to 2.3 grams of creatine per pound. Herring contains the most creatine at 3 to 4.5 grams per pound.

Restrictions of Sodium, Potassium, and Phosphorus Intake Per Day

Sodium: A major mineral, or macromineral, sodium levels should be monitored, especially by people with kidney disease. High sodium levels will further damage the kidneys and retain water in the body that may cause edema or water retention in the feet and legs and other parts of the body, including the abdomen.

According to the U.S. Food and Drug Administration (FDA), if you have kidney disease, you should limit your sodium level to 1,500 mg per day,

Other guidelines say the limitation should be 2,000 mg daily. Read the levels. According to Cleveland Clinic, you may limit sodium intake to 300 mg sodium per serving or 600 mg for a complete frozen dinner.

Potassium: Government guidelines recommend that healthy men and women over the age of 19 eat at least 3,400 mg and 2,600 mg of potassium daily, respectively.

However, potassium restrictions for people with third-stage CKD or above stages, limit is below <2,000 mg per day.

The three levels of potassium are as follows:

- Safe zone: 3.5 to 5.0 mmol/L
- Caution: 5.1 to 6.0 mmol/L
- Danger zone: >6.0 mmol/L or higher

But generally, when you have third-stage kidney disease, you don't have to limit your blood potassium intake unless it exceeds the normal range of 3.6 to 5.2 millimoles per liter (mmol/L). Of course, references to potassium ranges differ from lab to lab.

However, it would be best to avoid a very low potassium level (less than 2.5 mmol/L) because it will be life-threatening and require urgent medical attention. A high potassium level, as indicated above, is not good, too.

Phosphorus: Food experts advise that for phosphorus intake per day, you should limit your dietary phosphorus to 800-1,000 mg/ per day. Also, you must avoid foods with phosphorus additives. A very high phosphorus level leads to hyperphosphatemia, which often leads to bone disease.

Eating More Plant Protein than Animal Protein

The most important thing is to eat more plant protein than animal protein. Animal protein is hard on the kidneys. And another thing, protein produces a waste product, the BUN, that is difficult for the kidneys to process.

For more foods appropriate for kidney disease, go to Chapter 12: *Semi-Plant-Based Diets: Best Diets for Meat Eaters with Diabetes, Kidney, and Heart Diseases.*

Foods for People With CKD to Limit or Avoid

- Canned foods
- Sugary beverages
- Red Meat
- Dairy products
- White potatoes
- Bananas
- Avocado
- Egg yolks
- Alcohol

Other Sources of High Proteins and Creatine

Red Meat: It consists of the meat of mammals, including beef, pork, and sheep. Beef has a high protein and creatine content, particularly the steak, which has 5g per kilogram of uncooked beef.

Chicken: A great source of high protein and creatine, a 100 g of chicken has 23.2g of protein and 3.4kg of creatine.

Mutton (Sheep meat): This meat is rich in quality proteins. The creatine content is about 5kg of uncooked mutton.

Venison (Deer meat): Venison has 50% less fat than beef, but it's high in protein and creatine. A 100g of venison provides 4-5g of creatine.

People with more advanced kidney disease, like those in the third stage or above, may limit their intake of phosphorus-rich and potassium-rich foods, including meat, legumes, and vegetables.

You may ask your doctor or dietitian if some foods are limited for you based on your kidney condition

Limiting or Avoiding Fish With Highest Proteins and Creatine

If you have kidney disease but are not on dialysis yet, you should limit or avoid fish species with the highest protein and creatine. Why? Because they will worsen your kidney damage.

Let me remind you that the body uses muscle metabolism and that creatine turns into a waste product known as creatinine upon cooking.

Creatinine is the protein that fuels muscle metabolism. Therefore, too much animal proteins can produce extra BUN and other waste products.

13 Fish With Highest Proteins and Creatine

1. Anchovy (Canned in oil): A 4-oz serving delivers 52g of protein.
2 **Sardines**: You can get 50g of protein from a 6-oz serving.
3. **Trout**: A 6-oz serving delivers 40g of protein.
4. **Salmon**: A 6-oz serving gives 38g of protein.
5. **Yellowtail**: A 4-oz serving has 34 grams of protein.
6. **Haddock** (Wild): Has 34g of protein from a 6-oz serving.
7. **Mackerel**: A 6-oz serving gives 32g of protein.
8. **Perch** (Wild): A 6-oz serving delivers 32g of protein.
9. **Cod**: A 6-oz serving gives 30g of protein
10. **Bluefish**: A 4-oz serving delivers 29g of protein.
11. **Grouper**: It has 28 grams of protein per 4-oz serving.
12. **Pollock**: A 4-oz serving has 29g of protein
13. **Flounder** (Wild): You can get 22g of protein from a 6-oz serving of this fish

Source: *Men's Magazine*

Herring: Contains Highest Amount of Creatine?

An article by Anju Mobin, published on *Best for Nutrition,* says herring contains the highest amount of creatine among salt-water fishes, which is 3-4.5g per pound. It also has 20g of protein per 3-oz serving.

In other words, limit or avoid some fish, those with high protein and creatine.

Species of Fatty Fishes

Species of fatty fish are usually good for your health and heart because of their omega-3 acid content. However, there should be a limited amount of fish with high protein and creatine in your diet if you have kidney disease but is not on dialysis yet.

By way of explanation, you should not eat a lot of foods with high protein and creatine if you want to reverse your kidney disease, in case you have it. You will increase your BUN and creatinine levels if you eat a lot of them.

Best Foods for CKD Patients

- Blueberries
- Red grapes
- Bell peppers
- Apples
- Cauliflower
- Cranberries
- Salmon
- Sweet potatoes
- Onions
- Garlic
- Pineapple
- Turnips
- Macadamia nuts
- Lemon
- Arugula
- Buckwheat
- Avocado

My Journey

I limit or avoid the following foods with almost pure protein because of my kidney disease. Usually, high-protein foods have high creatine content. However, eggs don't have creatine.

- *Chicken breast*
- *Turkey breast*
- *Shrimp*
- *Halibut*
- *Tuna*
- *Cod*
- *Mackerel*

- *Tilapia*
- *Salmon*
- *Pollock*

I eat plant and animal foods (in small portions); I also eat whole grains, vegetables, some fruits, oats, meat, fish (not the fatty ones), shrimp, and a few kinds of seafood in limited quantity.

But I eat them in limited amounts or small portions; for example, red meat (including beef, pork, and lamb. I eat more chicken and fish.

The Right Exercise for CKD

The right exercise for improving kidney function is moderate-intensity walking. Also, you can do aerobic exercise, bicycling or swimming.

Wow! Walking Prolongs Life

The Clinical Journal of the American Society of Nephrology (CJASN) says that walking may help prolong life and reduce the risk of needed dialysis or a kidney transplant for individuals with kidney disease.

That's the conclusion of a study that appeared in an issue of *CJASN Journal.*

The study involved about 6,363 patients aged 70 years old with CKD stages 3 to 5 in the China Medical University Hospital's CKD program.

Over 21% of the participants said walking was their most common form of exercise. The study showed that those who walked most were 33% less likely to die and 21% less likely to undergo dialysis or a kidney transplant.

In a study published by BioMedicalCentral.com (BMC) in 2019 on its website, the researchers confirmed that moderate-intensity exercise benefits kidney function and BMI (body mass index) for patients with Stage 3-4 CKD.

The study showed that exercise therapy could modify lipid metabolism and improve the estimated glomerular filtration rate (eGFR).

That's why my moderate-intensity walking works. (See Chapter 9.) It has helped me to increase my GFR continuously and steadily.

Vigorous-Intensity Activity: A No-No!

It would be best if you don't do any vigorous or high-intensity exercise.

In a study published by the U.S. National Institute of Health on its website, it showed the following:

"Conclusion: A single high-intensity interval resistance training (HIIRT) session caused early and significant elevations in creatine kinase (CK), myoglobin, SCr (serum creatinine), microalbuminuria, and urinary biomarkers indicative of kidney tubular injury; thereby suggesting the occurrence of muscle and kidney damage."

My Journey: What Do I Eat?

I eat plant and animal foods; I eat whole grains, vegetables, fruits, oats, red meat, fish, shrimp, and other seafood. But I eat the beef, pork, and chicken in limited amounts or small portions.

I mix small meat pieces with plant-based foods and vegetables. Such vegetables are green beans, taro, eggplants, okra, chayote, squash, spinach, and other greens.

Sometimes, my daughter buys cooked vegetables from a Filipino restaurant. I like eating our native foods such as pork or chicken adobo and mixed vegetables called pinakbet, whose main ingredients are eggplants, beans, okra, ampalaya (bitter melon), and others.

I have reversed and put my kidney function into remission. But I continue to manage my renal disease with moderate-intensity walking, drinking a lot of fluids, and eating a semi-plant-based diet with a combination of small portions of meat, chicken, fish, or shrimp mixed with Basmati brown rice.

I figured out that water can be a "medicine" for reversing the condition in treating my kidney disease. You'll have lower creatinine and BUN levels. And the good news is that you'll have a higher GFR number, indicating increased kidney function.

I do not smoke, nor do I drink alcohol. That's my advantage over other people who do smoke and drink. I always have low creatinine and BUN numbers and a higher GFR number.

Treating myself for my diseases is an adventure, and I'm addicted to it. Life is worth living!

GFR Echocardiogram Test Results

Here are GFR test results from My Medical Chart at the website of a hospital in the suburbs of Detroit, Michigan, that shows that I have reversed and put my kidney disease into remission:

1. Hospital Laboratory Test Results (Hospital name withheld for privacy). From (My Chart, Hospital website)

COMPREHENSIVE METABOLIC PANEL (CMP) – Test Details
Collected on 09/21/2016; Resulted on 09/21/2016
GFR: 35%

Component Results

Component	Your Value	Standard Range	Flag
Sodium	138 mmol/L	135 to 145 mmol/L135 - 145 mmol/L	
Potassium	4.1 mmol/L	3.5 to 5.2 mmol/L3.5 - 5.2 mmol/L	
Chloride	99 mmol/L	98 to 110 mmol/L98 - 110 mmol/L	
Carbon Dioxide (CO2)	26 mmol/L	22 to 32 mmol/L22 - 32 mmol/L	

Anion Gap	13	5 to 17 5 - 17	
Glucose	170 mg/dL	60 to 99 mg/dL60 - 99 mg/dL	H
Fasting glucose 60-99 mg/dL			
Random glucose 60-139 mg/dL			
Blood Urea Nitrogen (BUN)	48 mg/dL	8 to 22 mg/dL8 - 22 mg/dL	H
Creatinine	1.78 mg/dL	0.60 to 1.40 mg/dL0.60 - 1.40 mg/dL	H
GFR Non African American	**35 mL/min/ 1.73m2**	>59 mL/min/1.73m2>59 mL/ min/1.73m2	L
GFR African American	40 mL/min/ 1.73m2	>59 mL/min/1.73m2>59 mL/ min/1.73m2	L

G1: Normal GFR: >=90
G2: Mildly decreased GFR: 60-89
G3a: Mildly to moderately decreased GFR: 45-59
G3b: Moderately to severely decreased GFR: 30-44
G4: Severely decreased GFR: 15-29
G5: Kidney failure GFR: <15

My Lowest GFR Number

This test shows a GFR of 35%, the lowest GFR I have had. My GFR improved to 54% in a test done on 09/15/2018, then my GFR sky-rocketed to 73% on December 4, 2020, the highest GFR number in my life as a kidney patient.

(In a Comprehensive Metabolic Panel (CMP) test taken on July 7, 2022, my GFR was 73%.)

Note: Estimated Glomerular Filtration Rate (GFR) is estimated from serum creatinine based on age, gender, and race using the CKD-EPI equation.

2. Hospital Laboratory Test Results (Hospital name withheld for privacy)

From My Chart Chart: Hospital |Website
Veltisezar B. Bautista
COMPREHENSIVE METABOLIC PANEL (CMP) - Details

Collected on 09/15/2018 7:10 AM
Resulted on 09/15/2018 11:27 AM
Veltisezar B. Bautista

Component Results

Component	Your Value	Standard Range	Flag
Sodium	138 mmol/L	135 to 145 mmol/L135 - 145 mmol/L	
Potassium	4.2 mmol/L	3.5 to 5.2 mmol/L3.5 - 5.2 mmol/L	
Chloride	102 mmol/L	98 to 110 mmol/L98 - 110 mmol/L	
Carbon Dioxide (CO2)	22 mmol/L	22 to 32 mmol/L22 - 32 mmol/L	
Anion Gap	14	5 to 17 5 - 17	
Glucose	85 mg/dL	60 to 99 mg/dL60 - 99 mg/dL	
Fasting glucose 60-99 mg/dL Random glucose 60-139 mg/dL			
Blood Urea Nitrogen (BUN)	32 mg/dL	8 to 22 mg/dL8 - 22 mg/dL	H
Creatinine	1.22 mg/dL	0.60 to 1.40 mg/dL0.60 - 1.40 mg/dL	
GFR Non African American	**54 mL/min/** 1.73m2	>59 mL/min/1.73m2>59 mL/min/1.73m2	L
GFR African American	62 mL/min/1.73m2	>59 mL/min/1.73m2>59 mL/min/1.73m2	

3. Hospital Laboratory Test Results (Hospital name withheld for privacy)

From My Chart: Hospital |Website
Veltisezar B. Bautista

COMPREHENSIVE METABOLIC PANEL (CMP) - Details

Component Results

Component	Your Value	Standard Range	Flag
Sodium	135 mmol/L	135 to 145 mmol/L135 - 145 mmol/L	
Potassium	4.1 mmol/L	3.5 to 5.2 mmol/L3.5 - 5.2 mmol/L	
Chloride	103 mmol/L	98 to 111 mmol/L98 - 111 mmol/L	
Carbon Dioxide (CO2)	25 mmol/L	20 to 29 mmol/L20 - 29 mmol/L	
Anion Gap	7	5 to 17 5 - 17	
Glucose	79 mg/dL	60 to 99 mg/dL60 - 99 mg/dL	
Fasting Blood Glucose: 60-99 mg/dL Random Blood Glucose: 60-139 mg/dL			
Blood Urea Nitrogen (BUN)	25 mg/dL	7 to 25 mg/dL7 - 25 mg/dL	
Creatinine	0.94 mg/dL	0.60 to 1.30 mg/dL0.60 - 1.30 mg/dL	
GFR Non African American	**73 mL/min/1.73m2**	>=60 mL/min/1.73m2>=60 mL/min/1.73m2	

Collected on 12/04/2020 7:24 AM from Blood, Venous (Blood)

Nothing to Worry About My Kidney Disease?

These days, my GFR levels remain at the remission stages. Remission stage ranges from 60% to any numbers above it.

Here's the summary of GFR test results until I got the 73% GFR when I reversed my kidney disease:

GFR: 35% - 09/21/2016
GFR: 54% - 09/15/2018
GFR: 73% - 12/04/2020
GFR: 73% - 07/19/2022
GFR: 71% - 04/22/2023
GFR: 72% - 12/09/2023

EGFR Dec. 9, 2023

eGFR By Creatinine
View trends
Normal range: above >60 mL/min/1.73m2
Value
72
Calculation based on the Chronic Kidney Disease Epidemiology Collaboration (CKD-EPI) equation refit without adjustment for race. Glomerular Filtration Rate is estimated from serum creatinine, age and gender using the CKD-EPI equation: G1: Normal GFR: >=90 G2: Mildly decreased GFR: 60-89 G3a: Mildly to moderately decreased GFR: 45-59 G3b: Moderately to severely decreased GFR: 30-44 G4: Severely decreased GFR: 15-29 G5: Kidney failure GFR: <15

To this day, my kidney disease is still in remission.

Hard copies of the above test reports are in my possession. I can also access my medical records in my hospital chart for the past many years, and I'm the only one who can access my chart at my hospital's website.

Chapter 8

Can You Reverse Your Heart Disease Severity & Stabilize It Into a Better Condition?

Brief Subject Summary

- Heart Failure Reversal
- Types of Heart Diseases
- What Is a Heartburn?
- What Is a Heart Attack?
- What Is a Stroke?
- Coronary Artery Disease (CAD) or Coronary Heart Disease (CHD)
- Congestive Heart Failure (CHF)
- Heart Failure Stages and Classifications
- Atrial Fibrillation (A-Fib)
- Controlling Cholesterol and Triglycerides
- High Blood Pressure
- Medical Procedures
- What Is Ejection Fraction?
- 7 Powerful Ways You Can Strengthen Your Heart
- Medical Devices for People with Heart Disease

Can you reverse the severity of your heart disease (or heart failure) and stabilize it into a better condition?

Yes, you can reverse the severity of the disease, although not in its totality. I know it; it's because I did it! I have reduced my heart failure's gravity and stabilized it into a better condition.

Heart Failure Reversal

Commenting on the reversal of heart failure, Mayo Clinic says, "Not all conditions that lead to heart failure can be reversed, but treatments can improve the signs and symptoms of heart failure and help you live longer. Lifestyle changes — such as exercising, reducing sodium in your diet, managing stress, and losing weight — can improve your quality of life."

The University of California San Francisco reports, "Although heart failure is a serious condition that progressively gets worse over time, certain cases can be reversed with treatment.

Even when the heart muscle is impaired, there are a number of treatments that can relieve symptoms and stop or slow the gradual worsening of the condition."

From the Providence Heart Institute in Portland, Oregon

"Certain types of heart disease can be reversible. In coronary artery disease, where there is cholesterol plaque buildup in the heart's arteries, healthy lifestyle changes, and medications (such as statins) can stabilize the condition, prevent additional plaque deposits and, in some cases, help reverse the severity of the disease."

So says Dr. Lori M. Tam, medical director for the Women's Heart Program at the Providence Heart Institute in Portland, Oregon.

She adds that you must understand the severity of your heart disease, starting with knowing your numbers about blood pressure, cholesterol, blood sugar, and body mass index (BMI).

Dr. Tam says understanding the severity of your heart disease starts with "knowing your numbers," which are key indicators of your heart health.

From the University of Alabama

As reported on the website, Myheart.Net, Dr. Mustafa Ahmed has stated this, "There is no miracle cure yet – I am sure to tell patients there is no miracle cure that will reverse heart disease. The key is to stabilize heart disease, and if we are fortunate, we may see a regression over time, although large regressions in blockages are not the goal, as there is no good evidence that can occur. Stabilization of disease is the key and can be achieved through a combination of lifestyle changes and currently available treatments."

Dr. Ahmed is a structural heart specialist, interventional cardiologist, and scientist. He is the director of the Structural Heart Disease Program at the University of Alabama at Birmingham.

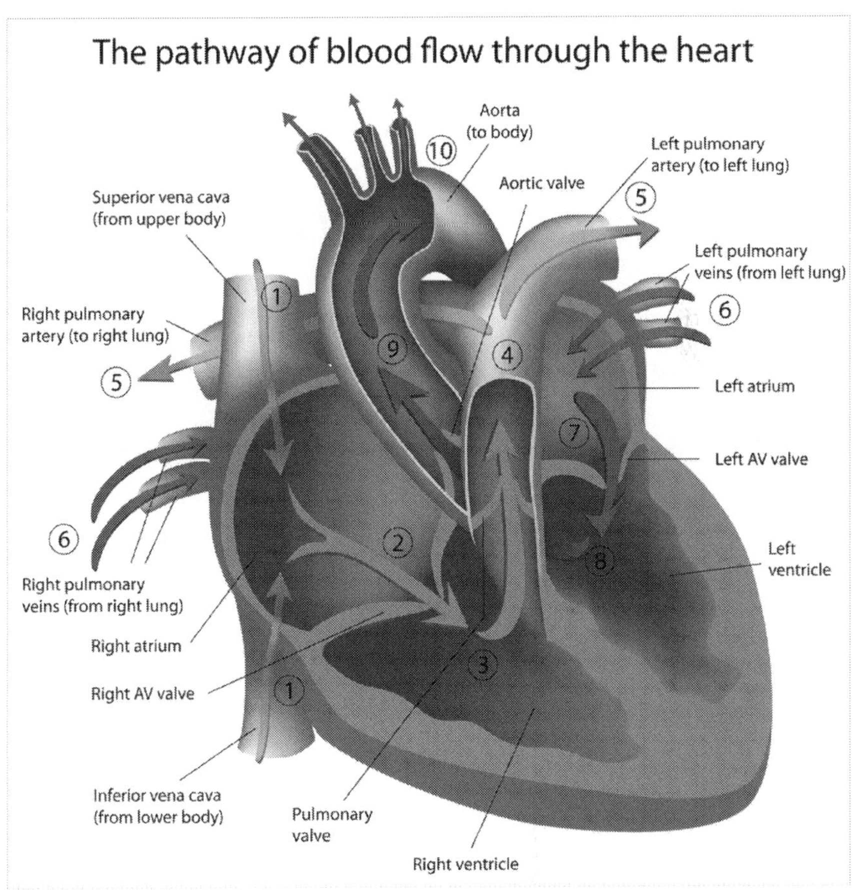

Photo Source: Shutterstock

How Does Blood Flow Through the Heart?

MedlinePlus says, "The heart is a large muscular organ which constantly pushes oxygen-rich blood to the brain and extremities and transports oxygen-poor blood from the brain and extremities to the lungs to gain oxygen."

On the other hand, according to Michigan Medicine of the University of Michigan, blood flows through the heart and lungs in 4 steps, which are:

- "The right atrium receives oxygen-poor blood from the body and pumps it to the right ventricle through the tricuspid valve.
- "The right ventricle pumps the oxygen-poor blood to the lungs through the pulmonary valve.
- "The left atrium receives oxygen-rich blood from the lungs and pumps it to the left ventricle through the mitral valve.
- "The left ventricle pumps the oxygen-rich blood through the aortic valve out to the rest of the body."

I. Types of Heart Diseases

The Centers for Disease Control and Prevention (CDC) says, "The term 'heart disease' refers to several types of heart conditions. The most common heart disease type in the United States is coronary artery disease (CAD), which affects the heart's blood flow. Decreased blood flow can cause a heart attack."

It adds, "Over time, high blood sugar can damage blood vessels and the nerves that control your heart. People with diabetes are also more likely to have other conditions that raise the risk of heart disease."

Several types of heart diseases include the following:

- Coronary artery disease (CAD) or Coronary heart disease (CHD), blood vessel disease
- Congestive heart failure (CHF) or simply heart failure (a chronic progressive condition affecting the pumping power of the heart muscle)
- Atrial Fibrillation: the most common arrhythmia (irregular heartbeat)
- Congenital heart defects (the disease that anyone is born with)
- Dilated cardiomyopathy (heart chamber dilation)
- Myocardial infarction (heart attack)
- Hypertrophic cardiomyopathy (genetic problem)
- Mitral valve regurgitation (mitral valve does not close tightly enough and allows blood to flow back into the heart)
- Mitral valve prolapse (valve flaps the mitral valve, causing it not to close properly, producing a heart murmur)
- Aortic stenosis (the valve does not open properly, making it difficult for the heart to pump blood from the right ventricle into the pulmonary artery

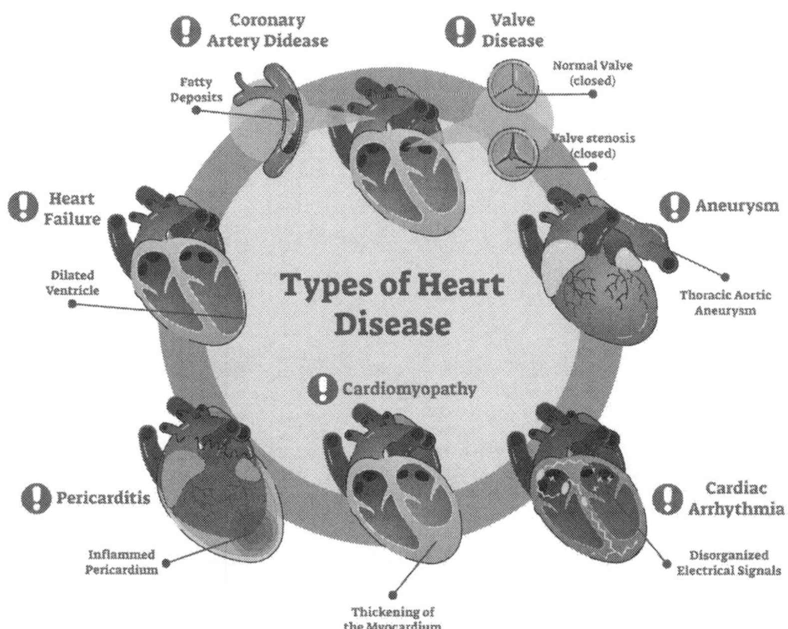

II. Heartburn

What Is Heartburn?

The Cleveland Clinic defines heartburn as "a symptom of many different conditions, including acid reflux and GERD. It typically feels like a burning in the center of the chest, behind your breastbone."

What Causes Heartburn Pain?

Heartburn or acid reflux is a gastroesophageal reflux disease (GERD).

The food passes down a long tube called the esophagus, connecting the mouth to the stomach when you eat. The esophageal sphincter, a valve, opens when food comes in and closes to push and keep the contents down in the stomach. Once inside the gut, acidic chemicals start to digest the food.

However, some stomach acidic elements go back up the esophagus if the esophageal sphincter doesn't close properly. Then the acid hurts the esophagus, which becomes inflamed. Prolonged irritation and inflammation of the esophagus can lead to ulcers and possible serious bleeding.

Also, changes in the types of cells lining the esophagus may cause a disorder called Barrett's esophagus, which will increase your risk of esophageal cancer.

Symptoms of Heartburn

The typical symptoms of heartburn include:

- Tightness in your chest
- Pain in your chest when you bend over or lay down
- Burning feeling in your throat
- Coughing and wheezing
- Acidic, sour, or salty taste in the back of your throat
- Shortness of breath
- Hoarse, sore throat
- Excessive burping (if you swallow air along with your food or drink something like a soda or beer, with bubbles in it can come back upward through your esophagus, producing an unusual sound that is a burp.

III. Heart Attack

What Is a Heart Attack?

The American Heart Association (AHA) says, "A heart attack occurs when the blood flow that brings oxygen to the heart muscle is severely reduced or cut off completely."

When an artery blocked by plaques ruptures, oxygen to the heart will be interrupted, causing an inadequate blood flow, resulting in a heart attack.

This blockage happens because fatty deposits build up over the years, forming plaques in the heart's arteries. For example, if a plaque ruptures, a blood clot can form. Then the clot blocks the arteries, causing a heart attack.

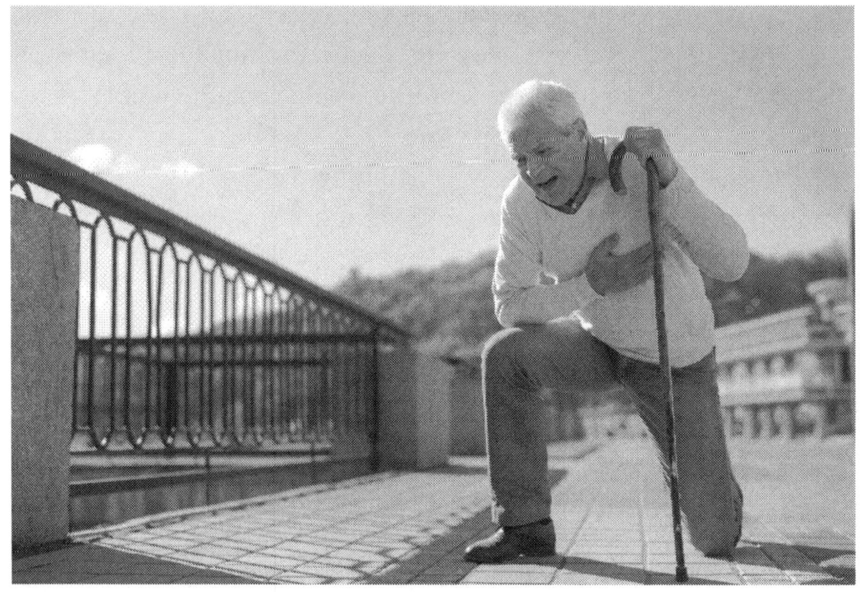

When Heart Attack Strike
s

(Photo Credit: Shutterstock)

Major Symptoms of a Heart Attack

- Discomfort in the center or left side of the heart, feeling like uncomfortable pain, squeezing, fullness, or alarming pressure
- Pain in the jaw, neck, or back
- Weakness, lightheadedness, dizziness, or fainting
- Pain or discomfort in one or both arms or shoulders
- Shortness of breath
- Heart palpitations
- Sweating or having cold sweet
- Heartburn-like pain in the center, above the stomach
- Nausea or vomiting

For women:

- Shortness of breath with or without chest discomfort
- Cold sweat, nausea. dizziness or lightheadedness
- Pain in one or both arms, back, stomach, or jaw
- Nausea or vomiting
- Upper back pressure and jaw pain

Factors That May Trigger a Heart Attack

For those people who are already under treatment for CAD may have a heart attack triggered by several factors, including:

- Extreme cold weather
- Very hot weather
- Pollution and vehicle exhaust
- Strong emotions
- Sudden or intense exertion
- Stress
- Major disasters
- Smoking
- High lipids, fatty substances that include cholesterol and triglycerides
- Age: Men, age 45 or older, and women age 55 or older are more likely to have a heart attack than are younger men and women.

In Case of an Emergency Open Heart Surgery

After a heart attack, cardiologists perform balloon angioplasty or coronary artery angioplasty in case of an emergency bypass surgery. The doctors insert a mesh cage called a stent into the blocked blood vessels to keep the artery open.

In 2003, medical doctors started to use a new generation of stents. Instead of bare metal, they now use drug-coated stents.

But plaque, in a process called restenosis, can gradually clog the inserted stent. To help keep such arterial passageways clear, scientists have developed drug-coated stents.

Usually, this cardiac incident is the first heart attack of a person who doesn't know coronary artery disease. Once you have had a heart attack, it may be possible that you may suffer from another or more heart attacks in the future, depending on your heart condition involving metabolic syndrome.

What Is It: Heartburn or Heart Attack?

If you think you have heartburn, drink a lot of water to push back the acid to the stomach. If the discomfort and pain in the chest don't go away, most probably, it's a heart attack.

I did this procedure when I felt discomfort But the condition didn't disappear. Yet I didn't call 911 emergency medical service (EMS) to rush me to the hospital. What misjudgment on my part!

Now, I know what a heart attack is. I didn't have any second heart attack. Many years have passed since then.

Call the EMS wherever you are if you're not sure what's causing your chest discomfort and pain.

Similarities and Differences Between Heart Attack and Heartburn

Similarities: Both heartburn and heart attack usually cause discomfort and pain in the center of the chest. Both of them can happen after eating.

Differences: Heart attacks usually occur in the early morning, which is the most dangerous. (My heart attack happened between 4 a.m. and 5 a.m.)

- Heart attack can also cause pain in the left chest and the center of the chest.
- Heartburn occurs after eating, usually after 1 hour up to 4 hours.

One Million Heart Attacks Per Year

According to the Cleveland Clinic, coronary artery disease (narrowing of the arteries supplying blood to the heart) causes about one million heart attacks each year.

Research shows that 220,000 people with heart attacks may die even before reaching the hospital.

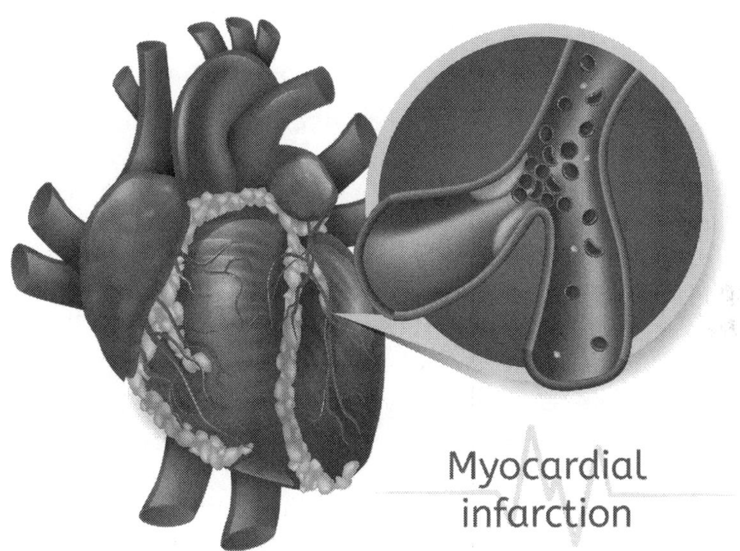

Heart Attack (Myocardial Infarction). 3d Realistic Illustration of Human Heart with Blocked Coronary Artery. Vector Plaque

Photo Credit: Shutterstock

My Journey: An Unforgettable Incident

One early morning, maybe at 5:30 a.m., February 1996, I woke up with discomfort and tightness in the middle part of my chest. I felt a little shortness of breath but not excruciating chest pain. It was like a strong pressure inside my chest.

I presumed the chest tightness was due to heartburn or acid reflux, known as gastroesophageal reflux disease (GERD) because I used to have the same feeling before. It occurs when your stomach acid

flows back into the esophagus, a tube connecting your mouth and stomach.
I drank a lot of water, which I would always do when I experienced heartburn: pushed back the acid to the stomach, and it would usually go away.

But the discomfort didn't disappear; I continued to be restless, going to bed and getting up again to find comfort. Immediately, I drove to my doctor's clinic, and I had an ECG or EKG test.

The clinic called the EMS that rushed me to the nearest hospital.

In the emergency room, I was given the necessary protocols to alleviate my condition. The medical team hooked me to several machines, and the emergency doctor did an angioplasty on me to open the blocked artery that caused the heart attack.

Afterward, the doctor told me, "About 40% of your heart was damaged." What did I do? I asked myself. I should have called 911 after I felt the feeling of discomfort in my chest. What a mistake, presuming that chest pain was due only to heartburn or acid reflux. What an unforgettable incident!

I cannot undo the damage to my heart that has been done. Although 26 years had passed, those memorable moments are still fresh in my mind.
Later, upon research, I learned that heart attacks and heartburns have the same symptoms in some ways. It's no wonder I committed a terrible mistake that nearly cost my life.

What Is Sudden Cardiac Arrest (SCA)?

Sudden cardiac arrest is a condition in which the heart suddenly stops beating. When this happens, immediate action is needed to restart the heart because blood stops flowing to the brain and other vital organs.

Cardiopulmonary resuscitation (CPR) is a lifesaving procedure useful for heart attacks or cardiac arrest emergencies. The American Heart Association recommends starting CPR on a patient with hard and fast chest compressions. The recommendation applies to both untrained bystanders and first responders in a cardiac arrest situation.

Of course, the first thing to do in a medical emergency is call 911. CPR should be done immediately by anyone who can do it on the patient while waiting for an ambulance to arrive.

Difference Between Heart Attack and Cardiac Arrest

Heart attack is a circulation problem. On the other hand, cardiac arrest is an electrical issue caused by disrupting the heart's rhythm.

IV. Strokes

What Is a Stroke?

Stroke, the No. 5 cause of death in the United States, is a condition that affects the arteries leading to and within the brain. A stroke happens when a blood vessel that carries oxygen and nutrients to the brain is blocked, or a clot or a blood vessel ruptures, stopping the blood flow to the brain and causing the death of cells.

Types of Stroke

The three main types of stroke are:

- Ischemic stroke
- Hemorrhagic stroke
- Transient ischemic attack (TIA), a warning or a "mini-stroke")

Ischemic Stroke

Blood clots often cause blockages in the arteries that lead to ischemic strokes.

Hemorrhagic Stroke

When an artery ruptures, it leaks blood that will put too much pressure on brain cells, causing damage. That's called a hemorrhagic stroke.

Strokes can also happen due to the following:

- Heart Attack
- High blood pressure, causing arteries to rupture
- Aneurysm balloon-like bulges in a blood vessel that can stretch and burst

Transient Ischemic Attack (or Stroke)

A transient ischemic attack (TIA) is considered a mini-stroke. It happens when a part of the brain temporarily lacks blood flow. A mini-stroke on its own doesn't cause lasting symptoms or disabilities.

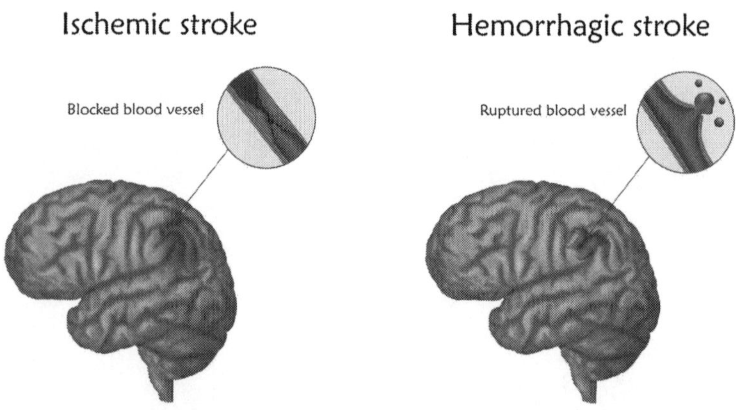

Types of Stroke: Ischemic Vs. Hemorrhagic

Photo Credit: Shutterstock

Causes of Stroke

- **High blood pressure:** The biggest cause of stroke
- **Medicines:** Some medicines can cause a stroke
- **Family:** Strokes can run in families
- **Gender:** Men are more likely to have a stroke than women who have the same age
- **Race:** African-Americans, Spanish Americans, and Asian Americans are more likely to have strokes than any ethnic group in the U.S.

Symptoms of Stroke

- Dizziness or feeling of falling
- Not capable of talking
- Double or blurred vision at least in one eye
- Numbness or weakness on one side of the body

Heatstroke: Another Type of Stroke

Heatstroke results from prolonged exposure to high temperatures with dehydration, failing the body's temperature control system. If you have a heat stroke, your body's temperature should be more than 104 degrees Fahrenheit.

Symptoms Of Heat Stroke

- Seizures
- Nausea
- Confusion
- The possible occurrence of loss of consciousness or coma

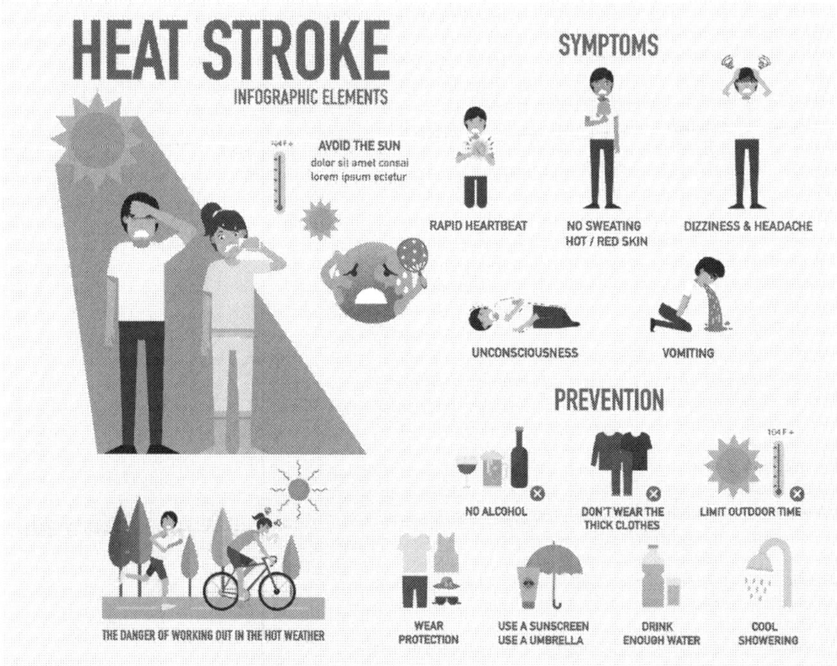

Photo Credit: Shutterstock

V. Coronary Artery Disease (CAD); Also Called Coronary Heart Disease (CHD)

Because of diabetes, you increase your risk of developing heart and blood vessel disease. Coronary artery disease, also called coronary heart disease (CHD), is the most common.

Causes of CAD

- Diabetes
- Smoking
- High blood pressure
- High LDL (bad) cholesterol, high triglycerides levels, and low HDL (good) cholesterol

- Obesity
- Lack of exercise
- High saturated fat diet
- Family history

Symptoms of CAD or CHD

Symptoms of coronary heart artery disease (CAD), also known as coronary heart disease (CHD), in the beginning, may involve only light stabbing pain in the chest and shortness of breath once in a while. But once you have a heart attack, all the symptoms appear.

You should quickly call the medical emergency service in your area in your country. In the United States, you call the EMS number, 911, if you think you have symptoms of a heart attack.

The symptoms include:

- Pain or discomfort in the chest and other areas of the upper body, including the arms, jaw, neck, stomach, and left shoulder
- Choking feeling (may feel like indigestion or heartburn)
- Sweating
- Shortness of breath
- Nausea or vomiting
- Lightheadedness or dizziness
- Irregular heart beat

Treatment of CAD

Medicines: If you have coronary disease, your primary doctor or cardiologist will prescribe for you a list of medications, which may include medications for high blood pressure, diabetes, high cholesterol, and triglycerides.

Lifestyle Changes: As a part of treatment for CAD, you may make some lifestyle changes, involving:

- Eating a heart-healthy diet
- Doing exercise
- De-stressing
- Quitting smoking
- Limiting or avoiding alcohol consumption

- Eliminating high intake of salt and canned foods
- Decreasing LDL (bad) cholesterol triglycerides and increasing HDL (good) cholesterol
- Limiting or avoiding saturated fats, and trans fat
- Eating foods with healthy oil, such as olive oil and avocado oil
- Having a good night's sleep
- Losing 5% to 10% of your body weight, if you're overweight
- Getting enough exercise that makes your body more sensitive to insulin (the hormone that allows cells in your body to use blood sugar for energy).

The Bautista Treatment System

Lifestyle changes that can help you lower your risk for heart disease or keep it from getting worse are as follows:

- Following a semi-plant-based diet, composing whole grains, vegetables, legumes, and fruits
- Doing a moderate-intensity walking exercise or any other aerobic exercise such as walking, bicycle riding, stationary bike, and swimming
- Limiting or eliminating red meat such as pork, beef, and lamb with high saturated fats and trans fats
- Avoiding smoking
- Reducing or avoiding alcohol intake
- Having a healthy weight: if you're overweight, losing 5% to 10% of your body weight

VI: Congestive Heart Failure (CHF)

What Is Heart Failure?

The American Heart Association says, "Heart failure is a chronic, progressive condition in which the heart muscle is unable to pump enough blood to meet the body's needs for blood and oxygen. The heart can't keep up with its workload."

The Cleveland Clinic has this comment on heart failure:

"The term 'heart failure' can be frightening. It doesn't mean the heart has 'failed' or stopped working. It means the heart doesn't pump as well as it should."

Statistics

About six million Americans are afflicted with congestive heart failure, and there are about 550,000 new cases of heart failure every year.

Heart failure is a leading cause of death for 1 in 9 Americans, according to the U.S. Centers for Disease Control and Prevention (CDC). About half of them who are diagnosed with heart failure pass away after 5 years.

Types of Congestive Heart Failure (CHF)

The left ventricle gives more pumping power, so it's larger than the other chambers, the right ventricle, and the left atrium and right atrium (upper chambers).

Each of the valves of the four chambers only permits blood to flow in one direction. The left ventricle is considered the strongest among the four chambers because it pumps blood out to the entire body.

There are two types of heart failure:

- Left-sided heart failure
- Right-sided heart failure

Left-Sided Heart Failure

There are two types of left-sided heart failure:

Heart failure with reduced ejection fraction (HFrEF): Also called **systolic failure,** this heart condition occurs when the left ventricle fails to contract normally. So the level of force available to push blood into circulation is reduced.

Heart failure with preserved ejection fraction (HFpEF): Also called **diastolic failure**, this heart condition happens when the left ventricle loses its ability to relax normally due to muscle stiffness. Therefore, the heart can't properly fill itself with blood while resting between every beat.

Right-Sided Heart Failure

Right-sided or right ventricular heart failure also called cor pulmonale or pulmonary heart disease, causes the right side of the heart to lose its power to pump normally.

As a result, fluid flows back through the lungs, weakening the heart's right side leading to right-sided heart failure. Also, the condition usually occurs as a result of left-sided heart failure.

Causes of Heart Failure

- Diabetes
- Ischemic heart disease
- Heart attack
- Heart valve disease
- Cardiomyopathy, a disorder of the heart muscle
- Congenital heart defect
- Certain types of arrhythmias, or irregular heart rhythms
- High blood pressure
- Other heart diseases or conditions

Symptoms of Heart Failure

- Fatigue and weakness
- Shortness of breath
- Inactivity
- Rapid or irregular heartbeat
- Chest pain if heart attack caused the heart failure
- Frequency of urination
- Fluid retention (edema) in your feet, legs, and ankles
- Palpitations or irregular heartbeat
- Reduced ability to exercise
- Lack of appetite

Treatments of Heart Failure

The treatments include:

- Taking medicines, some vitamins, and minerals
- Eating heart-healthy foods and avoiding foods with lots of saturated fat, such as canned foods
- Eating more plant protein than animal protein
- Consuming a flexible mini-plant-based diet consisting of whole grains, vegetables, fruits, and nuts (good for diabetes, kidney disease, and heart disease)
- Doing low-intensity or moderate-intensity walking for 20 minutes one hour after each meal of the day, reducing blood sugar (if you have diabetes), and achieving a 64% to 76% target heart rate of your estimated maximum heart rate
- Drinking enough water, from 8 to 10 cups or glasses of water (8 ounces) or more based on your condition to dilute blood sugar (if you have diabetes), dissolves creatinine and blood urea nitrogen (BUN) if you have kidney disease (but avoiding a lot of water intake, if you have advance kidney disease and heart failure with water restrictions)
- Getting enough sleep, at least 7 to 9 hours at night
- Loss of 5% to 10% of body weight, if needed
- Eating fatty fish, if you don't have kidney disease
- Quitting smoking
- Managing stress
- Controlling blood pressure
- Managing cholesterol levels and limiting or avoiding alcohol
- Implantation of an (ICD), CRT-P or CRT-D, if needed
- Standard treatment system recommended by a doctor

VII. Heart Failure Stages and Classifications

What Are the 4 Heart Failure Stages?

The four heart failure stages are Class I, Class II, Class III, and Class IV.

A doctor may determine patients' heart failure classifications based on their symptoms and functional limitations. The heart failure condition depends on how well your heart can pump blood to your whole body.

In general, physicians use the NYHA (New York Heart Association) Class guidelines as the most common measure to determine the severity of heart failure.

NYHA Functional Classifications

NYHA Class: Patients with Cardiac Disease (Description of HF Related Symptoms):

Class I (Mild): Patients with cardiac disease but without resulting in limitation of physical activity. Ordinary physical activity does not cause undue fatigue, palpitation (rapid or pounding heartbeat), dyspnea (shortness of breath), or anginal pain (chest pain).

Class II (Mild): Patients with cardiac disease resulting in slight limitation of physical activity. They are comfortable at rest. Ordinary physical activity results in fatigue, palpitation, dyspnea, or anginal pain.

Class III (Moderate): Patients with cardiac disease resulting in marked limitation of physical activity. They are comfortable at rest. Less than ordinary activity causes fatigue, palpitation, dyspnea, or anginal pain.

Class IV (Severe): Patients with cardiac disease cannot carry out any physical activity without discomfort. Symptoms of heart failure or anginal syndrome may be present even at rest. If any physical activity is undertaken, discomfort is increased.

(The Criteria Committee of the New York Heart Association. Nomenclature and Criteria for Diagnosis of Diseases of the Heart and Great Vessels. 9th ed. Boston, Mass: Little, Brown & Co; 1994:253-256.)

Source: CHF Solutions: https://www.chf-solutions.com/heart-failure-classifications/

My Journey: Water Intake

I have a history of heart failure. Cardiac patients, based on the heart's condition, may have water restriction intake. Doctors recommend that these patients drink only 6 to 8 cups or glasses (8 oz) of water daily.

A heart failure incident happened to me in the early part of 2017. Doctors extracted too much fluids my lungs by giving me large dosages of diuretics. I stayed in the hospital for about three days. Although my doctors say I had a heart failure event, I had it only once throughout my life since I had a heart attack in 1996.

I had a fluid overload. My weakened heart had a hard time pumping the fluids and it flowed back to the lungs and other organs instead of sending the bulk of blood to all parts of the body because the damaged heart could not handle the too much fluids in the body. So there was an abnormal buildup of fluid in the lungs leading to shortness of breath. That was why my daughter rushed me to the hospital nearby.

Before the heart failure event happened, I had drunk a high amount of fluids, which caused the buildup of too much liquid in the lungs, causing pulmonary edema. Medline Plus says, "Pulmonary edema is often caused by congestive heart failure. When the heart cannot pump efficiently, blood can back up into the veins that take blood through the lungs."

I learned a lesson from the cardiac incident. However, I little by little, I increased my fluid intake. Now, I consume enough water (but not in excess) to dilute my blood sugar, creatinine, and blood urea nitrogen (BUN), which are all water-soluble.

My water intake? Currently, I consume 9 to 10 cups or glasses of water (8 ounces of water each glass) per day. I have not had, with this quota, any accumulation of fluids (called pulmonary edema) in my lungs.

If you have heart failure, you may ask your physician how much water (including coffee or tea) you can consume. My case is different from yours.

My regular cardiologist has told me that my congestive heart failure falls under Class I or Stage I. Before, I had Class 3 (Stage 3) heart failure.

My Journey: CRT-D Biventricular Pacemaker

A cardiologist/electrophysiologist implanted a Biventricular pacemaker (CRT-D) in my left chest in 2018. A CRT-D delivers small electrical impulses to the heart's left and right ventricles to help them contract simultaneously. Up to now, my new CRT-D pacemaker has not fired yet, to indicate any irregular heartbeat.

In a summary discharge prepared by my cardiologist-physiologist who did the implantation of a new pacemaker in my left chest at a hospital in Pontiac, Michigan, he said:

"The patient is an 84-year old Filipino male with a remote history of coronary artery bypass grafting and ischemic cardiomyopathy with an ejection fraction of around 30%, left bundle branch block with QRS duration of 160, msec and chronic Class 3 congestive heart failure despite a good medical regimen. He received a single-chamber ICD in the remote past. It is now dead. He was brought in electively for an upgrade to a biventricular system, and this was completed on the day of admission."

As you can see, the cardiologist-electrophysiologist stated that my heart failure condition was at Class 3 (Stage 3) before my CTR-D biventricular pacemaker was installed. Then after 2 years, my ejection fraction increased to 47% in 2020, and my heart disease has improved and my regular cardiologist toled me that my heart failure falls under Class 1 (Stage 1) mild. Up to now, my heart disease is still in a good shape.

Living into the 90s

I still remember that many years ago, a fortune-teller told me that I would live up to 75. When I reached that age, I could not sleep on the night of my birthday. I asked myself: "Would I wake up tomorrow?" I didn't die.

The next morning, I set a new goal: I wanted to live up to 85. When I reached 85, I thought of another intent: to live up to the 90s. Well, I am in the 90s now. Wow! And who knows, as a friend told me, "I think you'll be living up to 100." Why not?

Yes, dreams come true. That's why I'm continuing to dream dreams. Tomorrow is forever. Sometimes you may say, "I will do this thing tomorrow."

Heart Failure Medications

ACE) Angiotensin-conversing enzyme inhibitors or **angiotensin receptor blockers (ARBs):** ACE and ARB medicines help treat high blood pressure and congestive heart failure, preventing kidney failure and reducing the risk of stroke.

Anticoagulants or antiplatelets: Doctors use anticoagulants and antiplatelets, two types of blood thinners, to prevent blood from clotting that can result in artery blockages, strokes, and heart attacks.

Diuretics: Diuretics, known as water pills, help the kidneys release more sodium into the urine. Thus, more water flushes out of your body. So they reduce the fluid from your body, decreasing blood pressure.

Vasodilators: Doctors use a group of medicines that dilate (open) blood vessels, known as vasodilators. They prescribe them to prevent or treat high blood pressure, angina, and heart failure.

Digitalis glycosides: Physicians use cardiac glycosides to treat heart failure and several irregular heartbeats. They are for people with atrial fibrillation (a distinctive and often rapid heart rate) and atrial flutter (a type of abnormal heart rhythm or arrhythmia).

Aldosterone inhibitors: They allow the kidneys to pass out more fluid and keep the body's potassium. In other words, these aldosterone antagonists spare potassium in getting out of the body.

Beta-blockers: Beta-blockers are a group of medicines used to block the effects of stress hormones, such as adrenaline and cortisol, the primary hormone, on the heart.

List of Medicines and Supplements I take:

Prescribed Medicines

- Carvedilol tab, 6.25mg (twice a day)
- Atorvastatin Calcium tab, 20mg
- Isosorbide Mononirate ER tab, 30mg
- Losartan Potassium tab, 25mg
- Furosemide tab, 20mg
- Niacin ER tab, 500m (twice a day)
- Digoxin tab, 0.125mg
- Clopidogrel tab, 75mg
- Omega-3-Acid Ethyl Esters cap, 1gm (2 capsules, twice a day)
- Ecotrin, 81mg

Self-Prescribed Supplements

- High Absorption magnesium
- Magnesium taurate
- Magnesium orotate
- Qunol Ultra CoQ10
- Ubiquinol QH absorb
- Vitamin B12
- Folic acid
- Omega-3-Acid Ethyl Esters capsules, USP
- Plus other supplements for my peripheral neuropathy and peripheral artery disease (PAD)

Those are my medicines, vitamins, and minerals; these apply to me only, based on my current conditions. You may ask your doctor what you can take for medications for you.

Magnesium Dosage

According to the National Institutes of Health (NIH), your magnesium needs depend on age and sex. Men over 70 and teenage girls are the most likely groups to be magnesium deficient. (See magnesium in Chapter 10.)

Suggested amounts of magnesium:

- 400–420 milligrams a day for men
- 310–320 mg a day for women
- 350–360 mg a day for pregnant women

Why Should Kidney Disease and Heart Failure Patients Limit Water Intake?

Doctors impose fluid restrictions on patients with heart failure as a way to avoid overloading your heart, as more fluids in your bloodstream make it harder for your heart to pump. Also, excess water can overload the diseased kidneys, depending on their condition.

The American Heart Association (AHA) says that you should limit your total fluid intake to 2 quarts (64 oz or 8 cups) or less per day, depending on the heart failure stage. The limitation is to help keep your body from retaining fluid.

However, some sources opine that if your heart failure is not very bad, you may not have to limit your fluids too much. It would best to restrict your water intake as advised by your physician to avoid a heart failure event to be hospitalized to remove the excess fluids from around your lungs and heart, causing you shortness of breath and other symptoms.

VIII. Atrial Fibrillation (A-Fib): Most Common Type of Arrhythmia

According to the CDC, "Atrial fibrillation, often called AFib or AF, is the most common type of treated heart arrhythmia. An arrhythmia is when the heart beats too slowly, too fast, or in a weird way."

On the other hand, Johns Hopkins Medicine describes atrial fibrillation as "the most common type of sustained cardiac arrhythmia. It occurs when there are too many electrical signals that normally control the heartbeat, causing the upper chambers of the heart (the atria) to beat extremely rapidly (more than 400 beats per minute) and quiver (fibrillate)." Luckily, I don't have this condition.

What Is Cardiac Arrhythmia?

Cardiac arrhythmia refers to a group of conditions that cause the heart to beat irregularly, too slowly, or too quickly.

- Bradycardia, or a slow heartbeat
- Tachycardia, or a fast heartbeat
- Irregular heartbeat, also known as a flutter or fibrillation early heartbeat, or a premature ventricular contraction

Causes of Atrial Fibrillation (A-Fib)

Any interruption to the electrical impulses that stimulate heart contractions may result in arrhythmia.

Several factors can cause the heart to work incorrectly, including:

- Diabetes
- Heart attack
- Drinking too much caffeine and alcohol
- Heart disease, such as congestive heart failure
- High blood pressure
- Overactive thyroid gland
- Stress
- High blood pressure
- Structural changes in the heart

Symptoms of Atrial Fibrillation (A-Fib)

Symptoms may include:

- Weakness or fatigue
- Shortness of breath
- Chest pain or tightness
- Sweating
- Anxiety
- Blurry vision
- Palpitations
- Blurry vision
- Dizziness or lightheadedness
- Fainting

Treatment for Atrial Fibrillation

The first line of treatment for A-Fib will be medications. They help make the symptoms less bothersome, but they don't cure them.

Here are the procedures to treat A-Fib:

Catheter ablation: Ablation is a non-surgical treatment option that locates and destroys abnormal electrical pathways in the heart that cause atrial fibrillation.

Doctors use radio frequency ablation heat to destroy abnormal electrical pathways. On the other hand, the so-called cryoballoon ablation freezes the abnormal pathways.

Left atrial appendage closure: Doctors close the left atrial appendage, a pocket-like section in the heart's left atrium (upper chamber). Why? Because the left atrial appendage is often the source of blood clot formation. One of the treatments is the Watchman procedure. This process is considered minimally invasive.

Total Thoracoscopic Modified Maze (TT Maze) Procedure

Considered a minimal procedure, a cardiac surgeon makes small cuts or incisions on the sides of the chest to gain access to the heart. Afterward, the doctor makes scar patterns on the outside of the heart to disrupt the uneven flow of electricity that causes atrial fibrillation.

If atrial fibrillation doesn't stop, a cardiac electrophysiologist will have to do a catheter ablation, as described above.

IX. Omega-3 Polyunsaturated Fatty Acid (PUFAs)

Health Benefits Of MUFAs And PUFAs

Omega 3 fatty acids possess strong anti-inflammatory properties that lower the risk of heart disease, and Alzheimer's, promote vision, and boost brain health.

Monounsaturated fatty acids (MUFAs) are a healthy type of fat. that replaces less healthy fats, including saturated fats and trans fats, with unsaturated fats. MUFAs and polyunsaturated fats offer health benefits.

You may choose MUFAs and PUFAs-rich oils instead of saturated fats and other unhealthy fats because they can reduce the risk of heart disease.

MUFA oils are good in improving insulin levels and keeping blood sugar under control, thereby avoiding instances of prediabetes symptoms.

Evidence has proven that regular usage of MUFA oil lowers the bad cholesterol and improves the level of good cholesterol. Omega 3 fatty acids rich in PUFAs promote mood and alleviate depression and anxiety.

MUPAs and PUFAs intake help in cell and nerve maintenance and aid indigestion.

The key is moderation, as excessive fat intake can increase the risk of chronic ailments.

Benefits of Omega-3 PUFAs

Omega-3 polyunsaturated fatty acids (PUFAs) have many benefits, including:

- Lowering blood pressure slightly
- Reducing blood clotting
- Decreasing the risk of strokes and heart failure
- Reducing irregular heartbeat

- Increasing high-density lipoprotein (HDL), the good cholesterol
- Decreasing platelet aggregation

PUFAs: Good for Type 2 Diabetes, Kidney Disease, and Heart Disease

Omega-3 FUPA supplements are beneficial to type 2 diabetes, kidney disease, and heart failure (HF) patients, especially dilated cardiomyopathy patients.

In diabetic patients, they have a positive effect on insulin sensitivity. Studies have shown that PUFAs may reduce the so-called wave velocity, blood pressure, and triglyceride levels in patients with CKD. It also reduces the risk of vascular disease.

X. Controlling Cholesterol and Triglycerides

If you have any of these diseases: diabetes, kidney disease, and coronary artery disease (CAD), it's best if you would try your best in:

- Lowering your LDL (bad cholesterol) and triglycerides
- Increasing your HDL (good cholesterol
- Lowering creatinine and blood urea nitrogen (BUN)
- Raising your eGFR or GFR
- Reducing your blood pressure
- Increasing your ejection fraction
- Eating a semi-plant-based diet, not necessarily being a vegetarian or vegan

My Journey: Eating More Eggs?

Yes, eggs are controversial. Many doctors and even government and private institutions say that an individual needs only 3 whole eggs a go, because of its high content of cholesterol.

But I should tell you, eattng more eggs don't affect blood cholesterol. In fact, I eat 3 eggs daily, Monday to Sunday, and my experiment shows that eggs doesn't blood cholesterol. And you know what, since I started 3 whole eggs daily, my hdl (good) cholesterol has increased from 32 to 48 (current). That's good because hdl

(good cholesterol) sweeps eat or sweep away LDL (bad cholesterol). What a miracle for me. Before, I had a hard time raising my hdl cholesterol. Not anymore! Eating more eggs increase hdl cholesterol levels.
Below are the results of my Lipid Panel Tests before we went to press:

LIPID PANEL - Details
Veltisezar B. Bautista

Results
Dec. 9, 2023

Lab tests - Blood (Blood Venous)

Results

Compare result trends

Cholesterol
View trends
Normal range: below <200 mg/dL
Value
112
<200 mg/dL Desirable 200-239 mg/dL Borderline High >=240 mg/dL High
Triglycerides
View trends
Normal range: below <150 mg/dL
Value
47
<150 mg/dL Normal 150-199 mg/dL Borderline high 200-499 mg/dL High >=500 mg/dL Very High
HDL Cholesterol
View trends
Normal range: above >=40 mg/dL
Value
48

LDL Cholesterol, Calculated
View trends
Normal range: below <=129 mg/dL
Value
55
<70 mg/dL Desirable if very high risk <100 mg/dL Desirable if high risk 100-129 mg/dL Above desirable 130-159 mg/dL Borderline high 160-189 mg/dL High >=190 mg/dL Very high
Non-HDL Cholesterol, Calculated
View trends
Normal range: below <=159 mg/dL
Value
64
<130 mg/dL Desirable 130-159 mg/dL Above desirable 160-189 mg/dL Borderline high 190-219 mg/dL High >=220 mg/dL Very high
Cholesterol/HDL Ratio
View trends
Normal range: 1.8 - 4.9
1.84.9

XI. High Blood Pressure

What Is High Blood Pressure?

In its description of high blood pressure, Johns Hopkins Medicine says: "Blood pressure is the force of the blood pushing against the artery walls. Each time the heart beats, it pumps blood into these arteries, resulting in the highest blood pressure when the heart contracts and pumps the blood."

High blood pressure can lead to stroke or heart disease. High blood pressure is twice as likely to strike a diabetic person than an individual without prediabetes or type 2 diabetes.

2 Numbers to Remember

There are 2 numbers involved in blood pressure:

- The number on the top is called systolic pressure. It measures the pressure inside the artery when the heart contracts and pumps the blood throughout the body.
- The bottom number, called diastolic pressure, measures the pressure inside the artery when the heart is resting and fills itself with blood.

Causes of Hypertension

Age: Due to the natural hardening of the arteries, known as arteriosclerosis, with age, a kidney or heart patient experiences an increased blood pressure flow. Two out of three people over the age of 75 suffer from hypertension.

Family History of Hypertension: One study showed that an individual with a family history of high blood pressure who doesn't exercise regularly would have a chance to have hypertension.

High Intake of Salt: According to the Institute of Medicine, now named the National Academy of Medicine, a diet high in salt content is the cause of approximately 20% to 40% of cases of hypertension (high blood pressure) in the United States.

Smoking: If you smoke, you'll increase your risk of suffering from high blood pressure.

Obese or Overweight: People who are obese or overweight occasionally have high blood pressure as they grow older and practice a sedentary lifestyle and an unhealthy diet.

Stress: Stress can be a big factor in developing hypertension. With emotional stress, you can put yourself at a higher risk of high blood pressure.

Sleep Apnea: It's a condition by which, if you have it, you'll wake up if your oxygen supply in the body decreases. That can put a strain on your heart and blood vessels causing elevated blood pressure.

Alcohol intake: If you drink alcohol, you may limit it or avoid it. Drinking can cause your blood pressure to rise.

Symptoms of High Blood Pressure

Persistent high blood pressure is bad for diabetes, kidney disease, and heart disease because it greatly impacts them. Controlling high blood pressure is a must for you and me.

Generally, there are no noticeable symptoms of high blood pressure unless it's exceptionally elevated, causing a person to experience the following:

- Blurry vision
- Dizziness
- Headache
- Nosebleed
- Face flushing
- Loss of balance
- Floaters in the eyes (small flecks of a protein called collagen), being part of vitreous, a gel-like substance in the back of your eye, brought about by eye problems

Treatments

According to the American Diabetes Association, there are several ways to prevent occurrences of high blood pressure, which include:

- Exercising regularly
- Reducing salt intake
- Engaging in stress-relieving activities
- Quitting smoking, if you smoke
- Avoiding excessive alcohol intake
- Monitoring your blood pressure regularly
- Getting to and staying at a healthy weight based on your age, height, and body mass index (BMI)

  To calculate your BMI, you may go to: https://www.nhlbi.nih.gov/health/educational/losewt/BMI/bmicalc.htm. Or google another BMI calculator.
- Consuming a healthy diet rich in grains, fruits, vegetables, and low-fat dairy products
- Losing at least 5% to 7% of your current body weight
- Cutting back on caffeine intake

The Silent Killer

High blood pressure is frequently called the "silent killer" in America; it happens without notice. High blood pressure and high cholesterol are bad for diabetes, kidney disease, and heart disease, increasing their progression.

What are the possible complications of high blood pressure? High blood pressure may cause the following:

Stroke: A stroke occurs when the brain cannot get an adequate blood supply due to a blood vessel blockage.

Heart Attack or Heart Damage: A person may have a heart attack because of high blood pressure. If not, the heart may be damaged by high blood pressure, including injury to coronary arteries. That will result in several other heart conditions.

Kidney Damage: High blood pressure may damage arteries in the kidneys. If damaged, the kidneys can't do their job of filtering toxins out of the bloodstream. If not treated, you may damage your kidneys.

Vision Loss: If you have high blood pressure, there will be a strain on the blood vessels of your eyes. Because of this, high blood pressure may lead to permanent problems in your vision.

Erectile Dysfunction (ED): High blood pressure can restrict the blood flow needed for an erection resulting in Erectile Dysfunction (ED).

High Blood Pressure Guidelines: Europe Vs. U.S.
Blood Pressure Goals in Patients with Hypertension According to Clinical Conditions

Category	ESC/ESH 2018	ACC/AHA 2017
Age ≥65 yrs	130 to <140/70 to 79 mm Hg	<130/<80 mm Hg
Diabetes	Close to 130 (or lower if tolerated/70 to 79 mm Hg	<130/<80 mm Hg
Coronary artery disease	Close to 130 (or lower if tolerated/70 to 79 mm Hg	<130/<80 mm Hg
Chronic kidney disease (eGFR <60 ml/min/1.73 m2)	130 to <140/70 to 79 mm Hg	<130/<80 mm Hg
Post-stroke	Close to 130 (or lower if tolerated/70 to 79 mm Hg	<130/<80 mm Hg

eGFR = estimated filtration rate; other abbreviations
ESC/ESH: European Society of Cardiology/European Society of Hypertension
ACC/AHA: American College of Cardiology/American Heart Association (Source: Journal of American College of Cardiology (JACC)

Does Not Getting Enough Sleep Increase Blood Pressure?

If you don't have enough sleep at night, two major reactions can occur, high blood pressure and high blood sugar. These can happen if you sleep only for 6 and below hours per day.

Why does it happen? If you have sleep deprivation, the hormone levels in your body can also become irregular, and there will be swings in hormone activities.

What Are Hormones?

Imbalance hormones, particularly cortisol, a stress hormone that keeps your body awake and increases blood pressure and blood sugar levels, may lead to heart attack or stroke risk factors.

The hormones act as chemical messengers in the body. They play an important role in regulating the body's many processes, systems, and functions.

Indeed, sleep affects many hormones in the body, including those connected to stress or hunger. The endocrine system, a network of organs and glands, releases hormones.

The body needs different hormones to function properly. Hormones include:

- Cortisol
- Growth
- Heart rate
- Body temperature
- Blood pressure
- Sleep-wake cycles
- Metabolism
- Hunger

Functions of Cortisol

Cortisol works with a certain part of your brain to control your mood, fear, and motivation. The adrenal glands are triangle-shaped organs at the top of your kidneys that produce cortisol.

Cortisol's functions include:

- Controlling sleep/wake cycle
- Regulating blood pressure
- Keeping inflammation in the body down
- Managing the body's use of carbohydrates, proteins, and fats
- Boosting energy for handling stress

Sleep: Hormone Regulator

"Getting enough sleep can help with hormone regulation," says Abhinav Singh, MD, the medical director of Indiana Sleep Center.

Additionally, Kristen Knutson, Ph D. says, "We think whatever is happening in the brain, in the body, is sort of helping to maintain a multitude of processes -- endocrine, metabolic, cardiovascular." Knutson is a sleep researcher at the University of Chicago.

Also, research has shown that sleep deprivation contributes to over-activation in the sympathetic nervous system triggering the so-called fight-or-flight response.

How Many Hours of Sleep Time Should You Have?

According to a 2016 report from the American Heart Association, 7 to 9 hours of sleep per night is enough. Additionally, the American Academy of Sleep Medicine recommends 7 or more hours per night for adults, whether you have heart disease or none.

A report from the National Sleep Foundation that did a two-year study on sleeping said that the researchers found out that:

- Older adults, 65+ years, need 7 to 8 hours of sleep
- Adults, 26 to 64 years: require 7 to 9 hours of sleep

XII. Medical Procedures

Balloon Angioplasty

The process involves opening narrowed arteries by a cardiologist doing the angioplasty, using a long, thin tube called a catheter with a small balloon on its tip. The purpose is to compress the plaque against the artery wall as the doctor continues the procedure. Next, the cardiologist inserts a mesh cage called a stent into the artery. The mesh forms a scaffolding around the balloon to open the blood vessel. With the stent in the artery, the blood vessel stays open for a short or long time.

Later, in restenosis, plaque can gradually clog the stent. Restenosis means that a section of the blocked artery opened up with angioplasty, and a stent has narrowed again.

That's why doctors put drug-coated stents in the blood vessel to help clear such blood vessels

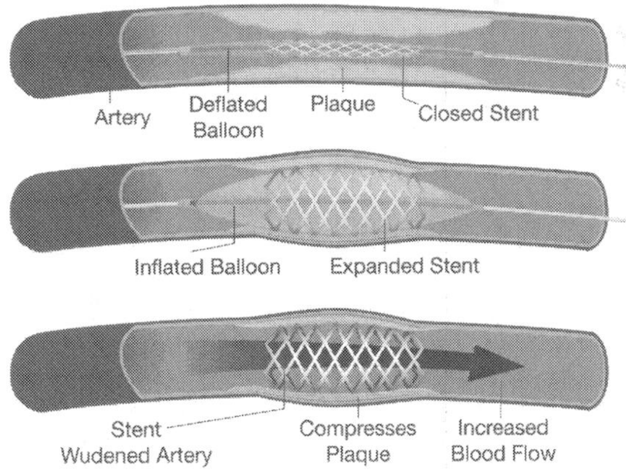

Another Procedure: Atherectomy

This cleaning procedure is done through a rotating shaver to remove plaque from the blocked artery.

Coronary Artery Bypass Graft Surgery (CABG) or Heart Bypass Graft Surgery

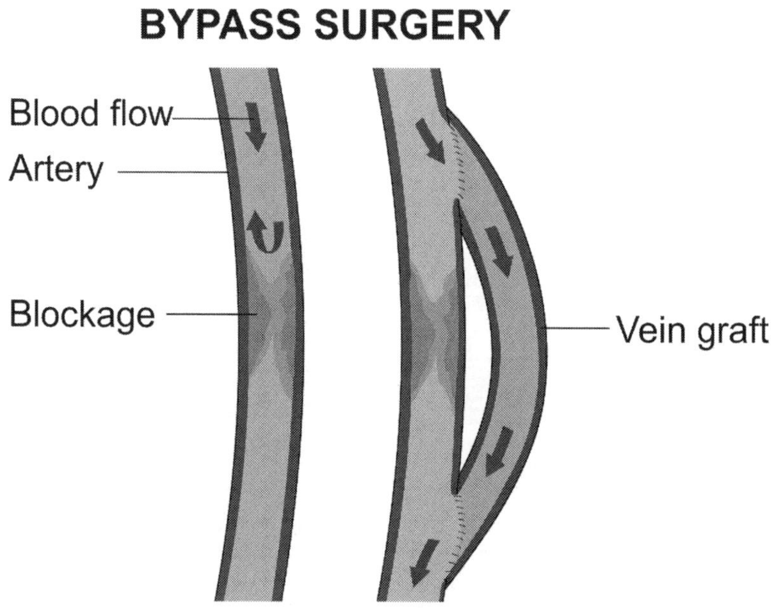

Bypass Surgery Procedure

Photo Credit: Shutterstock

What Is a Coronary Artery Bypass Graft Surgery?

Johns Hopkins Medicine describes coronary artery bypass graft surgery as "a procedure used to treat coronary artery disease."

If an artery or arteries become narrowed and blocked due to heart artery disease, the patient risks having a heart attack.

CABG surgery is an open heart surgery that requires opening the chest and repairing the heart's arteries. Depending on the operation, the incision will be about eight to ten inches long.

The surgery involves taking healthy blood veins depending on the number of blocked arteries from another or parts of the body.

Then the surgical team will use these blood vessels to bypass the blocked artery or arteries and graft them to the unblocked artery or arteries.

Doctors will stop the heart in bypass surgery, and the surgical team will connect you to a heart-lung machine or a bypass pump during the operation.

My Journey: Open-Heart Surgery

I had an open-heart CABG surgery in 2003, seven years after my first and only heart attack. It was quadruple bypass surgery. At the same time, the surgeon did the so-called Dor procedure on my heart,

Dor Procedure: Surgical Treatment of Ischemic Heart Failure

The Dor procedure, developed and practiced by Dr. Vincent Dor, MD, in the 1980s, is called left ventricular reconstructive surgery. In other words, besides doing the cardiac coronary surgery, the surgeon reshaped and rebuilt my heart to its normal size after slashing away the dead, scarred tissues.

In rebuilding my heart, seven years after my heart attack, the purpose of the operation was to avoid the occurrence of an aneurysm and return the left ventricle to a more normal shape. In doing the procedure on me, the heart became lighter and more efficient in pumping blood without the dead tissue, which can burden contraction.

What Is Left Ventricle Aneurysm?

A left ventricle aneurysm is a balloon-like bulge in a damaged blood vessel wall. There will be a big problem, and it will be deadly if the wall blood vessels burst due to too much stretching.

How Dor Procedure Treatment Process Works

During any procedure, the surgeon makes a small incision in the left ventricle and finds the scarred or dead tissue location. He has to place two or more rows of circular stitches around the dead tissue. The purpose is to separate the scarred muscle from the healthy ones.

There are times when the surgeon first removes the dead muscle before he pulls the stitches together. He places a patch if he thinks the stitches are not strong enough to exclude the area. Afterward, the surgeon reinforces the location with a row of stitches.

My Journey: Robotic-Like Pacemaker

With a reconditioned heart, now I have a robotic-like pacemaker device prolonging my life. A CRT-D (cardiac resynchronization therapy) device commands the left and right ventricles to contract simultaneously for pumping blood.

The CRT-D or any ICD, is a device placed under your he chest skin. It also contains a computer that tracks your heart rate and rhythm. The main difference is that if your heart beats way too fast or is very out of rhythm, the ICD sends out a shock to get it back into rhythm, CRT-D (defibrillator) commands itself to fire or strike to normalize irregular heartbeat or prevent a cardiac death.

In pumping blood, the right and left ventricles work this way: The right ventricle pumps the oxygen-poor blood to the lungs through the pulmonary valve. Then the left atrium receives the oxygenated blood or oxygen-rich blood from the lungs and pumps it to the left ventricle through the aortic valve.

So far, as I have said, my CRT-D (Defibrillator) has not fired itself yet, because it has not detected an irregular heartbeat or arrhythmia. A defibrillator, built in the pacemaker, restores an abnormal heartbeat by sending electric pulses or shocks to the heart for automatic actions: to prevent or correct an unusual heartbeat, called arrhythmia. Sometimes an arrhythmia is either a too slow or too fast heart rate.

XIII. Ejection Fraction

What Is Ejection Fraction?

According to the American Heart Association (AHA), "Ejection fraction (EF) is a measurement, expressed as a percentage, of how much blood the left ventricle pumps out with each contraction. An ejection fraction of 60 percent means that 60 percent of the total amount of blood in the left ventricle is pushed out with each heart-beat."

Ejection Fraction Tests

The tests for ejection fraction include the following tests:

- **Echocardiogram**: The most common test for measuring ejection fraction uses sound waves to produce images of your heart and the blood pumping through your heart. You can undergo an echocardiogram test once a year only.
- **Cardiac catheterization**: During this test, a thin plastic tube (catheter) is inserted into a blood vessel in your arm, leg, or arm and then carefully guided into your heart to take images. The images measure the ejection fraction.
- **Magnetic resonance imaging (MRI)**: This test uses a magnetic field and radio waves to produce cross-sectional photos of specific parts of your body.
- **Computerized tomography (CT)**: This test uses x-rays to take images of specific body parts.
- **Nuclear medicine scan**: In this test, the technician puts trace amounts of radioactive material and injects them into your blood-stream. The technician detects the radioactive material in your blood with special cameras as it goes through your lungs and heart.

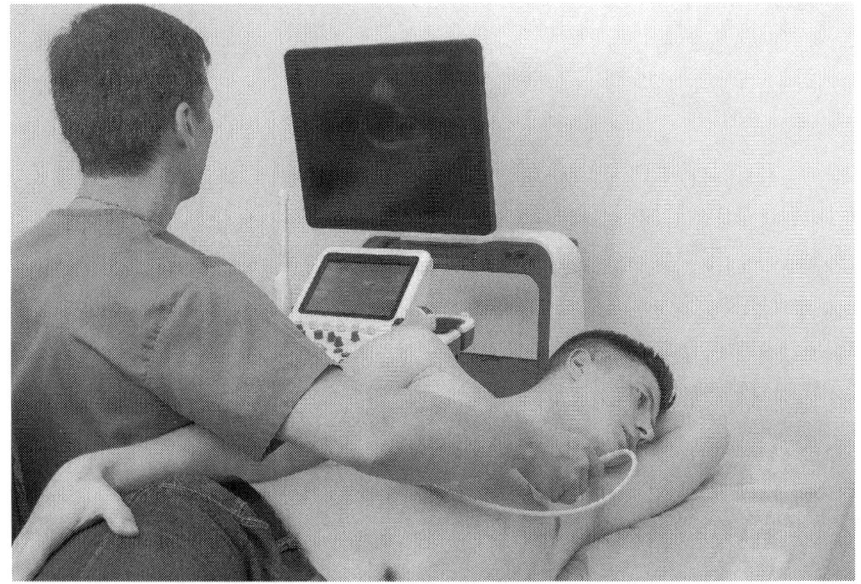

Echocardiogram Test: Determines Ejection Fraction

Photo Credit: Shutterstock

Types of Ejection Fraction

A healthy heart contracts, emptying blood and relaxes, refilling blood 60 to 80 times per minute. The heart pumps blood from the left and right ventricle in each heartbeat.

For example, an ejection fraction of 50% means the ventricle pumps out 50% of blood each heartbeat.

There are two types of ejection fraction, which are:

- **The left ventricular ejection fraction** measures how much blood gets pumped from the left ventricle with each contraction. In other words, the left ventricular ejection fraction (LVEF) is the central measure of left ventricular systolic function. Generally, ejection fraction refers to the left ventricle.

- **The right ventricular fraction** measures how much blood the right ventricle pumps out to the lungs. The right ventricular dysfunction is a strong, independent predictor of any arrhythmic events that may come.
- What Do Ejection Fraction Numbers Mean?
- 50% to 70%: Normal heart function
- 40% to 55%: Below normal heart function. It can indicate previous heart damage from a heart attack or cardiomyopathy.
- Higher than 75%: This can signify a heart condition like hypertrophic cardiomyopathy, a common cause of sudden cardiac arrest

Less than 40% – May confirm the diagnosis of heart failure.

My Journey: Medical Records

I have successfully maintained the stability of my heart disease into a better condition.

Blood tests results and reports of echocardiogram tests prove that I have reversed my heart failure severity from Class 3 (stage 3) to Class 1 (stage 1) and put it into a better shape. I can access any of my medical test results, laboratory tests, and medical procedure reports in my medical chart on my hospital's website.

Results of Lab Test

Below are the results of a 2D Ecjp (Transthoracic) W Doppler-Test done in my hospital, showing that I had only a 15% ejection fraction in 2016.

1. 2016: 2D ECHO (TRANSTHORACIC) W -DOPPLER - Details

An excerpt from the report says:

"Findings Left Ventricle: The left ventricular chamber size is severely enlarged. There is normal wall thickness. There is a severely decreased left ventricular ejection fraction. **The visually estimated ejection fraction is 15%."**

September 21, 2016 - 15%

Note: Ejection fraction of 15% in 2017 increased to 47% in 2020.

2. March 28, 2017: MYOCARDIAL PERFUSION IMAGING MULTIPLE STUDY SPECT W WALL MOTION AND EJECTION FACTOR - Details

Study Result

Excerpts from the study are as follows:

TR MYOCARDIAL PERFUSION IMAGING STUDY w/GATING with pharmacologic administration

"The gated images exhibit a markedly dilated LV chamber. There is hypokinesis-akinesis in the septal and anterior walls and apex. The average LVEF from 2 separate computer programs is **23% (ejection fraction.)"**

March 28, 2017 - 23%

ECHOCARDIOGRAM/DOPPLER REPORT

Patient Name: Veltisegar Bandisda Date of Service: 3/16/19
Ordering Physician: Date of Birth:
Daianoses/IN

Left Ventricular Dimension		Mitral Valve		Tricuspid Valve	
Diastole (3.5-5.7)	5.9	Peak Velocity (0.6-1.3/sec)		Peak Velocity (0.3-0.7m/sec)	
Systole (less than 4 cm)	4.2	Regurgitation		Regurgitation	
Septal wall (0.6-1.1 cm)	1.9	Pressure ½ time		RVSP	
Posterior wall (0.6-1.1 cm)	1.4	Mean Gradient			
%FS (>50%)		Mitral Valve Area			
EF (>50%)	30%				
Aortic Valve		**Aortic valve**		**Pulmonary Valve**	
Aortic Root (2.0-3.7 cm)	3.0	Peak Velocity (1-1.7m/sec)		Peak Velocity (0.6-0.9/sec)	
Cusp Separation (1.5-2.6 cm)	2.0	Regurgitation		Regurgitation	
		Peak Gradient			
LAD (1.9-4.0 cm)	5.3	Mean Gradient		RVD (0.7-2.6)	

3. Echocardiogram/Doppler report showing the ejection fraction of 30% (with arrow.)That was done in 2019.

ECHOCARDIOGRAM/DOPPLER REPORT

Patient Name: [illegible] Date of Service: 8.22.20
Ordering Physician: Date of Birth:
Diagnoses/In

Left Ventricular Dimension		Mitral Valve		Tricuspid Valve	
Diastole (3.5- 5.7)	6.3	Peak Velocity(0.6-1.3/sec)		Peak Velocity(0.3-0.7m/sec)	
Systole(less than 4cm)	5.07	Regurgitation		Regurgitation	mild
Septal wall(0.6-1.1cm)	1.0	Pressure 1/2 time		RVSP 31 mm Hg	
Posterior wall(0.6-1.1cm)	1.0	Mean Gradient			
%FS(>50%)	24%	Mitral Valve Area			
EF(>50%)	47%				
Aortic Valve		**Aortic Valve**		**Pulmonary Valve**	
Aortic Root(2.0-3.7cm)	3.85	Peak Velocity(1-1.7m/sec		Peak Velocity(0.6-0.9/sec)	
Cusp Separation(1.5-2.6cm)	1.68	Regutgitation	mild	Regurgitation	mild
		Peak Gradient			
LAD(1.9-4.0cm)	4.9	Mean Gradient		RVD(0.7-2.6)	
		A1 Pressure 1/2			
		Aortic Valve Area			

Summary and Interpretation:
1. Left Ventricle: dilated severe to moderate
2. Right Ventricle: – pacemaker
3. Left Atrium: – mod to sev. dilated

4. Echocardiogram/Doppler test results report on EF of 47%, 2020

Summary of My Ejection Fraction Numbers, leading to heart failure reversal

September 21, 2016 - 15%
March 28, 2017 - 23%
March 16, 2018 - 30%
August 22, 2020 - 47%
August 27, 2022 - 44% (see page 398, Chapter 23)
August 28, 2023 -43%

My regular cardiologist has told me that my heart failure condition falls under Class 1 (mild), based on the guidelines of the New York American Heart Association NYAHA), the most used guidelines by physicians in determining stages of heart failure in the U.S.

XIV. 7 Powerful Ways You Can Strengthen Your Heart

1. Adopting a Semi-Plant-Based Diet or a Flexible Semi-Plant-Based Diet

Eat more plant proteins than animal proteins. Plant proteins have no saturated fats compared to animal proteins that clog your arteries with plaques that may lead to heart attack or stroke. This diet is appropriate for diabetes, kidney disease, and heart disease.

Among the popular diets in the U.S. are the Mediterranean Diet, Flexitarian Diet, Ornish Diet, and the DASH Diet. For winners of Best Diets for 2022 for diabetes, heart disease, and other healthy diets, go to Chapter 11.

2. Exercising 3 to 7 Days a Week?

Government guidelines recommend aerobics exercises which are enough, particularly if you are an older adult. They may include walking, biking or stationary biking, swimming, stretching, tai chi (a Chinese exercise), etc. According to government guidelines, if you can't do it daily, you may do your exercise three to five times a week.

The Bautista Walking System

My walking system is different. My 20-minute three-walking sessions per day, every day, are ideal for diabetes, kidney disease, and heart disease. If you have diabetes, you may do moderate-intensity walking (or brisk walking) one hour after each meal of the day to reduce blood sugar and make your kidney and heart stronger.

If you can't do moderate-intensity walking, you may do the low-intensity walk due to your old age or disability. (See Chapter 9.)

3. Losing Some Weight

The CDC recommends that a person lose 5% to 10% of his or her body weight which is enough to decrease A1C.

The step should involve 150 minutes of exercise per week as per government guidelines. (I walk 420 minutes per week.) Weight loss can reduce the heart's work because the lighter you are, the easier it is for the heart to pump blood throughout your body.

4. Quitting Smoking

According to the CDC, chemicals in cigarette smoke can cause the blood to thicken and clog the veins and arteries of the body, especially the heart.

In other words, smoking can increase plaque formation in your blood vessel, which may result in you having coronary heart disease. If you have heart disease and still smoke, it will worsen your condition.

It's because nicotine can cause an increase in blood pressure, heart rate, and blood flow to the heart. It also can harden the arterial walls, leading to coronary artery disease or heart attack.

Did you know that you may suffer from a heart disease called alcoholic cardiomyopathy if you are a heavy drinker? Alcohol can weaken and thin heart muscle, affecting blood pumping throughout the body. If this happens, then you can have heart failure.

5. Having Enough Sleep

Go back to page 159 in this chapter.

6. Reducing Stress

Everybody gets stressed: in their jobs, in society, in love affairs, and at home about money, family relationships, and bad things happening throughout the world.

But you and I should minimize stress because it will ruin our lives, cause us diseases, deprive us of happy moments, and subject us to endless worries and problems.

When stressed, the body releases the hormone cortisol in response to anxiety and emotional tension.

Studies have shown that long-term worries increase blood sugar, cholesterol, triglycerides, and blood pressure. And you know what? Stress can affect you, making your blood stickier and raising the risk of stroke or heart attack.

You may take steps to reduce mental tension that may ruin you physically and mentally. You may do the following:

- Get plenty of exercises, especially moderate or low-intensity walking, depending on your physical condition or disability.
- Listen to music.
- Do yoga, tai chi (a Chinese form of exercise), or meditation.
- Travel and see exotic places and know different cultures and experience them.
- Limit or avoid listening to bad news because it can make you sad, anxious, nervous, hopeless, and depressed. Anyway, we can't control what's happening in the world!
- It would be best to disregard the bad things you and I have no control over. I always try to avoid listening to or watching news broadcasts.

7. Installation of a Medical Device

There are three medical devices that doctors can implant under the skin in your chest if needed. They are:

- Implantable Cardioverter Defibrillator (ICD)
- Cardiac Resynchronization Therapy Pacemaker (CRT-P)
- Cardiac Resynchronization Therapy Defibrillator (CRT-D)

XV. Medical Devices for People with Heart Disease

There are three basic kinds of pacemakers:

Single chamber: One lead attaches to the upper or lower heart chamber.

Dual-chamber: Uses two wires, one for the upper and the other for the lower chamber.

Biventricular pacemakers: Uses three leads or wires.

1. Implantable Cardioverter Defibrillator (ICD)

An ICD is a battery-powered device implanted under the skin of your chest to monitor your heart rate. The ICD system consists of the generator (typically referred to as the "ICD") and at least one lead (wire), usually a right ventricular defibrillation lead. Two small wires and thin leads connect the machine to the heart. If this device detects an abnormal heart rhythm, it delivers electric pulses or shocks to your heart to restore a normal heartbeat.

The machine can also prevent sudden death if you have a cardiac arrest. It normalizes the rapid and irregular heart rate when the heart's two upper chambers experience chaotic electrical signals.

2. Cardiac Resynchronization Therapy (CRT)

Doctors use two CRTs (cardiac resynchronization therapy) devices to treat the delay in heart ventricle contractions in some people with heart failure.

The two CRTs are the CRT-P (with a peacemaker) and the CRT-D with a pacemaker and a defibrillator. A defibrillator apparatus controls heart fibrillation by applying an electric current to the chest wall or heart. Each device has 2 or 3 leads (wires) placed in the right atrium, right ventricle, and left ventricle.

CRT-P: Like a normal pacemaker, a CRT-P, also called "biventricular pacemaker," is used to treat slow heart rhythms. It also delivers small electrical impulses or shocks to the left and right ventricles to aid them in contracting together simultaneously for more efficient blood pumping.

CRT-D: A CRT-D is a pacemaker with a built-in cardioverter defibrillator that can save heart failure patients from cardiac arrest death if it occurs.

A CRT (whether a CRT-P or CRT-D) has three wires connected to three heart parts.

If the device senses dangerously fast heart rhythms, it delivers a shock to the heart. Then the shock stops the abnormal heartbeat and prevents the patient from dying from cardiac arrest.

Surgeons program the CRT and implant the leads through a vein in the right atrium and right ventricle and into the coronary sinus vein of the left ventricle. The purpose is to synchronize the contraction of the right and left ventricles, meaning doing it simultaneously.

If you are eligible to get any of these three medical devices, you may ask your doctor about implanting one in your chest if you have heart disease or heart failure depending on your needs.

If you are in the early stage of your heart disease, including an irregular heartbeat, you may have the ICD or CRT-P, but if you already have heart failure, more so, with left bundle branch block (LBBB), then it's best to get the CRT-D), because this is one of the treatments for heart failure.

The devices, powered by a battery, are implanted under the skin in the chest, usually on the left side.

In a report, Johns Hopkins Medicine says that CRT therapy works in about 7 out 10 cases of heart failure.

When any machine detects an abnormal heart rhythm, the three devices can fire and send electrical shock (impulses) to the heart.

The CRT-D is ideal for heart failure because people with heart failure most often have the so-called left bundle branch block (LBBB).

The LBBB affects the heart's electrical conduction system. It may be partially or completely blocked. When this happens, the left ventricle contracts a little later than it should, in coordination with the action of the right ventricle as they pump blood. In simple words, they don't beat simultaneously, resulting in the lack of enough volume of blood throughout the body.

According to a study published by the National Institute of Health on its website, 30% of patients with heart failure have LBBB, and they are the ideal candidates for the implantation of a CRT-D or the CRT-P.

The researchers also found that LBBB occurred in 1/5 of HF patients requiring hospitalization and was associated with very high mortality.

Eligibility for ICD, CRT-P, or CRT-D

Among others, heart patients with a left ventricle ejection of <35% and below are the ideal candidates for implantation of CRT devices. Also, doctors allocate CRT devices for heart failure, particularly those with LBBB.

CRT is a treatment for people with so-called impaired cardiac pump function (left ventricular ejection fraction (<35%) and a wide QRS complex. Despite maximum tolerated medical therapy, these patients remain symptomatic of heart failure, meaning with symptoms.

However, despite improving CRT devices, 30% of patients implanted with these machines do not respond to this therapy.

Research shows that to optimize the CRT therapy, the patients should complement the machine with lifestyle changes and exercise to reap the benefits of having a CRT.

However, those with advanced heart failure may not likely respond to the CRT-D (defibrillator). Those who don't need the CRT-D can get the CRT-P, a CRT device with a peacemaker without a defibrillator).

However, those with advanced heart failure may not likely respond to the CRT-D (defibrillator). Those who don't need the CRT-D can get the CRT-P, a CRT device with a peacemaker without a defibrillator).

Requirements for Installation of CRT Machines

Patients who can be eligible for getting the ICD or CRT devices must have the following:

- You have moderate to severe heart failure, with an ejection fraction of <35% and below.
- Tests show that your heart is enlarged and weak.
- The left and right ventricles don't contract simultaneously; the left ventricle is always late in contraction.
- Medicines and lifestyle changes, including exercise, are not improving the heart condition.

3. Left Ventricular Assist Devices

A left ventricular assist device (LVAD) is a mechanical pump implanted in severe heart failure patients.

Also known as a mechanical circulatory support device, an LVAD helps the left bottom chamber of your heart (left ventricle) pump blood out of the ventricle to the aorta through the so-called aortic valve and the rest of the body.

The aorta is the largest artery in the body. It begins at the top of the left ventricle, the heart's main pumping chamber.

Candidates for LVAD Implantations

- Heart failure patients who are waiting for a heart transplant
- Patients who are not candidates for a heart transplant but may want long-term treatment for heart failure

My Journey: ICD Pacemaker

In 2011, when I suffered from episodes of an irregular heartbeat, doctors implanted an ICD (implantable cardioverter device). It was a regular single-chamber (only one lead or wire) device with a defibrillator in my left chest.

In 2018, my old ICD ran out of battery after seven years of being my guard and friend. It was always on guard to protect me from any cardiac event. So a cardiologist-physiologist implanted a CRT-D into my left chest under the skin instead of the ordinary ICD. The purpose of the implant was to enable my left and right ventricles to contract simultaneously.

My CRT-D Biventricular Pacemaker

A CRT-P or CRT-D is an ideal machine for heart failure patients, especially those with left bundle branch block (LBBB). An LBBB is a problem with the heart's electrical wiring (conduction) system. I have this condition.

My Journey: That Was Then; This Is Now!

Now I have a robotic-like pacemaker device to protect and prolong my life with a reconditioned heart. A CRT-D (cardiac resynchronization therapy) device can send signals to the left and right ventricles to contract simultaneously for pumping blood. The device is also called a biventricular pacemaker.

The CRT-D or any ICD (an implantable cardioverter device with a pacemaker) can fire or strike with electrical impulses to normalize irregular heartbeat or prevent a cardiac arrest death. So far, the CRT-D has not taken any action yet; no arrhythmias.

Chapter 9

Walking System: Why It Works for Diabetes, Kidney Disease, and Heart Disease

Brief Subject Summary

- What Does Moderate-Intensity Walking to Brisk Walking Mean?
- Timing, Speed, and Duration of Exercise
- Measuring Physical Activity Intensity
- Blood Glucose Levels Peak within 70 to 90 Minutes After Meal
- Walking Techniques
- How Does Exercise Affect Your Digestion
- How Does Walking Affect Heart Rate
- Target Heart Rate
- What Does Walking Do to Reduce Blood Sugar
- Don't Have Time to Exercise?

Have you struggled with lowering your blood sugar to treat your diabetes and jump-starting your weak heart to make it stronger? No problem.

Here's my proven strategy: Low-intensity to moderate-intensity walking to brisk walking at the right time, speed, and duration, one hour after each meal every day can lower your blood sugar (glucose) by 30-60 points or 30 mg/dl to 60 mg/dl in just a 20-minute exercise session without taking any medications.

Not only that. You can achieve 64 to 76% of your estimated maximum heart rate. Also, exercise can make your kidney disease healthy. Also, exercise can make your kidney disease healthy. Moderate-intensity walking to brisk walking works!

How do I know this system is effective? Because I have done it, I am still doing it and will continue doing it. I'm confident that it may work for you, too!

What Does Moderate-Intensity Walking to Brisk Walking Mean?

Well, it all depends on your age and physical fitness. Yes, for me, moderate-intensity walking is the best speed to reduce blood glucose.

According to the Center for Disease Control and Prevention (CDC), moderate-intensity walking ranges from miles to 3.5 miles per hour (mph), while a brisk walk is 3.5 to 4 miles.

You can elevate your heart rate during walking and also burn more calories than walking at your usual pace. Moderate-intensity walk, which checks in at 3 to 3.5 or more miles in an hour.

In a way, it's because the pace may depend on the rate of your metabolism acts to let the muscles get blood glucose from the blood stream.

An older adults, like me, 90, with type 2 diabetes, kidney disease, may choose to a moderate-intensity walking of 3 to 3.5 miles per hour, as recommended. I do this very day, covering a distance of 3.3 to 3.5 miles in hour hour.

Yes, I walk outdoor at moderate-intensity speed on the flat surface or paved roads. And I walk on the treadmill a little faster than the speed of 3.3 to 3.5 miles per hour outside.

Why? It's much easier to talk on the treadmill because the rolling belt is somewhat pushing you forward, remaining at the same position because you're not going forward. I usually have extra walking to and from the mall or elsewhere.

Timing, Speed, and Duration: How fast should be walking pace decrease blood sugar? For instance, how long should be the walking be, or at what time should you walk after each meal? Different studies showed mixed results. For example, you should walk for 10, 15 or 20 minutes per walking session.

Maybe the duration of walking should depend on your ability to walk. For instance, which speed are you comfortable with? And how far can you do a 15-minute to 20-minute walk without rest or stop?

If you're still not so old yet (or even old, depending on your physical fitness), maybe you cn do moderate-intensity walking of the required 3 to 3.5 miles per hour.

I'm a living testimony tht an older adult, (actually I'm an oldest old), I still walk from 3 to 4 miles per hour, in three 20-minute session.

Measuring Physical Activity Intensity: According to the CDC, the easiest way to measure any physical activity is by knowing intensity and how walking, for instance, affects heart rate and breathing.

The CDC says, "The talk test is a simple way to measure relative intensity. In general, if you're doing moderate-intensity walk, you can talk but not sing during the activity."

Slow Walkers: Does Low-intensity Walking Work?

If you're an older adult, you may do low-intensity walking instead of moderate-intensity exercise. Or you may stroll if that's the only way you can do it. Remember, it is also an effective way to lower blood sugar, if you have diabetes.

Does slow-walk work? According to a study in 2018 published only by the U.S. National Institute of Health on its website, yes, it works.

Yes, it's never too late to reap the benefits of walking or any activity, whether you're 50, 75 or 90.

Low-Intensity Walking

What is the walking pace of slow walkers? The walking speed should depend on your physical condition, age, and body build, especially the elderly.

While 3 miles per hour (mph) which is the minimum walking speed for a moderate-intensity walking, your pace may fall under 3 miles mph, if you're an older adult with a disability.

Moderate-Intensity Walking or Brisk Walking

Usually, moderate-intensity walking is at least 100 meters per minute.

If you're doing moderate intensity-walking, you should be able to cover a minutes 3 mph to 4 mph to follow the government's guidelines.

Vigorous-Intensity or High-Intensity Walking or Any Activity

As a rule, if you're doing a vigorous-intensity or high-intensity waking or any activity, you may not be able to say more then a few words without pausing for a breathe. Your speed will be from 4.6 mph to 5 mph and over.

Samples of vigorous-intensity activities:

- Hiking uphill or with a heavy backpack
- Swimming laps
- Heavy gardening (digging or hoeing)
- Race walking, jogging, or running
- Aerobic dancing

My Journey

I do my moderate-intensity walking in three 20-minute moderate-intensity walking sessions each day, one hour after each meal from Monday to Sunday, including holidays; I cover 3 to 4 miles of walking to lower levels of my blood sugar, blood pressure, creatinine, and BUN, and increase my heart rate to strengthen the heart muscles and make my human machine stronger.

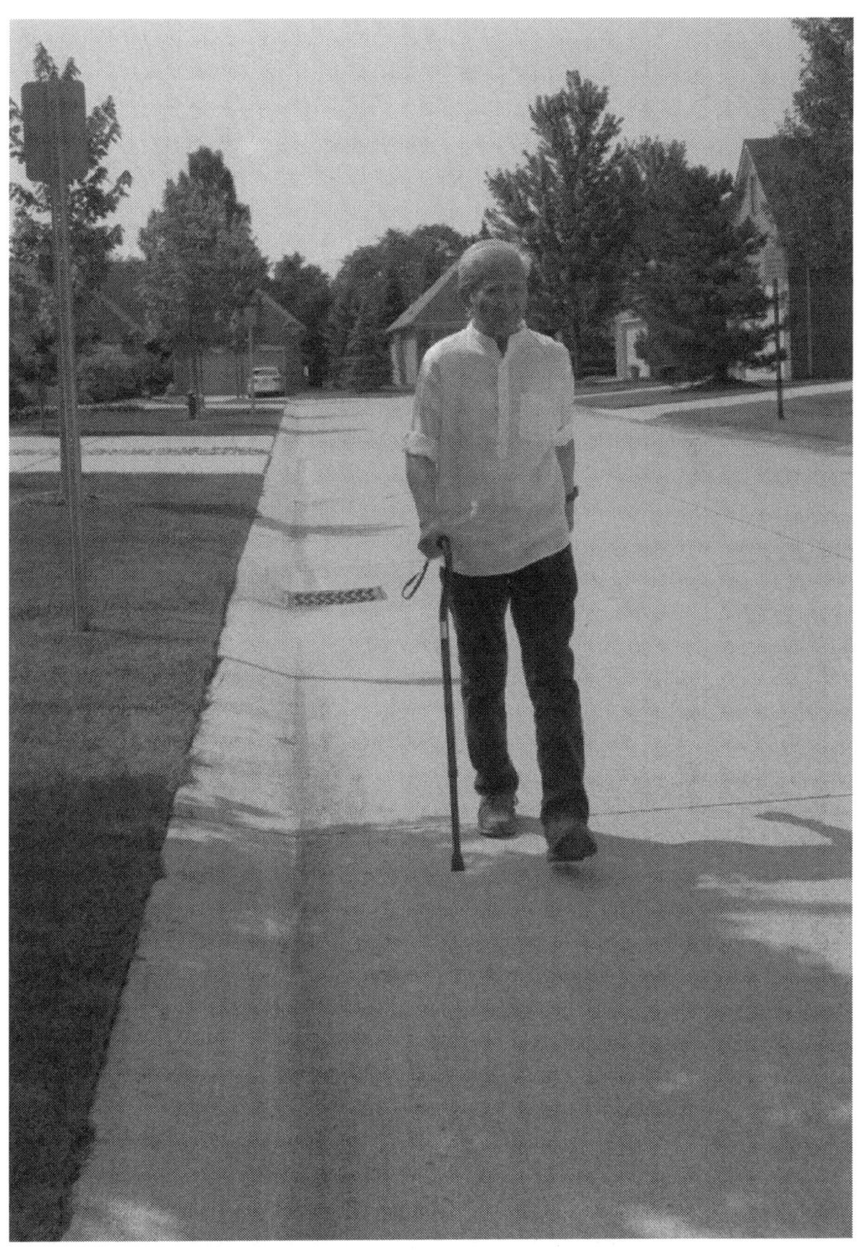

Author Does Moderate-Intensity Walking

What Does Walking Do to the Body?

When you do moderate-intensity exercise (3 to 3.5 mph), your heart beat maybe faster, and your breathing may be a little harder.

Then the muscle use4 more glucose, taking in the sugar from your blood stream. Of course, this can reduce the glucose, making the insulin in your body work better.

"The muscles we use to walk use glucose as energy, drawing it out of circulation," says Andrew Reynolds, a postdoctoral research fellow at the University of Otago in New Zealand.

"Italians have been walking after meals for centuries, so it must be good," says Loretta DiPietro, a professor of exercise science at George Washington University's Milken Institute School of Public Health."

Meanwhile, here's another comment: "Exercising is the most underused treatment, and it's so powerful," says Sharon Movsas, RD, a diabetes nutrition specialist at the Clinical Diabetes Center at Montefiore Medical Center in New York City.

On the other hand, Sheri Colberg-Ochs, diabetes and exercise research at Old Dominion University in Virginia, explains, "Exercise stimulates peristalsis, which is the process of moving digested food through the GI tract."

Colberg-Ochs also says glucose tends to peak 90 minutes after a meal.

Warning: Exercising Outdoor

When you go outside to do your walking, be sure that the weather temperature is not more than 80°F.

When the temperature is 81°F or more, the arteries and veins will dilate and stress. Yes, high temperature causes them to expand and allows opre to flow into the legs.

If this happens, you'll have pain in your legs, resulting in your being tired. Due to the damaged veins, fluids may leak out to your tissues an stay there, causing edema or swelling

This can happen to you, if you have the so-called chronic venous disease (CVD), which is the result of poor blood circulation in your veins.

In the United Sates, weathermen use the Fahrenheit scale in measuring temperatures. On the other hand, most countries that use the metric system use the Celsius scale to measure temperature.

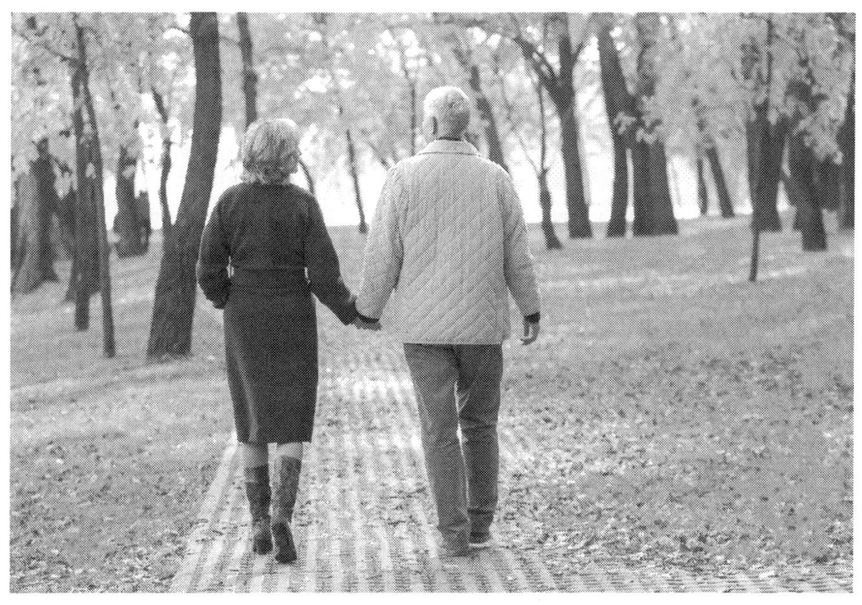

A Couple Walking Outdoor

Photo Source: Shutterstock

I. Walking Outside

Can Walking Immediately After Meal Delay Digestion?

In a 2017 study, researchers discovered that walking 30-40 minutes after meals delayed food digestion.

Here's why: There's some evidence that forms of exercise of meals for a while. It's because exercising muscles pull more blood flow during any activity. As a result, the GI tract gets less blood flow. In that way, it slows down the digestion of food in the stomach.

When you walk abruptly after a meal, for instance, within 30 minutes, the body redirects the blood flow from the internal organs to the hands and legs' large working muscles to provide the necessary energy for muscle contraction.

Thus, there will be a delay in food digestion in the gut. hat will mean a temporary pause in food processing in the stomach. But in the end, more glucose enters the cells of the body.

Watch Out!

Don't do downhill running! Pretty sure, your levels of creatine kinase (CK) or phosphocreatine kinase (PCK) may be raised, resulting in burdening the kidneys. Thus, your GFR number will decrease. (See Creatine Kinase, Chapter 7.)

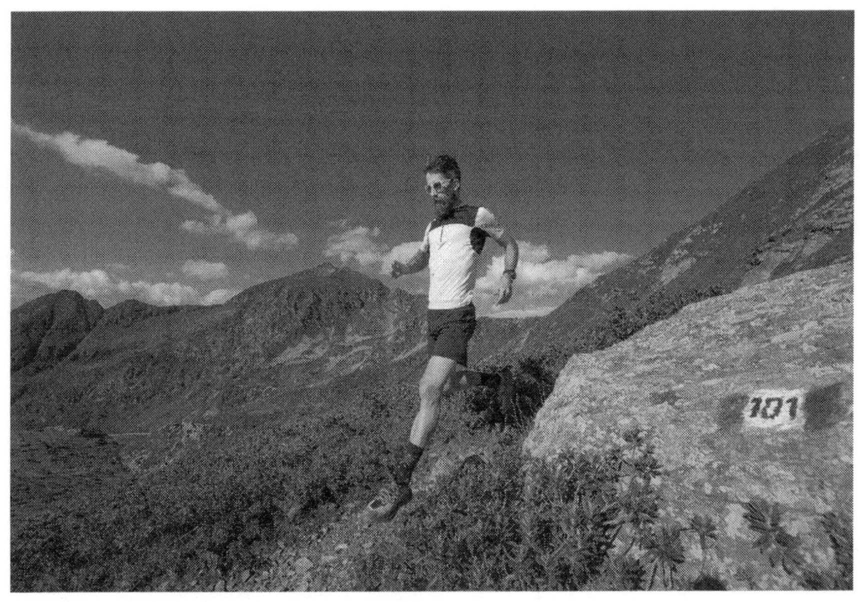

Running Downhill Elevates Creatine Kinase Levels

Photo Source: Shutterstock

Should Older Adults Walk with a Cane?

In the beginning, I could do moderate-intensity walking without a cane. But now I walk outside with a cane. It serves as good support. The cane on my right hand helps my body move forward. I also found out that with "three" feet, I'm steadier in my balancing as I walk.

For an older adult or even younger adult, a cane or stick can be a useful aid in walking. It helps you move your body forward, as your two feet do. Usually, I walk outside when the weather condition allows it. If it's too cold or hot, or when it's raining, I use my treadmill. I have a choice of indoor or outdoor walks. What a way to exercise!

My Journey: Minimum Speed Outside

Although I am 88, turning 89 this year, and have heart disease, my minimum speed in outdoor walking is 3.3 or more mph, and my maximum speed is 3.5 mph to 4 mph.

I walk faster on the treadmill, with less effort, covering a distance of 3.4 to 3.6 miles or more in one hour per day. So for a 20-minute exercise per session, I usually walk about 1.1 miles for that particular length of time per walking session.

When I walk outside, with an iWatch (pedometer) on my left hand and the right hand holding my cane, I do my exercise with both hands, swinging forward and backward, alternately, to give force to move my body forward.

In other words, I walk more than one mile in 20 minutes (three times a day), making an average of 7,000 to 8,500 steps per day.

Government Guidelines

Government guidelines stipulate that you should exercise for 150 minutes every week to be healthy. That is, 3 to 5 days of daily exercise. I do it differently: I walk for 420 minutes per week (60 minutes of three 20-minute walking sessions per day x 7 = 420 minutes.)

Walk, Walk, Don't Jog or Run!

S. Johnson, an award-winning blogger in a 2015 blog, reports that he learned that activity lowers blood sugar - but not always. He says, "Personally, I experienced this very early on and was extremely irritated! I just learned that exercise lowers blood sugar, but an intense 45-minute run consistently resulted in higher blood sugars than when I started! What in the world?"

And later, he learned the reason why.

I had that experience, too. After walking on the treadmill several years ago, I was surprised when I knew that my blood sugar had risen after the activity, much higher blood glucose before exercising. "It could not be that high!" I told myself.

Walking Pace: Why Did My Blood Sugar Increase?

What happened to my walking pace? And why did I increase my blood sugar? Instead of decreasing it?

Well, I didn't notice it: Instead of doing moderate-intensity walking on the treadmill, I unknowingly turned it into a vigorous-intensity exercise!

I learned these things after I did thorough research on the matter. My research has shown that:

- Exercise triggers the body to release stress hormones like adrenaline and cortisol.
- The adrenaline then stimulates the liver and the adrenal glands to release glucose and cortisol.
- The glucose and cortisol then make you more resistant to insulin.
- Any vigorous or strenuous activity triggers more stress hormones, increasing blood glucose (at least temporarily) in your bloodstream.

In other words, certain vigorous high-intensity exercises, like weight lifting, jogging, or running, can cause high blood sugar.

Why? Because there will be a burst of energy that will activate the body's response, causing a release of glucagon to power the muscles.

Generally, walking can effectively lower blood glucose from low-intensity to moderate-intensity walking. Increasing your heart rate is beneficial to the heart and will strengthen its pumping power.

Target Heart Rate and Estimated Maximum Heart Rate

According to the American Heart Association, you should achieve 50% to 85% of your estimated maximum heart rate during a moderate-intensity walk. (I'm getting 64% to 76% of my maximum heart rate.)

On the other hand, the U.S. Centers for Disease Control and Prevention (CDC) says a walker should set a target heart rate and estimated maximum heart rate.

The heart rate determines if your physical activity is within the target pulse or heart rate and the walking target zone.

Moderate-Intensity Physical Activity

CDC says our target heart rate should be between 64% and 76% of your estimated maximum heart rate. You can calculate your maximum heart rate based on your age.

To determine the maximum age-related heart rate, you may subtract your age from 220 (the standard number used). For instance, if you're 60 years old, calculate your estimated maximum age-related heart rate with this formula: 220 minus 60 years = 160 beats per minute (bpm). So 160 bpm is your estimated maximum heart rate. The 64% and 76% levels would be:

- 64% level: 160 x 0.64 = 102.4 bpm, and
- 76% level: 160 x 0.76 = 121.6 bpm

Thus, moderate-intensity physical activity for a 60-year older person should have a heart rate between 102.4 and 121.6 bpm during the walking.

My Moderate-Intensity Walk

I calculated my physical activity based on the following figures: 220 - 88 (my age) = 132 beats per minute (bpm), estimated maximum target.

The 64% and 76% levels would be:

- 64% level: 132 x 0.64 = 84 bpm (or 84.48 bpm)
- 76% level: 132 x 0.76 = 100 bpm (or 100.32 bpm)

Target Heart Rate

So it appears that my target heart rate should be from 84 bpm to 100 bpm. Walking outside or on the treadmill, I'm achieving the 64% to 76% of my estimated maximum heart rate of 132 bpm.

My average heartbeat while doing moderate-intensity walking ranges from 87 bpm to 93 bpm, numbers between my target heart rate of 84 to 100 bpm. That indicates that I'm achieving my target heart rate. On one occasion, I was able to have a heartbeat of 101 bpm.

My oxygen saturation is always 98% to 99% (mostly 99%), whether my body is at rest or in motion. Not bad for an older adult.

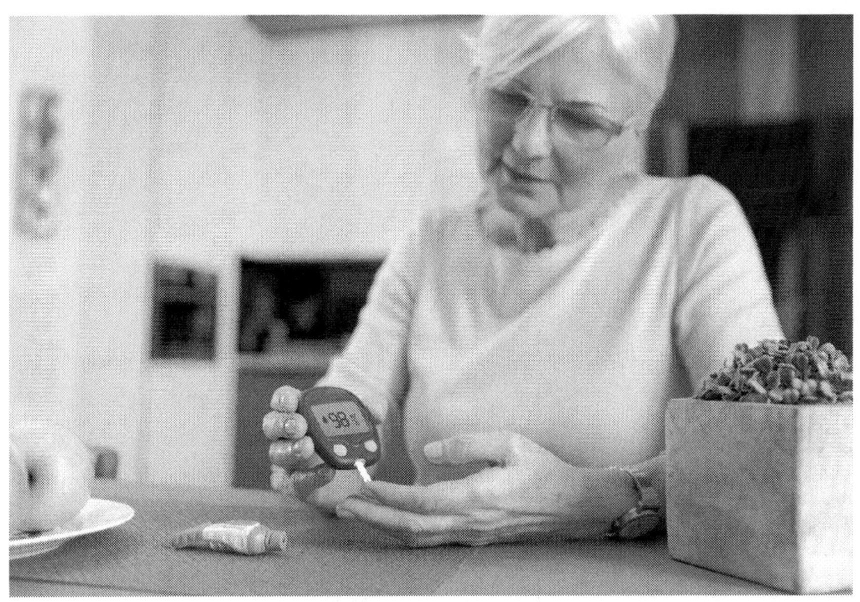

Blood Sugar Tests: Before and After Walking

Photo Credit: Shutterstock

Simple Formula

Just use a simple formula: Blood sugar number "before" the walk minus the number of the blood sugar "after" the exercise.

For example:

150 mg/dl blood sugar (one hour after a meal before exercise) minus 105 mg/dl (after exercise blood sugar) = 45 points decrease or 45mg/dl decrease.

Here are the actual numbers I got from my record book of blood sugar test results:

Walking duration: 20 minutes

Blood sugar before walking: 143
Blood sugar after walking: 105
143 - 105= 38 points decrease or 38 mg/dl decrease

Walking duration: 20 minutes

Blood sugar before walking: 138 mg/dl
Blood sugar after walking: 78 mg/dl
138 - 78 = 60 points decrease or 60 mg/dl decrease

Walking duration: 20 minutes

Blood sugar before walking: 132 mg/dl
Blood sugar after walking: 95 mg/dl
132 - 95 = 37 points decrease or 37 mg/dl decrease

Walking duration: 20 minutes

Blood sugar after a meal before walking: 119 mg/dl
Blood sugar after walking: 87 mg/dl
119 - 87 = 32 points decrease or 32 mg/dl decrease

Walking duration: 20 minutes

Blood sugar after a meal before walking: 155 mg/dl
Blood sugar after walking: 105 mg/dl
155 – 105 = 50 points decrease or 50 mg/dl decrease

Walking duration: 20 minutes

Blood sugar after a meal before walking: 157 mg/dl
Blood sugar after walking: 89 mg/dl
157 – 89 = 68 points decrease or 68 mg/dl decrease

People's Average Walking Speed By Age

Age	Sex	Meters/second	Miles/hour
20 to 29	Male	1.36	3.04
	Female	1.34	3.0
30 to 39	Male	1.43	3.2
	Female	1.34	3.0
40 to 49	Male	1.43	3.2
	Female	1.39	3.11
50 to 59	Male	1.43	3.2
	Female	1.31	2.93
60 to 69	Male	1.34	3.0
	Female	1.24	2.77
70 to 79	Male	1.26	2.82
	Female	1.13	2.53
80 to 89	Male	0.97	2.17
	Female	0.94	2.10

Source: *Healthline*

II. Treadmill Walking

Walking on the treadmill does not require maintaining your body mass forward momentum, like real walking outdoors. As a result, you can walk faster and cover more distance with the same effort on the treadmill than walking on a flat or rough road outside.

Why?

Because the machine is doing part of the work for you, bringing the road to you inside. It forces your legs and body to move forward, although you are in the same position.

Walking on the treadmill makes it easier because the rolling belt helps me push forward, although I stay in the same spot. I set the machine at a certain speed and walk, with my left hand with my I-Watch, hanging and swinging back and forth.

On the other hand, my right hand holds the treadmill's handrail.

Holding the Handrail or Console

If you're an older adult, you may think of your safety and stability while walking on the treadmill or the ground outside.

In that case, you may hold the treadmill handrail with one hand to protect yourself from any possible falls while balancing your body as you walk.

You can use the right or left handrail if you have a balance issue or a significant disability, with an i-Watch or pedometer on the other hand to count the steps or distance you're trying to achieve.

As an elderly, I hold on to the right handrails with my right hand while I swing my left arm with an iWatch on it, serving as my pedometer as my body moves. The iPhone records my steps and miles walked.

Chapter 10

6 Nutrients That Make You Alive

Brief Subject Summary

- Categories of Nutrients: Macronutrients and Micronutrients
- Carbohydrates
- Proteins
- Fats
- Vitamins
- Minerals
- Water
- Types and Forms of carbohydrates
- Two Types of Sugars
- Government Guidelines on Fiber Intake Daily
- Amino Acids: The Building Blocks of Protein
- Classifications of Amino Acids
- Types of Proteins
- Different Types of Fats
- Different Types of Vitamins
- What Are Minerals?
- Is Water a Macronutrient?

Nutrients are substances obtained from food that provide nourishment and energy for daily activities. They are essential for growth, the repair of muscles and tissues, and good health.

There are six major types of nutrients that your body needs:

- Carbohydrates
- Proteins
- Fats
- Vitamins
- Minerals
- Water

The World Health Organization (WHO) divides the nutrients into two categories:

1. Macronutrients: They consist of carbohydrates, proteins, and fats to provide energy in the form of calories for maintenance of growth, body functions, and daily activities. As the name "macro" implies big, macronutrients are consumed in large amounts. They are measured in calories per gram.

2. Micronutrients: They comprise vitamins and minerals essential in the production of enzymes, hormones, and other substances critical for growth and development. Deficiencies in them can cause serious or even life-threatening consequences. As the name "micro" implies small, micronutrients are consumed in small quantities.

They are measured in milligram, a thousandth of a gram, and a microgram, a millionth of a gram. One thousand micrograms are equal to 1 milligram.

I. Carbohydrates (Macronutrients)

What Are Carbohydrates?

Carbohydrates, or carbs, are molecules that have carbon, hydrogen, and oxygen atoms.

In nutrition, the word “carbs” refers to one of the three macronutrients. The other two are proteins and fats.

Carbohydrates, along with proteins and fats, are an essential macronutrients that provide nutrition and energy to the body by converting the carbs into glucose during the process of digestion. The bloodstream absorbs and uses it as a primary source of energy for the body. At the chemical level, they contain carbon, hydrogen, and oxygen.

Carbohydrates are comprised of the simple form of sugars with one (monosaccharide) and two (disaccharide) sugar molecules and the complex forms, which are starches and fibers. In caloric intake, there are calories per gram in carbohydrates.

Forms of Carbohydrates

The forms of carbohydrates are classified into two groups: simple carbohydrates and complex carbohydrates.

Simple carbohydrates

They are simple structures that contain one or two sugar molecules linked together.

Simple carbohydrates are broken down and absorbed by the body quickly for use as energy because they comprise shorter sugar chains. They are found in various natural food sources such as milk, fruits, and vegetables.

Simply put, simple sugars are made up of shorter chains of molecules and are quicker to digest than complex carbohydrates. For this reason, you'll have immediate spikes of sugar after you eat a meal.

Examples of simple carbs are white rice, bread, honey, syrups, and sugary drinks.

As a general rule, if you have prediabetes, type 2 diabetes, or type 1 diabetes, you should limit or avoid simple carbohydrates such as white rice, white bread, and white pasta to prevent an upsurge of blood sugar after a meal. People should avoid overly processed products that contain white flour and foods with added sugar.

Complex Carbohydrates

Complex carbohydrates, composed of fibers and starches, support the immune system, nervous system, digestive function, brain function, and the body's energy for performing tasks.

Dietitians and nutritionists recommend complex carbohydrates for a healthy body.

Carbohydrate Intake Requirements or Restrictions for Diabetics

How many grams of carbohydrates should you eat if you have prediabetes, type 2 diabetes, or type 1 diabetes? There is no "one size fits all" Why? Because different bodies react differently to carb requirements.

On average, CDC says people with diabetes should get about 45% of their calories from carbohydrates. A carbohydrate serving is about 15 grams. But, of course, if you want a low-carbohydrate diet, you can reduce the amounts of carbohydrates in your diet, depending on your diabetic condition.

ADA Recommendation

The American Diabetes Association (ADA) recommends that people with diabetes consume carbohydrates derived primarily from fresh fruits, vegetables, legumes, and whole grains.

For type 1 diabetics, the ADA suggests that a flexible approach to carbohydrate intake be matched with intensive insulin therapy, as published on the U.S. National Institute of Health website.

Low Carbohydrate Diet

Requirements for a very low-carbohydrate diet, a low-carbohydrate diet, and a moderate-carbohydrate diet:

- A very low-carbohydrate diet consisting of only 30 grams or less per day (which is hard to accomplish because carbs are the primary energy source)
- A low-carbohydrate diet with 130 grams or fewer daily
- A moderate-carbohydrate diet with carbs between 130 and 225 grams each day

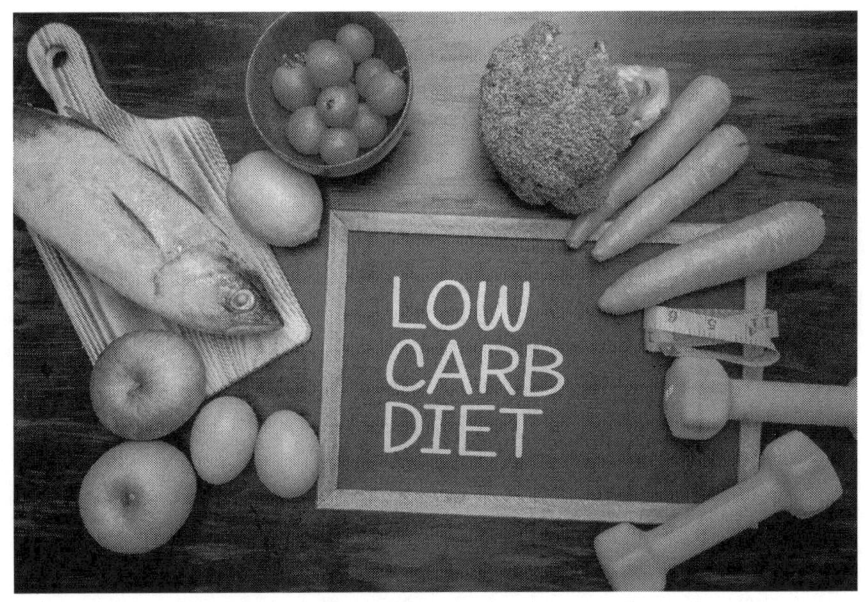

Low Carb Diet

Photo Credit: Shuterstock

3 Main Categories of Dietary Carbohydrates

Dietary carbohydrates have three main categories. They are:

Sugars: These are sweet, short-chain carbohydrates found in foods. Examples are glucose, fructose, galactose, and sucrose.

1. Sugars

Sugars are a class of carbohydrates that taste sweet, which the body converts to glucose, the energy source of cells in the body.

Sugars are categorized into single sugars and double sugars. Single sugars, called monosaccharides, include glucose, fructose, and galactose.

Meanwhile, double sugars, called disaccharides, include sucrose (table sugar), lactose, and maltose.

Monosaccharides

Glucose: A monosaccharide, glucose is the primary source of energy for the body, the end product after carbohydrate consumption and the main circulating sugar in the bloodstream.

Fructose: A monosaccharide, fructose is found in fruits, sugar cane, honey, and vegetables. It is often used as a preservative in food and can be converted to glucose.

Galactose: A monosaccharide, galactose is found in dairy products, fruits, sugar beets, and mucilages. Mucilages are thick, gluey substances produced by nearly all plants and some microorganisms. Galactose is combined with glucose to form lactose. Once consumed, it converts to glucose.

Disaccharides

Sucrose: Commonly known as table sugar, sucrose is a disaccharide found in sugar cane and sugar beets. Manufacturers use it as a sweetener in the manufacture of syrups and confections as well. Upon consumption, it is converted to glucose and fructose.

Lactose: A disaccharide, lactose is found in milk and milk products, food for infants and convalescents, and pharmaceutical preparations. When digested, it converts to glucose and galactose.

Maltose: A disaccharide, maltose is found in germinating grains and other plants and vegetables. It results from the breakdown of starch and composed of two glucose units.

To further explain them:

Monosaccharides (meaning single sugar)

- Fructose: fruit sugar
- Glucose: the body's blood sugar
- Galactose: part of milk sugar

Dissaccharides (meaning double sugars)

- Sucrose: fructose plus glucose = table sugar
- Lactose: galactose plus glucose = milk sugar
- Maltose: glucose plus glucose = malt sugar

Two Classifications of Sugars: Natural Sugar and Added Sugar

There are two types of sugar in human diets which are:

- Natural sugars which are found in foods such as fructose in fruits and vegetables, and lactose in milk
- Added sugars which include any sugars or caloric sweeteners added to foods or beverages during food processing, cooking, or eating, such as honey, corn syrup, white sugar, and brown sugar

After being eaten, digested, and broken down into glucose, these sugars serve as energy for red blood cells, the brain, and the central nervous system.

Sugar is added to foods to enhance their taste and prolong their shelf life.

Added Sugar When Consumed in Excess

If you eat too much sugar, it can harm your body, causing you some diseases or conditions such as the following:

- Obesity
- Diabetes
- Cardiovascular disease
- Non-alcoholic liver disease (NALD)
- Cognitive decline
- Some cancers

How Much Added Sugar Is Enough?

In its most recent dietary guidelines, the Food and Drug Administration (FDA) recommends that added sugars make up no more than 10 percent of your daily calories.

Maxine Yeung, MS, RD, CPT, and founder of The Wellness Whisk, says that as a general rule, a person eating 2,000 calories daily should consume no more than 50 grams of added sugar per day.

2. Added Sugar Recommendations

As a general rule, following this theory, your sugar intake for a different number of calories every day (if you have no major diseases yet, such as diabetes) should be as follows:

- 1,200 calories: 30 grams of added sugar
- 1,500 calories: 37 grams of added sugar
- 1,800 calories: 45 grams of added sugar
- 2,000 calories: 50 grams of added sugar
- 2,200 calories: 55 grams of added sugar

These calories and sugar intake refer only to healthy people. If you have prediabetes, type 2 diabetes, type 1 diabetes, kidney disease, and heart disease, added sugar should be lower than mentioned above.

On the other hand, the American Heart Association recommends limiting added sugar to 36 grams (9 teaspoons) per day for men and 25 grams (6 teaspoons) of added sugar daily for women.

3. Starches

Starches are a class of polysaccharide carbohydrates extracted from agricultural raw materials found in thousands of foods.

The starch molecules in any food consist of many glucose units joined by the so-called glycosidic bonds. Rich in nutrients, starches are an important source of energy.

These starches are produced by vegetables, such as beans, butternut squash, chickpeas, peas, potatoes, and grains, particularly corn, wheat, and rice. Unripe bananas, prunes, and raisins are also high in starch.

Starches are formed by longer saccharide chains. They take longer to break down, so the blood sugar levels are raised slowly upon their consumption. They refer to whole grain foods and starchy vegetables, which slowly absorb simple or refined carbohydrates.

They may include whole grains such as brown or black rice, steel-cut oats, barley, whole grain bread, and pasta.

Dietitians and nutritionists recommend complex carbohydrates for a healthy body.

4. Fibers

Fibers: Humans cannot digest fiber, but the bacteria in the digestive system can make use of some types. Plus, eating fiber is vital to your overall health.

Unlike other carbohydrates that can be broken down into sugar molecules, fibers are carbohydrates that cannot be broken down into sugar molecules and absorbed by the body. They pass through the gastrointestinal tract undigested by gastrointestinal enzymes and end up in the intestines, mostly intact. Fibers regulate the body's use of sugar.

2 Types of Fibers: Soluble Fiber and Insoluble Fiber

Soluble fiber means it dissolves in water, while insoluble fiber does not dissolve in fluids.

Different Types of Soluble Fibers

Soluble fiber dissolves in water and other fluids in your body. As it passes through the body, it forms into a gel-like substance. When it's already in the colon, the fiber feeds the good bacteria in the gut.

Soluble fiber is found in oats, peas, lentils, beans, apples, citrus fruits, carrots, barley, and psyllium

There are several types of soluble fiber, including the following:

Pectin: A long chain of sugars found in plants, pectin is a soluble fiber known as a polysaccharide. Expanding when heated, the fiber forms into a gel-like substance and blends with water in the gut.

Psyllium: A soluble fiber derived from the seeds of Plantago ovata, is grown exclusively in India. It is a dietary supplement in the form of husk, powder, or granules. Psyllium husk is the main ingredient of Metamucil, a fiber supplement that alleviates constipation.

Beta-Glucan: Beta-glucan is a soluble fiber found in cereal grains such as oats and barley plant cell walls. Yeasts and mushrooms also contain beta-glucans.

Pectins and gums: A combination of pectin and gums are known as polysaccharides. Food manufacturers use them as gelling agents, stabilizers, and thickeners. They come from constituents of plant tissues consisting of complex molecules.

Benefits of Soluble Fiber

- Soluble fiber lowers LDL (bad cholesterol) and triglycerides.
- It lowers blood pressure.
- It reduces the overall risk of cardiovascular diseases.
- It increases healthy gut bacteria, lowering inflammation in the body.
- It reduces the body's ability to absorb fat.
- It lowers the risk of occurrence of diverticulitis and hemorrhoids.

Good Sources of Soluble Fiber

- Psyllium
- Barley
- Carrots
- Peas
- Beans

Different Kinds of lnsoluble Fibers

The insoluble fiber doesn't dissolve in water and other liquids because it absorbs the water and sticks it to the other substances to form stools. In this way, there will be softer and bulkier stools.

In wheat bran, vegetables, and whole grains, insoluble fiber helps promote bowel health. It attracts water into your stool, making it softer and more comfortable to pass on to your bowel with less straining.

In wheat bran, vegetables, and whole grains, insoluble fiber helps promote bowel health. It attracts water into your stool, making it softer and more comfortable to pass into your bowel with less straining. They also improve insulin sensitivity.

Types of Insoluble Fibers

Cellulose: Cellulose, the substance made up of a plant's cell walls, is considered one of the most abundant organic compounds. It has many uses. Factories can use it in making plastics, paper, and explosives. It is a vital source of fiber for human consumption in your diet.

Hemicellulose: Hemicellulose is a collective term for non-digestive polysaccharides. They are large molecules made of many smaller monosaccharides. Monosaccharides are simple sugar, like glucose.

Lignin: Lignin is a complex organic polymer deposited in many plants' cell walls, making them rigid and woody.

Lignin, found in cell walls and between plant cells, transports liquid throughout the plant and keeps the plants upright. It is the only fiber not composed of carbohydrate (sugar) monomers.

Humans can't digest lignin because we lack the enzymes needed to break the so-called glycosidic bonds (the bonds between sugars in the polysaccharides).

Benefits of Insoluble Fibers

- Insoluble fiber helps promote bowel health
- It aids in controlling body weight
- It helps in controlling high blood pressure
- It attracts water into your stool, making it softer and more comfortable to pass into your bowel with less straining

- It can prevent and treat constipation
- It improves insulin sensitivity

Good Sources of Insoluble Fibers

- Wheat bran
- Whole-wheat flour
- Potatoes, nuts, and cauliflower
- Green beans

Dietary Fiber Intake

The American Heart Association Eating Plan recommends eating various food fiber sources., totaling the dietary fiber intake from 25 to 30 grams per day from foods, not supplements.

Based on statistics, the dietary fiber intakes among adults in the United States average about 15 grams a day, nearly half of the government guidelines on eating fiber.

Government Guidelines on Fiber Intake Daily

- Men, age 50 and under: 38 grams per day
- Women, age 50 and under: 25 grams per day
- Men, over 50: 30 grams per day
- Women, over 50: 21 grams per day

II. Proteins (Macronutrients)

Proteins are the basis of life. They are made up of many amino acids attached in long chains.

Each protein has its specific number and sequence of amino acids. The cycle of amino acids combination and their resulting shape determines the particular functions of the protein.

The body uses amino acids to make proteins to help the body do its functions: break down food, grow, repair body tissue, and perform many other functions. In caloric intake, proteins provide four calories per gram, the same amount as carbohydrates but less than fats.

Types of Proteins

There are 7 types of proteins, including

- Antibodies
- Contractile proteins
- Enzymes
- Hormonal proteins
- Structural proteins
- Storage proteins
- Transport proteins

Amino Acids: Building Blocks of Proteins

Amino acids are organic compounds that have a critical role in creating proteins and synthesizing hormones and neurotransmitters.

The following are the 20 amino acids:

- Alanine (ala)
- Arginine (arg)
- Asparagine (asn)
- Aspartic acid (asp)
- Cysteine (cys)
- Glutamine (gln)
- Glutamic acid (glu)
- Glycine (gly)
- Histidine (his)
- lsoleucine (ile)
- Leucine (leu)
- Lysine (lys)
- Methionine (met)
- Phenylalanine (phe)
- Proline (pro)
- Serine (ser)
- Threonine (thr)
- Tryptophan (trp)
- Tyrosine (tyr)
- Valine (val)

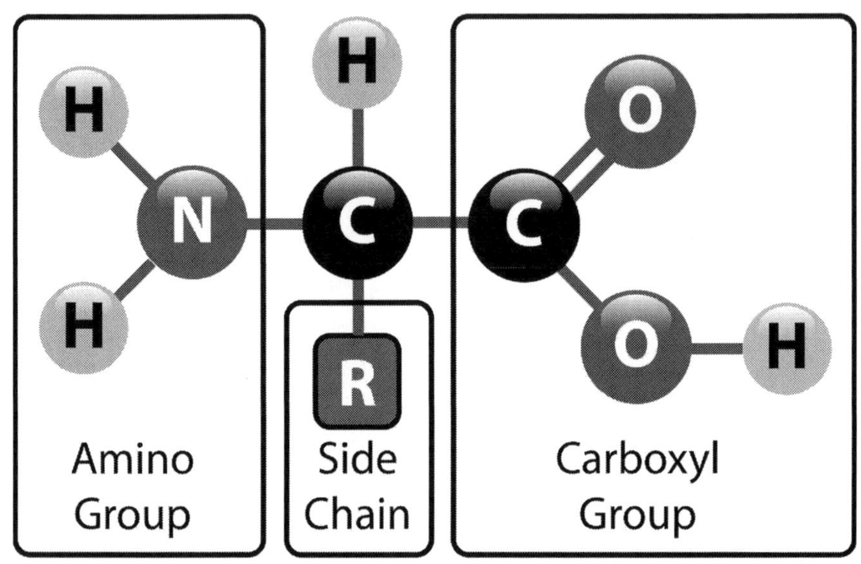

Amino Acid Structure

Photo Source: Shutterstock

What Are Amino Acids?

As the building blocks of proteins, amino acids are small organic molecules composed of an alpha (central) carbon atom connected to an amino group, carboxyl group, hydrogen atom, and a so-called side chain.

The components of amino acids are nitrogen, carbon, hydrogen, and oxygen.

Amino Acid Synthesis

Amino acid synthesis (the composition or combination of parts or elements to form a whole) is the biochemical processes (metabolic pathways) that produce amino acids. These amino acids, through biochemical processes, are joined by peptide bonds that make a polypeptide chain.

The chain then undergoes modifications and sometimes connects with other polypeptide chains to form a fully-functional protein.

About 500 amino acids have been identified in nature by scientists. However, humans use only 20 amino acids.

3 Classifications of Amino Acids

9 Essential amino acids: The body doesn't produce them, so you must take them from the foods you eat. They include histidine, isoleucine, leucine, lysine, methionine, phenylalanine, threonine, tryptophan, and valine.

11 Nonessential amino acids: The body produces them, so you don't need to take them into your diet. They include alanine, arginine, asparagine, aspartic acid, cysteine, glutamic acid, glutamine, glycine, proline, serine, and tyrosine.

6 Conditional amino acids: The six conditional amino acids are arginine, cysteine, glycine, glutamine, proline, and tyrosine.

That means that these amino acid syntheses are limited, such as in premature infants or individuals in severe catabolic distress. These amino acids are usually not essential, only used in times of illness and stress.

Protein Synthesis

Proteins are constantly being made, broken down, and remade. During the digestion process, enzymes, proteases, and peptidases digest and break down the protein into small peptide chains and into single amino acids, or small peptides that can be absorbed by the intestine and transported into the blood.

Amino acids are then consumed and used to make other proteins in the body. To have adequate proteins, replenish them by consuming foods that these macronutrients continuously.

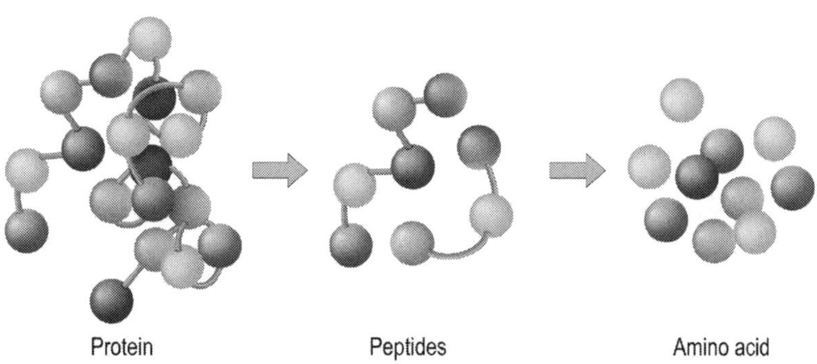

Digestion of Proteins

Photo Source: Shutterstock

Digestion of Proteins

The amino acids within a protein are considered the protein's primary structure. The human body consists of around 100 trillion cells, each of which has thousands of proteins.

The human body uses amino acids to make proteins to help them function.

Classes of Proteins

There are two classes of proteins, namely: complete proteins and incomplete proteins:

Complete Proteins: Complete proteins provide the essential amino acids that the body needs but cannot produce, so you must obtain them from foods. The primary sources of complete proteins include animal products, such as eggs, seafood (like tuna, salmon, mackerel), beef, pork, chicken, turkey, and eggs.

Incomplete Proteins: Incomplete proteins do not contain all the essential amino acids. The incomplete proteins mostly come from plants.

They may contain several amino acids, but sometimes the protein level is too low. Almost all plants don't contain complete proteins because they have only one or more of your body's nine essential amino acids.

However, there is a selection of plants that provide complete proteins. You may combine two incomplete proteins, and they can form complete proteins. Typical examples of the pairings are rice and beans, peanut butter and sandwiches, hummus and pitas, and pasta and peas.

Plants with Complete Proteins

- Grains (brown rice, black rice, wild rice, quinoa)
- Oats (rolled oats, steel-cut oats)
- Spirulina.
- Buckwheat
- Chia seed
- 6 Soybeans and soy products (tofu, tempeh, natto, soy yogurt, soy milk)

Functions of Proteins

Among the functions of proteins in the body are:

1. Building blocks: Form the building blocks of muscles and tissues of the body

2. Enhance immune health: Help form immunoglobulins, or antibodies, to battle infections invading the body

3. Reserved energy source: Serve as a valuable energy source in times of fasting, intensive exercise, or not enough calorie intake

4. Growth and maintenance: Provide help for the development and maintenance of tissues.

5. Transporter: Storage and transport of nutrient molecules in food that all organisms need to produce energy, grow, develop, and reproduce.

6. Chemical messengers: Some protein hormones act as chemical messengers of communication among your cells, tissues, and organs.

7. Proper pH maintenance: Proteins regulate the concentrations of acids and bases in your blood and other fluids, and they also maintain appropriate pH values of blood and other liquids.

8. Fibrous proteins: Give strength and elasticity to different body parts.

9. Protein hormones: According to *Healthline,* protein hormones are chemical messengers that help communication between cells, tissues, and organs.

The endocrine tissues or glands make these protein hormones and transport them to their target cells, tissues, and organs through the bloodstream. There, they bind to protein receptions on the surface of cells.

10. Antibodies: Proteins form antibodies that help fight infection, illness, and disease, assisting in destroying antigens such as bacteria and viruses.

11. Protein enzymes: Enzymes and globular proteins speed up the biochemical reactions.

12. Fibrinogen, a glycoprotein: Helps heal wounds, thus preventing blood loss and inhibiting the passage of germs. Fibrinogen is a specialized protein or clotting factor found in the blood. For example, thrombin, another clotting agent, is activated when any blood vessel is injured and changes fibrinogen to fibrin.

13. Building blocks of muscles and tissues: Protein's primary role isn't energy creation; instead, its amino acids form the building blocks for our muscles and tissues.

Protein Requirements

The National Academy of Medicine (formerly the Institute of Medicine) suggests that a man should eat at least 56 grams of protein per day.

On the other hand, a woman should consume at least 46 grams per day. A pregnant or nursing woman should eat at least 71 grams each day. But if you have kidney disease, the requirement may be different.

III. Fats (Macronutrients)

Macronutrients called fats are the primary form of stored energy essential for body functions. They are a type of lipids called triglycerides that are insoluble in water but soluble in organic solvents.

They are made up of a molecule of glycerol and three molecules of fatty acids. Glycerol is composed of three carbons, five hydrogens, and three hydroxyls (OH) groups.

At the same time, fatty acids have a long chain of hydrocarbons with a carboxyl group attached and composed of several carbons, most of which are between 12-18. In caloric intake, fats have 9 calories in each gram.

Functions of Fats

Fats have many functions in your body, which may include the following:

- **Neurotransmitter synthesizers:** Fats enhance the synthesis of many neurotransmitters, the brain's chemical messengers.
- **Brain health provider:** Because the brain consists of 60% fats, they serve as critical macronutrients for brain health and development.
- **Messengers:** Fats act as messengers, helping proteins do their jobs.
- **Chemical reactors:** Fats perform chemical reactions involved in growth, immune functions, reproduction, and other elements of primary metabolism.
- **Vitamin absorbers:** Fats help the body stock pile certain nutrients, such as the so-called "fat-soluble" vitamins, Vitamins A, D, E, and K. Fats store them in the liver and fatty tissues for future use.
- **Insulation and temperature maintainers:** Fat cells, stored in adipose tissues, or fatty tissues, insulate your body. They help in sustaining an average core body temperature. They also provide cushioning for the organs.

- **Hormone producers:** Fats assist the body in producing and regulating hormones, such as the hormone leptin, which regulates appetite.
- **Artery wall protectors:** Omega-3 fatty acids, a form of fats, protect the body through a wide range of mechanisms in promoting relaxation and contraction of artery walls.
- **Backup energy keepers:** Fats, like proteins, serve as a backup energy source for carbohydrates, the primary energy source.

Types of Fats

There are three major dietary fats that you get from the foods you eat, which include unsaturated fats, saturated fats, and trans fats.

1. Good Unsaturated Fats

The good unsaturated fats are monounsaturated and polyunsaturated. These healthy fats lower the risk of diseases. Foods high in healthy fats include vegetable and fruit oils, such as olive, canola, avocado, soy, corn, and sunflower), nuts, seeds, and fatty fish.

These healthy fats contain a high proportion of fatty acid molecules and are considered healthier than saturated fats.

2. Saturated Fats

What are saturated fats? The American Heart Association defines saturated fats as: "From a chemical standpoint, saturated fats are simply fat molecules that have no double bonds between carbon molecules because of the saturation of hydrogen molecules."

Usually, saturated fats in foods come from animal sources. They are naturally solid at room temperature. Examples of saturated fat sources are:

- Baked goods
- Beef, lamb, and chicken
- Yogurt, cheese, and ice cream
- Coconut and palm oils
- Fried foods
- Processed meats
- Whole milk and other dairy products

Harmful Effects of Saturated Fats in the Body

- **Risk of heart disease:** High saturated fats can cause cholesterol to accumulate in your arteries (blood vessels), raising your LDL (bad) cholesterol. Too much cholesterol increases your risk of cardiovascular disease, which may lead to a stroke or heart attack.
- **Weight gain:** Consuming too much saturated fats adds extra calories to your diet, causing weight gain.

3. Trans Fats

What are trans fats? Trans fats are composed of artificially-made fats produced through hydrogenation and those fats found in animal products such as meat and dairy. They are a form of unsaturated fat containing one or more double or triple bonds between the molecules.

The Mayo Clinic considers them the worst fat you can eat. Unlike other dietary fats, trans fats, also called trans-fatty acids, raise your LDL (bad cholesterol) and lower your HDL (good cholesterol).

How Are Trans Fats Created?

Most fats do their transformation through an industrial process called hydrogenation by which hydrogen is added to vegetable oil, making the oil solid at room temperature. The purpose is to have those foods have a longer shelf life.

FDA Prohibition

The US Food and Drug Administration (FDA) has already prohibited food manufacturers from adding the primary source of trans fat to beverages and foods.

Trans Fats in Foods

Known as partially hydrogenated oil, which is the manufactured form of trans fats, it may appear in different kinds of products including:

- Baked goods
- Stick margarine

Tips on Limiting or Avoiding Trans Fat in Cooking

Check food labels and look for the amount of trans fat as listed. Read the ingredient list for the term "partially hydrogenated." You can limit or eliminate trans fats in cooking by doing the following steps:

- Using oil instead of solid fats
- Sauteing foods with avocado oil or olive oil, instead of butter, and use canola oil when baking
- Trimming fat from meat, removing the skin from chicken and turkey
- Eating nuts, whole fruits, legumes, and vegetables for your snacks.
- Consuming fatty fish, like salmon, tuna, sardines, and mackerel (if you have no advanced kidney disease)
- Broiling lean meat and seafood instead of frying them

Harmful Effects of Trans Fats in the Body

If you overeat trans fats, here are some of the possible harmful effects of trans fats in your body, which include:

- Risk of a heart attack: In the Nurse Health Study, women who ate the highest number of trans fats in their diet had a 50% higher risk of heart attack than women who consumed the least trans fats.
- Risk of diabetes: Population studies indicate that trans fats may increase the risk of prediabetes or type 2 diabetes.

Foods with Nutrients to Replace Saturated and Trans Fats

- Whole grains like brown rice, black rice, barley, and steel-cut oats
- Fruits, legumes, and vegetables
- Fish, chicken, and turkey, without skin
- Healthy fats such as olive oil or avocado oil

Fats Daily Requirements

Since the body does not need trans fats, you should eat as little as possible. There is no specific amount. For total fats requirements, the 2010 Dietary Guidelines for Americans and the American Heart Association recommend the following:

- Limit to less than 1% of your daily calories
- To reduce the risk of heart disease, limit saturated fats to less than 7% of your diet's total daily calories

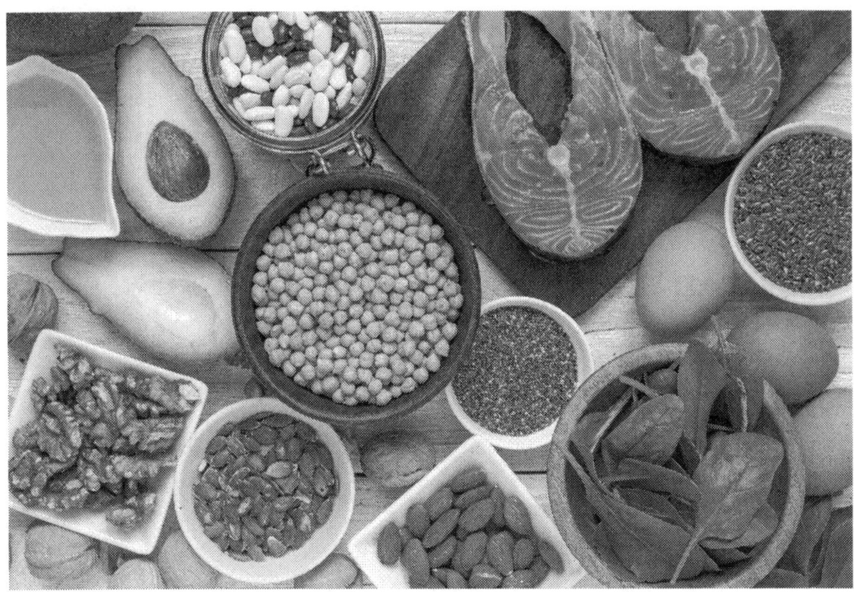

Foods With Omega-3 Acids & Healthy Fats

Photo Credit: Shutterstock

IV. Vitamins (Micronutrients)

What Are Vitamins?

According to the *MedlinePlus* website (a federal government website), "Vitamins are a group of substances that are needed for normal cell function, growth, and development."

There are 13 essential vitamins (meaning the body does not produce them.) You can have them by eating foods or taking vitamins.

There are two types of vitamins: fat-soluble vitamins and water-soluble vitamins.

Fat-Soluble Vitamins: They are absorbed by the body and stored in fatty tissues and the liver for long periods. Excess amounts of these vitamins can increase the risk of toxicity.

Water-Soluble Vitamins: They dissolve in water and cannot be stored. Because they exit the body through urine, constant replenishment through diet is required.

The following are the 13 essential vitamins that are important to maintain good health:

1. Fat-soluble Vitamins and Sources

- **Vitamin A**: Colored fruits and dark leafy greens, such as spinach and kale
- **Vitamin D**: Fortified milk and other dairy products, such as cereals
- **Vitamin E:** Nuts, seeds, fortified cereals, and leafy green vegetables
- **Vitamin K:** Beet greens, turnip, and dark green leafy vegetables

2. Water-Soluble Vitamin and Sources

- **Vitamin B1 (thiamine)**: Whole grains, nuts, seeds, and enriched grains
- **Vitamin B2 (riboflavin)**: Whole grains, enriched grains, and dairy products
- **Vitamin B3 (Niacin):** Meat, chicken, turkey, and whole grains

- **Vitamin B5 (Pantothenic acid)**: Vitamin B5 comes from various foods, such as beef, poultry, seafood, and organ meats; eggs and milk; vegetables such as mushrooms (especially shiitakes), broccoli, potatoes, avocados, and potatoes
- **Vitamin B6, or (Pyridoxine)**: Fortified cereals and soy products
- **Vitamin B7, or (Biotin)**: Fruits and meats
- **Vitamin B9, or Folic Acid (Folate):** Leafy vegetables
- **Vitamin B12**: Fish, poultry, meat, and dairy products
- **Vitamin C**: Citrus fruits and juices, such as oranges and grapefruits, and red, yellow, and green peppers

Functions of Fat-Soluble Vitamins and Sources

They include the following:

Vitamin A: An antioxidant, vitamin A is responsible for the growth and development, vision, cell recognition, immune function, and cell reproduction, including helping your heart, lungs, and kidneys do their jobs.

Vitamin D: The vitamin plays a vital role in body functions, absorbing the calcium you need and influencing cell growth and development. It thus monitors and keeps your nervous system working correctly and efficiently. A nutrient and a hormone, vitamin D is produced by the body. The skin can make its own vitamin D when exposed to the sun. It can also be derived from the foods that you eat and the supplements you take.

Vitamin E: An antioxidant, vitamin E helps your body form red blood cells and use vitamin K. Naturally contained in foods and available as a dietary supplement, this antioxidant protects your cells from damage. The term "vitamin E" describes eight compounds it has, the most active of which is *alpha-tocopherol.*

Vitamin K: Vitamin K, a group of compounds, the most important compounds of which are Vitamin K1 and vitamin K2, helps the blood clot, preventing excessive bleeding.

The synthesis of bacteria produces vitamin K in the large intestine. Vitamin K1, not typically used as a dietary supplement, is the main vitamin K supplement available in the U.S.

Functions of Water-Soluble Vitamins

Vitamin B1 (Thiamine): An essential nutrient, Vitamin B1 helps the body cells change carbohydrates into energy. It is vital for heart function and healthy nerve cells. It also helps the body make *adenosine triphosphate* (ATP), a molecule that transfers energy within cells. While nicotinic acid reduces cholesterol, the other form, niacinamide, doesn't lower cholesterol.

Vitamin B2 (Riboflavin): Vitamin B2, one of eight B vitamins that are essential for human health, among others, helps break down proteins, fats, and carbohydrates to maintain the body's energy supply. It also helps convert carbohydrates into adenosine triphosphate (ATP), vital for storing energy in muscles.

Vitamin B3 (Niacin): As a supplement and acting as an antioxidant, niacin can help reduce LDL (bad) cholesterol, and triglycerides and increase HDL (good) cholesterol.

Vitamin B5 (Pantothenic Acid): It is essential for the synthesis and metabolism of carbohydrates, fats, and proteins. It also helps in balancing hormonal production in the body. One of the vital vitamins for human life, pantothenic acid, helps make blood cells and aids your body in converting the foods you eat into energy.

Vitamin B6 (Pyridoxine): Vitamin B6 plays a significant role in protein, fat, and carbohydrate metabolism. It helps form red blood cells and maintain brain function. Your body does not produce vitamin B6.

Vitamin B7 (Biotin): Vitamin B7, also known as biotin, and co-enzymes for carboxylase enzymes, is needed by the body to metabolize fats, proteins, and carbohydrates.

Vitamin B9 (Folic Acid/Folate): Folic acid, one of the eight B vitamins, helps the body convert carbohydrates into glucose for the body's energy. Vitamin B9, like other vitamins known as B-complex, also aids the body synthesize fats and proteins efficiently. and helps the nervous system function effectively.

Vitamin B12 (Cyanocobalamin): Like other B vitamins, Vitamin B12 plays a vital role in metabolism and aids in forming red blood cells and maintaining the central nervous system. Red meat and fish contain Vitamin B12.

Plant foods do not have Vitamin B12. So for vegans and vegetarians, you may include some meat in your diet or take some Vitamin B12 and other supplements.

Vitamin C (Ascorbic acid): An antioxidant, Vitamin C is one of the biggest immune system boosters. It promotes healthy gums and teeth and also helps the body absorb iron, and maintains healthy tissues. It is also essential for wound healing.

More Facts on Vitamins

Fat-soluble vitamins A, D, E, and K and fat-soluble vitamin B12: Vitamins that can be stored in the body.

Vitamin D3, niacin, and Vitamin K: Vitamins that the body can produce. (There are two forms of Vitamin D: Vitamin D2 and Vitamin D3, but they can be called simply Vitamin D.) Vitamin K is produced by the synthesis of bacteria in the large intestine, while D3 is produced by the body using sunlight.

Nicotinic acid, nicotinamide, and nicotinamide riboside, are collectively referred to as niacin or vitamin B3. Niacin is also produced in the body from tryptophan, found in protein-containing foods.

Water-soluble vitamins, C and B-complex vitamins such as B6, B12, niacin, riboflavin, and folate: Vitamins that dissolve in water and the body can't store them.

Niacin: Vitamin that the body can produce but cannot store in the body.

V. What are Minerals?

Minerals are inorganic nutrients that do not contain carbon, and the body cannot make them on its own. They come from the foods you eat.

According to an article published online by Michigan Medicine, the body needs essential minerals to keep it healthy.

Scientists divide minerals into major minerals (macrominerals) and trace minerals (microminerals). Larger amounts are needed for macrominerals, while only small quantities for trace minerals.

The two groups of minerals are as follows:

Major Minerals (Macrominerals)

- Sodium
- Chloride
- Potassium
- Magnesium
- Calcium
- Phosphorus
- Sulfur

Trace Minerals (Microminerals)

- Iron
- Zinc
- Iodine
- Selenium
- Copper
- Manganese
- Fluoride
- Chromium
- Molybdenum

Functions and Sources of Major Minerals

1. Sodium: Sodium plays a vital role in proper fluid balance, nerve transmission, and muscle contraction. Sources of sodium include bread, processed meats, and canned goods.

2. Chloride: Chloride helps keep the amount of fluid inside and outside your cells in balance. It also helps maintain your body fluids' proper blood volume, blood pressure, and pH.

Most of the chloride in your body comes from the salt (sodium chloride) you eat. The intestines absorb the chloride you consume after food digestion. Excess chloride leaves your body in your urine.

3. Potassium: Potassium, a type of electrolyte, aids your nerves function and muscles contract. It helps your heartbeat stay regular. Sources include whole grains, legumes, vegetables, and milk.

4. Calcium: The most abundant mineral, calcium, is used structurally, building bones and teeth and serving as a signaling messenger.

Sources include milk and milk products.

5. Phosphorus: It has a vital role in proper balance, nerve transmission, and muscle contraction. Part of the system maintains acid-base balance. It is essential for healthy bones and teeth. Sources include body cells, eggs, milk and milk products, and processed foods.

6. Magnesium: Widely used for metabolic processes, magnesium maintains body functions, including energy production, synthesis of biomolecules, and as a component of cell membranes and chromosomes. It also helps in the normalization of heart rhythm.

Magnesium is a mineral used to regulate dozens of processes, from muscle functioning to synthesizing proteins and bones. Sources include legumes, leafy green vegetables, seafood, nuts, and seeds.

Magnesium, which does many functions in the human body, is the most underrated and neglected mineral. That's why people do not usually take it, compared to calcium and vitamin D. What a mistake!

According to the World Health Organization, as much as 75% of the U.S. adult population does not meet the FDA's Recommended Daily Intake of 420 mg of magnesium.

For its part, the U.S. National Institutes of Health Office of Dietary Supplements (ODS) recommends 400 to 420 mg of magnesium daily for men and 310 to 320 mg of magnesium per day for most women.

7. Sulfur: Sulfur is an integral part of several amino acids (the building blocks of protein), particularly methionine and cysteine. Key functions of sulfur include enzyme reactions and protein synthesis. It helps the body to resist bacteria, cleans the blood, and protects the protoplasm of cells.

Sources of sulfur include fish and other seafood (shrimp, scallops, mussels, prawns); legumes (soybeans, black beans); nuts and seeds (Brazil nuts, almonds, walnuts, peanuts and pumpkin, and sesame seeds); eggs and dairy (cow's milk, parmesan, gorgonzola cheese); and dried fruits (apricots, sultanas, figs, peaches).

The Functions and Sources of Trace Minerals (Microminerals)

1. Iron: A critical component of many metabolic proteins and enzymes, iron is part of a molecule (hemoglobin) in red blood cells to carry oxygen to body tissues. Iron found in the body is in the form of heme iron or non-heme iron. Sources include red meat, fish, shellfish, chicken, turkey, eggs, enriched bread, and fortified cereals.

2. **Zinc**: Zinc is involved in many cellular metabolic processes. It is essential for growth and development and reproduction, the immune system, and neurological functions. Sources include fish, vegetables, whole grains, chicken, and turkey.

3. Iodine: A component of the thyroid hormone, iodine is needed for normal thyroid function. Sources include seafood, iodized salt, foods grown in iodine-rich soil, meats, and dairy products.

4. Selenium: According to the United States Office of Dietary Supplements, selenium, an essential trace mineral, is vital in many bodily processes, including a healthy immune system, and cognitive function. It says, "Selenium contributes to thyroid hormone metabolism and DNA synthesis." Food sources include meats, eggs, Brazil nuts, some fish, and brown rice.

5. Copper: Copper is a soft and ductile metal (able to be deformed without losing toughness) with very high thermal and electrical conductivity. In its elemental form, copper is smooth and shiny. A part of many enzymes, copper is needed for iron metabolism. Sources include whole grains, organ meats, nuts, and seeds.

6. Manganese: Manganese is a trace mineral that contributes to many bodily functions. Its functions include the metabolism of glucose, cholesterol, carbohydrates, and amino acids. It also plays a role in bone formation, blood clotting, and reducing inflammation.

Manganese helps form an antioxidant enzyme called *superoxide dismutase (SOD)*. It also contributes to wound healing. Sources of manganese include beans, fruits, raw pineapple, pineapple juice, nuts, beans, spinach, oatmeal, and brown rice.

7. Fluoride: The main purpose of fluoride in the body is to mineralize teeth and bones. It also protects the teeth from decay and is also regularly added to almost all kinds of toothpaste. Fluoride, found naturally in soil, water, and foods, is also produced synthetically for drinking water, mouthwashes, and various products.

Fluoride comes from the word fluorine, which is a common, natural, and abundant element. The water supply adds fluoride to reduce the incidence of tooth decay. Sources include drinking water (either fluoridated or naturally containing fluoride), some teas, and some seafood.

8. Chromium: "Chromium is an essential trace mineral that can improve insulin sensitivity and enhance protein, carbohydrate, and lipid metabolism)," says the *Medical News Today*.

A metallic clement, chromium, is used by the body minimally. In other words, people need only minimal quantities of this trace mineral. There are risks when taken in abundance. Food sources include liver, broccoli, and brewers' yeast.

9. Molybdenum: An essential trace mineral, molybdenum, breaks down proteins and other substances. People mostly use molybdenum to treat the esophagus and different types of cancers and conditions. Sources of molybdenum include legumes, leafy vegetables, cereal grains, nuts, and beef liver.

My Journey: Vitamins and Minerals

I'm taking the following vitamins and minerals for the heart and general health: (Self-Prescribed)

- *Doctor's High Absorption Magnesium, 100% chelated, 100 mg daily (for diabetes, and kidney and heart diseases, and overall health)*
- *Cardiovascular Research's Magnesium Taurate, soft gel, 100 mg, taken once a day (for the heart)*
- *Qunol Ultra CoQ10, 100 mg per day (for heart and cholesterol)*
- *Jarrow Formula's Ubiquinol QH-Absorb, High Absorption/ Enhanced Stability, 100 mg, 120 Softgels (for heart and overall health)*
- *Omega-[3-Acid Ethyl Esters, Capsules (generic of Lovaza, first fish oil, approved by the U.S. Food and Drug Administration (FDA), taken 4,000 mg daily for the heart and high cholesterol and glycerides*
- *Swanson's Magnesium Orotate, 40 mg (for the heart)*
- *Vitamin D (helps in the absorption of iron and magnesium)*

Which Type or Brand of Magnesium to Take?

Regarding magnesium, the National Institutes of Health Office of Dietary Supplements (ODS) recommends that you consider taking magnesium aspartate, citrate, lactate, or chloride, which are absorbed better than magnesium oxide or sulfate.

Upon my research, I have concluded that the highly-absorbed types of magnesium are chelated magnesium, taurate magnesium, and orotate magnesium. So, to increase the absorption of magnesium, I'm also taking Vitamin D.

If you're interested in taking vitamins and minerals, you may ask your doctor which ones are right for you, based on your condition and the medicines you're taking, if any. Some vitamins and minerals interact with medications.

VI. Water

What Is Water?

Water in the aquifers (rock layers underground), lakes, rivers, and seas is a colorless, transparent, odorless liquid. It is in living organism fluids, such as plants, animals, and humans. A substance composed of hydrogen and oxygen, water exists in gaseous, liquid, and solid states.

Is Water a Macronutrient?

Water, consumed in large quantities, is often classified as a macronutrient. It's on the USDA's (US Department of Agriculture) Acceptable Macronutrient Distribution Range (AMDR). As listed on AMDR, the three main categories of macros are carbohydrates, proteins, and fats.

However, water does not have calories or carbon, so it does not provide energy directly. Still, when you drink water, it can help you eliminate the symptoms of dehydration with fatigue and tiredness, giving you vigor and vitality.

Water is the single largest component of the human body, consisting of about 50 to 70% of the body weight.

Functions of Water

The functions of water include:

- Providing liquid or fluid to prevent dehydration in parts of the whole body, including cells, organs, and tissues
- Dissolving vitamins, minerals, and other nutrients for body use
- Carrying nutrients and oxygen throughout the body
- Helping the kidneys and liver to flush out waste products
- Regulating body temperature and maintaining other bodily functions
- Enhancing brain function and mood
- Dissolving urea, nitrogen, creatinine, blood sugar, ammonia, and helping prevent heart attack or stroke at night

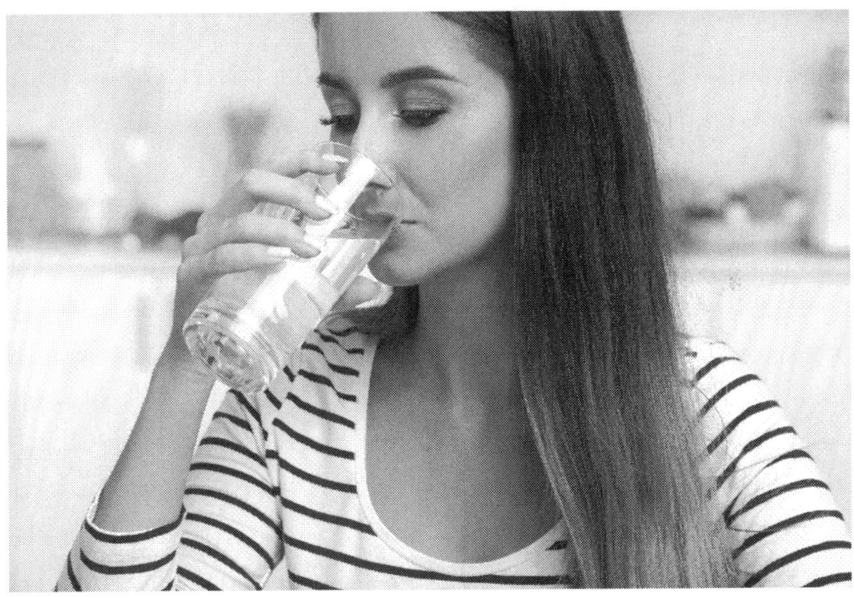

Drinking Enough Water to Dilute Blood Sugar, Creatinine, and Blood Urea Nitrogen (BUN), to Lower Their Levels in the Bloodstream

Photo Credit: Shutterstock

Chapter 11

Best Diets for 2023 for Diabetes, Heart Disease, Etc. --U.S. News & World Report

Brief Subject Summary

- I. The Mediterranean Diet
- II. The DASH Diet
- III. The Flexitarian Diet
- IV. The Vegetarian Diet
- V. The Vegan Diet
- VI. The Mayo Clinic Diet
- VII. The Ornish Diet
- VIII. The Nordic Diet
- IX. The MIND Diet
- X. The Ketogenic Diet

Whether you have prediabetes, type 2 diabetes, type 1 diabetes, kidney disease, or heart disease, you must know what foods to eat and not to eat. It would be best to have a balanced diet consisting of three macronutrients: carbohydrates, protein, and fats.

But as a guide to achieving a healthy diet for your particular disease or other diseases, you may select a specific diet appropriate for you to achieve your goal of lowering your blood sugar.

And of course, you should take the necessary steps to slow, stabilize, and reverse your disease.

It may be relatively easy for you to make a diet plan if you have only prediabetes or type 2 diabetes. But if you have several ailments like me, it is complicated and challenging.

Just look! I have type 2 diabetes, kidney disease, and heart disease (heart failure), and I have to adjust my diet, a semi-plant-based diet, not totally a whole plant-based diet.

Best Diet Rankings for 2023 by U.S. News & World Report

The U.S. News, the global authority in rankings and consumer advice, has announced its annual rankings of the year's best diets.

It formed a panel of top specialists in nutrition, diabetes, heart health, and weight loss to make the rankings. The 27 panelists extensively surveyed and scored 40 diets in several categories.

Best Overall Diets

The panel ranked the Mediterranean Diet as the sixth-year top overall diet for 2023. The DASH Diet and Flexitarian Diet tied for second place.

The Mediterranean Diet was also the top placer in five other diet categories.

The MIND Diet got 4th place in Best Diets Overall. And Mayo Clinic Diet, TLC Diet, Volumetrics Diet, and the WW (Weight Watchers) Diet were tied for 5th positions.

The top scorers in best diets for 2023 are as follows:

2023 Best Diets Rankings

Best Diets Overall

1. Mediterranean Diet
2. DASH Diet (tie)
2. Flexitarian Diet (tie)

Best Weight-Loss Diets

1. WeightWatchers (WW) Diet
2. DASH Diet
3. Mayo Clinic Diet (tie)
3. TLC Diet (tie)

Best Fast Weight-Loss Diets

1. Keto Diet
2. Atkins Diet (tie)
2. Nutrisystem (tie)

2. OPTAVIA (tie)
2. SlimFast Diet (tie)

Best Diets for Healthy Eating

1. Mediterranean Diet
2. DASH Diet
3. Flexitarian Diet

Best Heart-Healthy Diets

1. DASH Diet
2. Mediterranean Diet
3. Flexitarian Diet (tie)
3. Ornish Diet (tie)

Best Diabetes Diets

1. DASH Diet
2. Mediterranean Diet
3. Flexitarian Diet

Best Diets for Bone and Joint Health

1. DASH Diet (tie)
1. Mediterranean Diet (tie)
3. Flexitarian Diet

Best Family-Friendly Diets

1. Flexitarian Diet (tie)
1. Mediterranean Diet (tie)
1. TLC Diet (tie)

Best Plant-Based Diets

1. Mediterranean Diet
2. Flexitarian Diet
3. MIND Diet

Easiest Diets to Follow

1. Flexitarian Diet (tie)
1. TLC Diet (tie)
3. DASH Diet (tie)
3. Mediterranean Diet (tie)

Best Diet Programs

1. WeightWatchers (WW) Diet
2. Jenny Craig Diet (tie)
2. Noom Diet (tie)

For more information on the U.S. News Best Diets, explore Facebook, Twitter and Instagram using #BestDiets.

Media Contact: Michelle Day, mday@usnews.com, 202-955-2212

For a complete list of Best Diets for 2023, you may go to: https://health.usnews.com/best-diet

Media Contact: Sarah Javors, sjavors@usnews.com, 202-955-2153

I. The Mediterranean Diet

#1 for Best Diet Overall; Best Diet for Bone and Joint Health and tied with DASH for #1 position; Best Family-Friendly Diets, tied with Flexitarian Diet and TLC Diet for first place position; #2 for Best Diabetes Diets; #2 for Heart-Healthy Diets and #1 for Best Plant-Based Diets, and #3 for Easiest Diets to Follow, tied with DASH Diet.

For the sixth consecutive year, the Mediterranean Diet got the No. 1 spot for the Best Diet Overall. This diet emphasizes the eating of a lot of vegetables, fruits, olive oil and fish. This diet also claimed the top spot in Best Diets for Bone and Joint Health (tied at No. 1). Best Family-Friendly Diets (tied at No. 1), Best Diets for Healthy Eating and Best Plant-Based Diets. The DASH Diet and the Flexitarian Diet, tied at No. 2 for Best Diets Overall.

The Mediterranean Diet and Dash Diet tied for No. 1 for Best Diets for Bone and Joint Health. On the other hand, the Mediterranean Diet, Flexitarian Diet and TLC Diet tied for No. 1 position for Best Family Friendly Diets.

What Is the Mediterranean Diet?

The Mediterranean diet focuses on an active lifestyle, weight control, and a diet low in red meat, sugar, and saturated fat but high in healthy fats.

No Single Definition for the Mediterranean Diet

While there is no single definition of the Mediterranean diet, it is typically high in:

- Vegetables
- Legumes
- Fruits
- Whole grains
- Nuts and seeds
- Herbs
- Olives
- Olive oil
- Avocado oil

High in Monounsaturated Fat

According to a 2007 article in the Journal of Clinical Interventions in Aging, "The Mediterranean diet is high in monounsaturated fat from olive oil, low in saturated fat, high in complex carbohydrates from legumes, and high in fiber, mostly from vegetables and fruits."

The Mediterranean Diet

- Diet should be plant-based, not animal-based
- Limited intake of red meat Daily consumption of whole grains, fruits, whole grains, and healthy fats, such as olives, olive oil, avocado, or avocado oil
- Moderate portions of dairy products

- Intake every week of fish, seafood, poultry, eggs, and beans, such as pinto and black beans

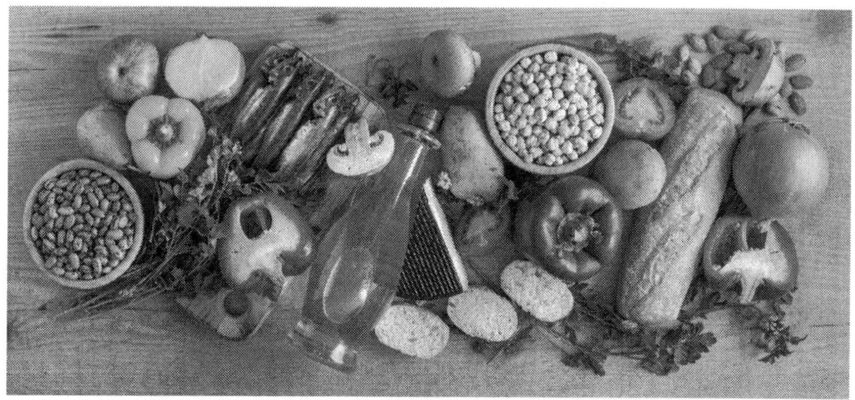

Mediterranean Diet

Photo Credit: Shuttershock.com

Healthy Foods to Eat

- **Whole grains:** Whole oats (such as steel-cut oats), brown rice, black rice, barley, rye, corn, buckwheat, whole wheat, whole-grain bread, and other foods
- **Vegetables:** Spinach, onions, cauliflower, carrots, broccoli, kale, spinach, onions, cauliflower, tomatoes, cucumbers, and Brussels sprouts
- **Legumes:** Beans, peas, lentils, pulses, peanuts, chickpeas, etc.
- **Fruits:** Pears, oranges, grapes, blueberries, apples, pears, strawberry, etc.
- **Nuts and seeds**: Walnuts, cashews, almonds, hazelnuts, walnuts, macadamia nuts, sunflower seeds, and pumpkin seeds
- **Tubers**: Potatoes, sweet potatoes, turnips, yams, and others
- **Fish and seafood:** Salmon, sardines, trout, tuna, mackerel, shrimp, oysters, crab, clams, and others
- **Poultry:** Chicken, turkey, and duck
- **Eggs:** Chicken, duck, and quail
- **Dairy:** Milk, cheese, yogurt, Greek yogurt, and soy yogurt
- **Herbs and spices:** Garlic, onion, sage, mint, nutmeg, cinnamon, pepper, and basil

- **Healthy Fats:** Olives, extra virgin olive oil, and avocado oil

What to Drink

- Water (the best drink)
- Moderate amounts of red wine, around one glass daily
- Coffee and tea are acceptable (but you must limit or avoid these if you have prediabetes or type 2 diabetes because caffeine increases blood sugar levels)

Foods, Drinks, and Ingredients to Avoid

- **Drinks and foods:** Hard alcohol, sugary drinks, and foods with added sugar, candies, ice cream, and many others
- **Trans fats:** Vegetable shortenings and some stick margarine.
- **Refined grains:** White bread, pasta made with refined wheat, pizza dough with white flour
- **Saturated fats:** Red meat and other processed meat foods

Possible Side Effects of the Mediterranean Diet

- Iron loss because a Mediterranean diet has an inadequate intake of red and processed meat, an important supply of bioavailable iron, requiring you to eat other foods rich in iron
- Calcium loss from eating fewer dairy products, which may need you taking a supplement with the approval of your doctor
- Weight gain from overeating fats in olive oil, nuts, and seeds

Health Benefits of the Mediterranean Diet

- Diabetes prevention and control: Lowers blood sugar and blood pressure
- Weight loss
- Low risks of heart diseases, such as coronary heart disease and other cardiovascular conditions
- Cancer prevention
- Prevention of other diseases

Following the Mediterranean diet may lead to more stable blood sugar, lower cholesterol and triglycerides, and lower risk for heart disease and other heart conditions.

II: The DASH Diet

#2, in Best Overall Diets, tied with Flexitarian Diet; #2 in Best Weight-Loss Diets; #2 in Best Diets for Healthy Eating; #1 in Best Diabetes Diets; #1 in Best Heart-Healthy Diets; #1 tied with Mediterranean Diet in Best Diets for Bone and Joint Health; and tied with Mediterranean Diet for #3 position for Easiest Diets to follow.

What Is the DASH Diet?

The DASH Diet, which stands for Dietary Approaches to Stop Hypertension, is promoted by the National Heart, Lung, and Blood Institute to stop (or prevent) hypertension, popularly known as high blood pressure.

The DASH Diet features:

- Eating more fruits, vegetables, and low-dairy foods
- Cutting back on foods that are high in saturated fat, trans fat, and cholesterol
- Limiting sodium, sweets, sugary drinks, nuts, and seeds
- Consuming low-fat and fat-free Greek and soy yogurt
- Eating greens and raw vegetables in the form of salads with olive oil and vinegar
- Reading food labels to choose products that are low in sodium
- Drinking low-fat or skim dairy products any time

Foods to Limit or Avoid on DASH Diet

- Limit or avoid alcohol
- Lean protein: 6 (or fewer) ounces a day
- Can eat chicken, fish, and lean red meats in moderation
- Salt should be limited to 1,500 to 2,000 mg daily

What the DASH Diet Recommends

- Low-fat or fat-free dairy products (such as yogurt): 2-3 servings per day
- Lean meat, fish, and poultry: 2 or fewer servings per day
- Unsalted nuts, seeds, and cooked dry beans
- Limited sweets
- Healthy fats, such as olives, extra virgin oil, and avocado oil

Grains: 7-8 servings per day

- Low-fat or fat-free dairy products (such as yogurt): 2-3 servings per day
- Lean meat, fish, and poultry: 2 or fewer servings per day
- Unsalted nuts, seeds, and cooked dry beans
- Healthy fats, such as olives, extra virgin oil, and avocado oil

Benefits of the DASH Diet

- Benefits patients with diabetes and kidney and heart diseases
- Promotes stoppage of smoking and moderate intake of wine
- Lowers blood pressure by losing weight, having exercise (such as moderate-intensity walking or brisk walking, and healthy low glycemic index and glycemic load foods
- Includes diet food nutrients such as calcium, potassium, and magnesium to help reduce blood pressure

III. The Flexitarian Diet

#2, tied with DASH Diet in Best Diets Overall; #1, the Best Weight-Loss Diets, tied with Volumetrics and WW (Weight Watchers); #2, tied with DASH Diet in Best Diets for Healthy Eating; #2 in Easiest Diets to Follow; #2, tied in Best Diets for Diabetes, with Vegan Diet; and #2 in Best-Plant-Based Diets

Flexitarian Diet: Easy to Follow?

The Flexitarian diet is easy to follow because the diet is adjustable. It's up to you to be a semi-vegetarian, eating plant-based foods and consuming meat a few times a week, which is beneficial to diabetes, kidney, and heart diseases.

I follow my semi-plant-based diet, with a ratio of 70% plant foods to 30% animal foods. It's somewhat similar to the Flexitarian diet, but I eat more animal foods than flexitarians.

Dawn Jackson Blatner, RD, LDN, a spokesperson of the American Diabetes Association, coined the word Flexitarian.

The word flexitarian is a combination of words "flexible" and "vegetarian." The diet explicitly intends to improve your health with a mostly vegetarian diet that includes some meat on certain days of the week, the amount of which depends on the dieter's liking.

Blatner's book, *The Flexitarian Diet,* contains tips and strategies for following it.

In other words, if you have an interest in a vegetarian diet but can't eliminate meat, you can have the many health benefits of following the Flexitarian diet without completely giving up your love for meat, although limiting its intake.

Vegans eliminate meat: fish, eggs, dairy, and animal-derived foods. On the other hand, vegetarians eliminate meat but sometimes consume animal foods.

Flexitarians consume individual meals with some animal products, so they are not considered vegetarians or vegans.

The flexible diet has no clear-cut rules or recommendations. There are no rules on how many calories or macronutrients to include in the diet.

Basic Principles of the Flexitarian Diet

- Focusing on eating mostly whole grains, legumes, fruits, and vegetables
- Getting more protein from plant protein than animal products
- Incorporating plant and animal products in weekly meals
- Eating mostly natural forms of foods and consuming least processed products
- Limiting or avoiding sweets and foods with added sugar

Benefits of the Flexitarian Diet

- Eating more plant-based foods may help you lower your risk for kidney disease and cardiovascular diseases
- Plant-based foods can help you get your daily dose of fiber, which is a significant part of a healthy diet
- Plant products provide many vitamins and minerals, including vitamins A, C, E. K, folate, minerals, potassium, magnesium, phosphorus, and manganese
- This diet may reduce your cholesterol, triglycerides, and blood pressure if it is high
- It may help you in losing weight and lowering your blood sugar if you have diabetes
- It's easier to follow than vegan, vegetarian, or any other diets

IV. The Vegetarian Diet

What Is a Vegetarian Diet?

Vegetarian is a general term for people who don't eat meat, poultry, or seafood.

Types of Vegetarians

- Vegans (total vegetarians): Do not eat meat, poultry, fish, or any products derived from animals, including eggs, dairy products, and gelatin

- Lacto-Ovo vegetarians: Do not eat meat, poultry, or fish but eat eggs
- Lacto vegetarians: Eat no meat, poultry, fish, or eggs, but consume dairy products
- Ovo vegetarians: Eat no meat, poultry, fish, or dairy products, but eat eggs
- Partial vegetarians: Avoid meat but may eat fish (pesco-vegetarian)

Vegetarians Vs Vegans

Vegetarians typically avoid all meats, poultry, and seafood but eat dairy-based products. Vegans avoid all animal products and eat only a diet of plant-based foods.

Vegetarians can lack enough proteins, essential vitamins (B12 and D), and minerals without meat, poultry, or seafood. So the vegans and vegetarians need to eat other foods, such as:

- Fruits and vegetables
- Legumes such as peas, beans, and lentils
- Quinoa
- Steel-cut oats and rolled oats
- Eggs and dairy products
- Soy protein, including soy yogurt, tofu, nuts and seeds, tempeh, veggie burgers, chicken substitute, and soy milk
- Legumes, vegetables, and beans, such as black beans, chickpeas
- Nuts, seeds, and peanut butter
- Whole grains, such as black rice, barley, and amaranth

Vegetarian and Vegan Diet Risks

Suppose you're a vegetarian or vegan. In that case, you may be at risk of nutrient deficiencies when you cut back on meat and its products, depending on your other foods' adequacy.

Vitamin Deficiencies in the Vegetarian Diet and Vegan Diet

Veggies, nuts, and other vegetarian diets come with plenty of micronutrients that your body needs to function at the highest level.

But iodine, zinc, and vitamin B-12 are hard to come by when you leave meat, seafood, and dairy products out of your meals. Without these nutrients, you can suffer from diarrhea, fatigue, goiter problems, loss of taste and smell, and even neurological damage.

Well, as a vegetarian, you have to take supplements and minerals. You have to find foods that can replace these micronutrients and add them to your diet. If not, you can take some supplements and minerals.

Nutrients Not Found in Plants

- Iron
- Zinc
- Calcium
- Omega-3 fatty acids
- Vitamin B-12
- Creatine
- Vitamin D3
- Carnosine
- Heme iron
- Taurine
- DHA (Docosahexaenoic acid)

Almost exclusively, animal foods provide the above nutrients lacking in plant foods. They include:

- Meat
- Fish
- Eggs and dairy products

In other words, you have to find foods that can replace the mentioned micronutrients and add them to your diet.

If you can't get all the nutrients from plant foods, you may have to take supplements and minerals.

V. The Vegan Diet

What Is a Vegan Diet?

A vegan diet is similar to a vegetarian diet, adhering to a plant-based diet. The vegans are the so-called total vegetarians. The different types of vegans are total vegetarians, *Lacto-Ovo* vegetarians, *Lacto* vegetarians, Ovo vegetarians, and *Partial* vegetarians.

Vegans do not eat meat, poultry, fish, or any products derived from animals, including eggs, dairy products, and gelatin. Other vegetarians do eat eggs and dairy products. (See the Vegetarian Diet in this chapter).

Deficiencies of the Vegan Diet (See the Vegetarian Diet)

There are possible deficiencies in selecting the vegan diet and the vegetarian diet. Animal foods provide, almost exclusively, the above nutrients that are nonexistent in plant foods.

Grains, Legumes, Nuts, and Seeds

To avoid such deficiencies, you may eat grains and legumes, which contain both iron and zinc. You may include nuts and seeds in your diet. You may add citrus fruits to get enough vitamin C.

Some flexitarians may limit dairy and need to eat plant-based sources of calcium to get adequate amounts of this nutrient.

Because vegans don't eat meat, poultry, seafood, eggs, and dairy products, they can be lacking enough proteins, vitamins (like Vitamin B-12), and minerals. So vegans may derive these nutrients from other foods, such as:

- Soy protein, including soy yogurt, tofu, nuts and seeds, tempeh, veggie burgers, and chicken substitute, and soy milk
- Fruits, vegetables, and legumes such as peas, beans, and lentils
- Legumes such as peas, beans, and lentils
- Quinoa
- Steel-cut oats and rolled oats
- Nuts, seeds, and peanut butter

- Whole grains, such as black rice, brown rice, barley, and amaranth

VI. The Mayo Clinic Diet

#3 Best Weight-Loss Diets, tied with TLC Diet and Mayo Clinic Diet, TLC Diet, Volumetrics Diet, and the WW (Weight Watchers) Diet were tied for 5th positions in Best Diets Overall.

What Is the Mayo Clinic Diet?

The Mayo Clinic Diet, a long-term weight management program created by a team of weight-loss experts at Mayo Clinic, is a lifestyle approach to weight loss that can help you maintain a healthy weight for a lifetime.

According to Mayo Clinic, among the benefits of a Mayo Clinic Diet are:

- Personalized Mayo Clinic-approved meal plans and recipes
- A diet you can stick with for life, not a fad or quick fix
- Dropping unhealthy lifestyle habits and gaining healthy ones
- Enjoying the types and amounts of food featured in the diet, including lots of fruits and vegetables
- Eating low-energy-dense foods that can help you lose weight by feeling full on fewer calories
- Meal plan options that include healthy Keto, higher protein, Vegetarian, and Mediterranean
- Healthy choices in each of the other food groups in moderate amounts make up the rest of the pyramid, including whole-grain carbohydrates, lean sources of protein, and heart-healthy unsaturated fats
- Increasing your physical activity daily for good health
- Knowing the natural sugar in fruits affecting your carbohydrate intake

VII. The Ornish Diet

#3, Best Heart-Healthy Diets, tied with Flexitarian Diet

What Is an Ornish Diet?

The Ornish Diet is a low-fat, lacto-ovo-vegetarian diet intended to promote weight loss and reverse the progression of chronic diseases such as prostate cancer, heart disease, and diabetes.

It is a plan developed by Dr. Dean Ornish, a physician, researcher, and founder of the Preventive Medicine Research Institute, in Sausalito, California.

The Ornish Diet tied with the Mediterranean Diet in the Heart-Healthy Diets category for the No. 1 position.

Plant-Based Foods

The plan focuses on plant-based foods such as:

- Whole grains
- Vegetables, legumes, fruits
- Soy products
- Limited amounts (4 grams) of high-fat foods like nuts, seeds, and vegetable oils
- Egg whites permitted
- Veggie burgers or whole-grain cereals in moderation, containing fewer than 3 grams of fat per serving
- Healthy fats of about 10% of the total daily calorie intake, mostly from fats in whole foods, such as legumes and whole grains
- Up to two daily servings of non-fat products, like animal milk and yogurt, or soy yogurt, and milk
- Three or fewer servings of foods like nuts and seeds per day

Note. The Ornish Diet does not include meat, poultry, fish, and any products made from these foods.

Benefits of Ornish Diet

- Aids in weight loss
- Helps in the prevention or treatment of chronic diseases, such as diabetes, kidney disease, heart disease, and different types of cancers
- Lowers levels of total cholesterol, triglycerides, LDL (bad) cholesterol, and inflammation in the body, all of which are risk factors for heart disease *(Trusted Source)*

VIII. The Nordic Diet

What Is the Nordic Diet?

The Nordic diet based on cuisine in Nordic countries, emphasizes cutting out processed foods and most high-fat meats like hot dogs, sausage, and bacon.

The diet focuses on fatty fish such as salmon, mackerel, herring, berries and other fruits, beans, nuts, seeds, legumes, leafy vegetables, and root vegetables, such as white or sweet potatoes and carrots and whole grains.

This diet features the local and seasonal foods from the Nordic region, Norway, Sweden, Denmark, Iceland, and Finland.

Benefits of the Nordic Diet

- Reduces LDL (bad) cholesterol
- Improves insulin resistance
- Promotes weight loss

X. The MIND Diet

#3, Best Plant-Based Diets

What Is the MIND Diet?

The MIND diet which stands for Mediterranean-DASH Intervention for Neurodegenerative Delay (but later changed to the DASH Diet), was developed by a team of researchers led by Martha Clare Morris, a nutritional epidemiologist at the Rush University Medical Center in Chicago, Illinois.

Specifically, the diet reduces the risk of dementia for older people, including Alzheimer's disease and a decline in brain functions.

9 Foods to Eat on the MIND Diet

- **Whole grains:** Include brown rice, black rice, quinoa, whole-wheat pasta, whole-wheat bread, barley, and steel-cut oats. You should eat at least 3 servings per day.
- **Green and leafy vegetables**: You may include kale, lettuce, spinach, collard greens, and salads. Have at least six or more servings of these veggies.
- **Nuts**: The nuts may include walnuts, almonds, pistachios, and cashews--at least 5 servings per week.
- The MIND diet deviates from the Mediterranean and DASH diet because it restricts the type and amount of fruits and vegetables, specifying eating berries but not other fruits.
- **Fish:** Choose fatty fish, such as tuna, trout, salmon, and mackerel, because of the omega-3 fatty acids they contain. Eat fish at least once every week.
- **Beans or legumes:** Eat at least 4 servings per week. Specifically, the diet encourages eating beans that may include kidney beans, pinto beans, chickpeas, lentils, peas, or soybeans in at least 4 meals per week.
- **Poultry**: You may eat chicken or turkey (but not the fried ones) at least two times a week.
- **Olive oil:** Use olive oil as your primary cooking oil.

- **Wine:** It is best to drink red wine, which has resveratrol compounds, because this may prevent you from having Alzheimer's disease. But white wine is okay, too. You must consume at least one glass of wine per day.

Benefits of the Mind Diet

- . Reduces the body's so-called oxidative stress and inflammation
- Decreases the potentially harmful beta-amyloid protein (protein fragments found in the body), resulting in increased brain health function
- Losing weight and lowering blood pressure, cholesterol, and triglycerides were shown in a study conducted at the Harokokia University in Athens, Greece

X. The Keto Diet

#1, Best Fast Weigh-Loss Diets

What Is the Keto Diet or Ketogenic Diet?

According to *Healthline,* "The keto diet is a low carb, high fat diet. It lowers blood sugar and insulin levels and shifts the body's metabolism away from carbs and toward fat and ketones."

It adds: "It involves drastically reducing carbohydrate intake and replacing it with fat. This reduction in carbs puts your body into a metabolic state called ketosis."

As a result, your body becomes effective at burning fat for energy.

Different Types of Ketogenic Diet The targeted ketogenic diet (TKD):

The Ketogenic Diet has several versions, including:

- **The standard ketogenic diet (SKD)**: It typically contains 75% fat, 20% protein, and only 5% carbs. *(Trusted Source)*
- **The cyclical ketogenic diet (CKD):** This diet involves eating clean carbohydrates for one or two days out of the week. The five or six

days will then follow a standard ketogenic diet consisting of very low carbohydrates, moderate protein, and high fats.

- **The targeted ketogenic diet (TKD):** This diet allows you to add carbs around workouts. It's like a regular keto diet, except eating carbs around your workout times.
- **High-protein ketogenic diet:** Like a standard ketogenic diet, a high-protein diet simply means including more protein in this diet. The ratio is about 60% fat, 35% protein, and 5% carbs.

Right Foods for Keto Diet

- **Red meat and poultry:** Beef, pork, lamb, venison, chicken, & turkey
- **Seafood:** Tuna, trout, salmon, sardines, mackerel, clams, oysters, octopus, and mussels
- **Eggs:** Preferably pastured or omega-3 whole eggs
- **Nuts and seeds:** Good fats to include in a keto diet
- **Healthy oils:** Extra virgin oil, and avocado oil
- **Low-carb vegetables:** Non-starchy veggies include green leafy vegetables, such as kale, spinach, cauliflower, broccoli, etc.
- **Berries:** Blueberries, raspberries, and strawberries
- **Drinks:** Water (No. 1 option), unsweetened coffee or tea, dark chocolate, and cocoa,

Benefits of Ketogenic Diet

- Significant reduction of blood sugar and the improvement of insulin sensitivity by 75% (Trusted Source)
- Beneficial to patients with diabetes, cancer, epilepsy, and Alzheimer's diseases *(Trusted Source).*

Chapter 12

Semi-Plant-Based Diet: Best for Meat Eaters with T2D, CKD, & Heart Disease

Brief Subject Summary

- What Are Plant-Based Diets?
- Popular Plant-Based Diets in the U.S.
- What They Say About Plant-based Diets?
- Why Do Many Japanese Reach the Age of 100 and Over?
- The Okinawa Diet
- Principles of Plant-Based Diets
- Plant Foods with Complete or Nearly Complete Protein Sources
- Focusing on Plant Proteins
- Plant-Based Diets: Good for Diabetes, Kidney, Disease, and Heart Disease
- My Semi-Plant-Based Diet
- You Are What You Eat

What Are Plant-Based Diets?

The Plant-based diets focus on limiting or avoiding eating red meat, animal products, and processed foods such as hot dogs, bacon, sausage, and canned meats.

The vegetarian or vegan diets limit or avoid all animal foods, depending on which diet. But you don't have to be a vegan or a vegetarian to enjoy eating plant-based foods with certain adjustments, you can eat meat with whole grains, fruits, legumes, vegetables, nuts, and seeds, which all come from plants.

For instance, the Flexitarian Diet, a semi-vegetarian diet, advocates a style of eating a few meals with meat in a week. My diet, which I call my semi-plant-based diet, is discussed later in this chapter.

Most Popular Plant-Based Diets in the U.S.

The most popular plant-based diets in the U.S. include:

- The Mediterranean Diet
- The Flexitarian Diet
- The Vegetarian Diet
- The DASH Diet
- The Ornish Diet
- The Vegan Diet
- The Mayo Clinic Diet

Clarification: My Semi-Plant-Based Diet

While many plant-based diets involve diets similar to Vegetarian and Vegan diets, I use a semi-plant-based diet and I recommend it for meat eaters.with diabetes, kidney disease, and heart disease.

My semi-plant diet consists of 70% plant-based foods and 30% animal foods. Why? Because I have loved meat since I was a little boy. I cannot eliminate meat from my diet, so I created my own style of eating. A semi-plant-based works for me. And I'm confident that it will work for you, too.

However for the purpose of discussion, let's talk about plant-based diets.

Do Plant-Based Diets Work?

Studies have shown that plant-based diets are healthy and good for diabetes, kidney disease, and heart disease.

That means to say that meat eaters should include a lot of vegetables, legumes, and fruits their their diets

Here's What They Say About Plant-Based Diets

Plant-Based Diets Are Associated With a Lower Risk of Cardiovascular Morbidity...

https://www.ahajournals.org/doi/10.1161/JAHA.119.012865

by H Kim · 2019 — Plant-based diets, diets that emphasize higher intakes of plant foods and lower intakes of animal foods are associated with a lower risk of cardiovascular morbidity and mortality in a general population.

National Institute of Health PMC Website

CFR Cardiac Failure Review

A Review of Plant-Based Diets to Prevent and Treat Heart Failure

https://www.ncbi.nim.nih.gov/pmc/articles/PMD5971679//

Conor P Kerly, in a study published on the website PMC of the National Institute of Health, concludes:

"The existing but limited human evidence suggests that a plant-based diet rich in fruit, vegetables, legumes, and whole grains is likely beneficial. The role of nuts, dairy, and poultry is controversial, while red/processed meats, eggs, and refined carbohydrates appear to be detrimental."

Why Do Many Japanese Reach the Age of 100 and Over?

Many centenarians live in Okinawa, the largest island of the Ryukyu Islands in Japan. It is called the "Island of Immortals." No, they have not found the fountain of youth; yet the elders of Okinawa island seem to know the secrets to a long, happy living.

The Okinawa Diet: 96% Plant-Based Diet

The Okinawa Diet has gained international fame as many people worldwide have been trying to adopt this diet. And reach the age of 100 and above.

The diet pertains to the traditional eating ways and lifestyle of the Okinawan inhabitants. Their traditional diet is low in calories and fat but high in carbs. The people eat a lot of vegetables, especially sweet potatoes and soy products, like tofu. However, they also eat other foods in small portions.

In a nutshell, the super-food rich cuisine diet involves eating:

- Locally available fresh and raw vegetables, such as sweet potato, bamboo shoots, radish, Chinese okra, pumpkin, papaya, and bitter melon
- Grains (33%): Rice, millet, wheat, and noodles
- Soy products, such as tofu, miso, natto, and edamame, which account for a larger portion of their meals for centuries
- Fish, noodles, and pork, in small portions
- Medicinal herb-rich foods
- Daily drinking of a lot of green tea, turmeric tea, and Jasmine tea, known as sanpin-cha, an antioxidant-rich form of Jasmine green tea.

The Okinawan Diet

The Okinawan Diet focuses on eating more low glycemic foods and less high glycemic foods. Heart disease, stroke, and cancer, the leading causes of death of people in the West, also occur in Okinawans but with the lowest frequency worldwide.

Centenarian Study Investigator

Dr. Craig Willcox, Professor of Gerontology and co-principal Investigator of the Okinawa Centenarian Study, says, “the Japanese diet, particularly the Okinawa diet, has always been a healthy diet.”

Dr. Willcox has been living in Okinawa and studying centenarians since 1994.

68 centenarians in Okinawa, Japan

For every 100,000 inhabitants, Okinawa has 68 centenarians – more than three times the numbers found in U.S. populations of the same size.

The Oldest Person in the World

Because of the traditional Japanese diet, it's not surprising that the current oldest person in the world, Kane Tanaka was born on Jan. 2, 1903. She celebrated her 118th birthday in southwestern Japan on Saturday, January 2, 2021, where she currently lives in her nursing home.

She was born in the former village of Wajiro, now part of the city of Fukuoka, Japan where she was born.

At her age, she still exercises, does calculations, and plays Reversi, a card game. When asked about her secret to living a long life, Tanaka replied, "Eating delicious food and studying." She aims to live up to 120.

On March 9, 2019, The Guinness World Records presented Tanaka with two certificates, the "World's Oldest Living Person"and "World's Oldest Living Woman" titles, at the age of 116 years old.

According to Guinness World Records, Jeanne Calment, from Arles, France, was the oldest person who ever lived. She died at the age of 122 years and 164 days old.

Oldest Person in America

According to the Gerontology Research Group, Thelma Sutcliffe became the U.S. oldest living person and seventh-oldest in the world on April 17, 2021, when Hester Ford, a 115-year-old woman, died in North Carolina.

Sutcliffe was 115 years and 108 days old at the time of her death on January 21, 2022.

Her secret to long life? A friend of her said Sutcliffe didn't believe in worrying at all. She resided in an assisted living facility in Omaha, Nebraska.

Luella "Lou" Mason said her friend had been in hospice care when she died. "She passed very peacefully", she said.

Principles of Plant-Based Diets

The principles of a plant diet may include the following features:

- Focuses on plants, including vegetables, fruits, whole grains, legumes, seeds, and nuts, emphasizing whole, minimally processed foods
- Limits or avoids animal products
- Promotes locally sourced and organic food whenever possible
- Recommends mostly plant-based proteins (especially for kidney disease patients)
- Eliminates refined foods with added sugar, white flour, and processed oils, such as margarine
- Encourages intake of healthy fats, such as extra-virgin oil, avocado oil, and avocado (whole)

Foods to Eat on a Plant-Based Diet

- **Whole grains**: Brown rice, black rice, red rice, barley, amaranth, etc.
- **Fruits**: Berries (blueberries and blackberries, pears, citrus, fruits, peaches, bananas, and pineapples
- **Non-starchy vegetables**: Green leafy vegetables, such as kale, spinach, tomatoes, broccoli, cauliflower, and asparagus
- **Starchy vegetables**: Roots or tubers, such as white potatoes and sweet potatoes
- **Legumes**: Peas, chickpeas, lentils, peanuts, and black beans
- **Healthy fats**: Extra virgin oil, avocado oil, and coconut oil
- **Seeds:** Nuts and nut butter of almonds, cashews, macadamia nuts, pumpkin seeds, chia seeds, sunflower seeds, and natural peanut butter
- **Unsweetened plant-based milk**: Soy milk, coconut milk, and almond milk
- **Spices, herbs, and seasonings**: Salt, vinegar, lemon (whole) or juice, sesame oil, turmeric, curry, and black pepper
- **Plant-based protein**: Tofu, tempeh, plant-based protein sources, or powders with no added sugar or artificial ingredients
- **Beverages**: Coffee, tea, and sparkling water

If you want to supplement your plant-based diet with 30% to 40% animal foods, you may choose the following:

- **Eggs**: Any chicken eggs, but pasture-raised is preferable, if available
- **Beef and pork**: Pastured or grass-fed when possible
- **Chicken and turkey:** (Organic if available)
- **Seafood**: Wild-caught seafood from sustainable fisheries if available
- **Dairy:** Organic dairy products if available
- **Natural sweeteners**: SweetLeaf Stevia, zero-carbohydrate, certified-paleo, and non-glycemic-response sweetener)

Foods to Limit or Avoid

- **Refined grains**: White rice, white pasta, white bread, and bagels
- **Fast foods**: Hot dogs, sausage, French fries, hamburgers, and chicken nuggets
- **Packaged foods**: Chips, crackers, cereal bars, and frozen dinners
- **Foods with added sugars and sweets**: Table sugar, soda, juice, sweet teas, pastries, cookies, candies, and sugary cereals
- **Refined grains**: White rice, bagels, pasta, and white bread
- **Processed animal products**: Lunch meats, sausages, bacon, corned beef, and lunch meat
- **Processed vegan-friendly foods**: Plant-based meats like veggie burgers and vegan butter

Benefits of a Plant-Based Diet

There are many benefits of a plant-based diet, whichever plant-based diet you are following:

- Causes weight loss (especially if you are obese)
- Lowers blood pressure that decreases the chance of kidney disease or heart disease, or slows the progression of any disease, if you already have it
- Improves cholesterol levels, lowering bad LDL (bad cholesterol) and triglyceride levels and raising HDL (good cholesterol)

- Diminishes the risk of prediabetes and type 2 diabetes or slows, stabilizes, or reverses diabetes; if you are diabetic
- Decreases risk of kidney disease, or slows, stabilizes, and reverses diabetic kidney disease

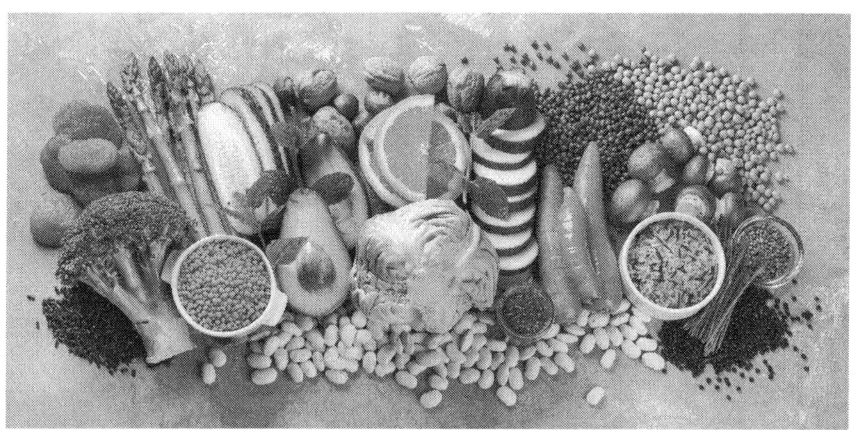

Different Plant-Based Foods

Photo Source: Shutterstock

Plant-Based Foods With Complete or Nearly Complete Protein Sources

If you have kidney disease, it's wise to limit the intake of animal products, especially those with high protein and creatine, whose waste product is creatinine.

When you eat meat, especially red meat or fish with high protein and creatine, you'll be eating a lot of creatine, thus giving you an elevated creatinine level, the byproduct.

For example, go to Chapter 15, and see the list of species of fish that have high protein and creatine.

The Importance of Proteins

Proteins are one of the macronutrients your body needs to form muscles and build and repair tissues. Also, they transport nutrients for the cells of all living things, including you and me. There are two classes of proteins, the complete protein and the incomplete protein.

What is a complete protein? Any food is considered a complete protein with the nine essential amino acids that the body cannot produce. The body naturally makes 13 amino acids, but you should eat nine others (as mentioned below) in your diet.

Focusing on Plant Proteins

Yes, animal foods provide the best sources of complete protein. In general, plants technically do not give complete proteins. However, there are exceptions. You can also combine incomplete plant food proteins to make them complete proteins.

Many plant foods also can provide complete proteins for vegans, vegetarians, and flexitarians (semi-vegetarians).

They are also sources of non-meat proteins such as fish, eggs, and dairies. If you don't eat them, you can also focus on soy products, such as tofu, soy yogurt, and soy milk.

Plants With High Proteins

There are several plants that provide high protein, including:

- Quinoa
- Buckwheat
- Amaranth
- Oats (Steel-cut oats, rolled oats or old fashioned, and instant oats)
- Soy products
- Lentils
- Spirulina
- Mycoprotein
- Seitan

The Benefits of Soy Products

Toby Smithson, on behalf of the Academy of Nutrition and Dietitians, cites the benefits of consuming soy products. In particular, she says, "It is absolutely safe to eat soy foods if you have diabetes. Soy foods can be used in the diet as a protein and carbohydrate source. Soy is a heart-healthy food which is an additional benefit for people with diabetes."

She adds, "In fact, there is a study that found that when soy foods replaced high saturated fat foods like red meat, cholesterol and inflammation were decreased, and insulin sensitivity was increased."

My Journey: How Semi-Plant-Based Diet Works

I'm following my semi-plant-based diet. Basically, like the Flexitarian Diet, it's flexible. I call it a semi-plant-based diet because I'm eating more plant foods than animal foods: the ratio being 70% plant foods to 30% animal foods.

If you wish, you might select a diet that you enjoy eating from the following options or ratios:

- *70% plant foods vs. 30% animal products*
- *60% plant foods vs. 40% animal products*
- *50% plant foods vs. 50% animal foods*

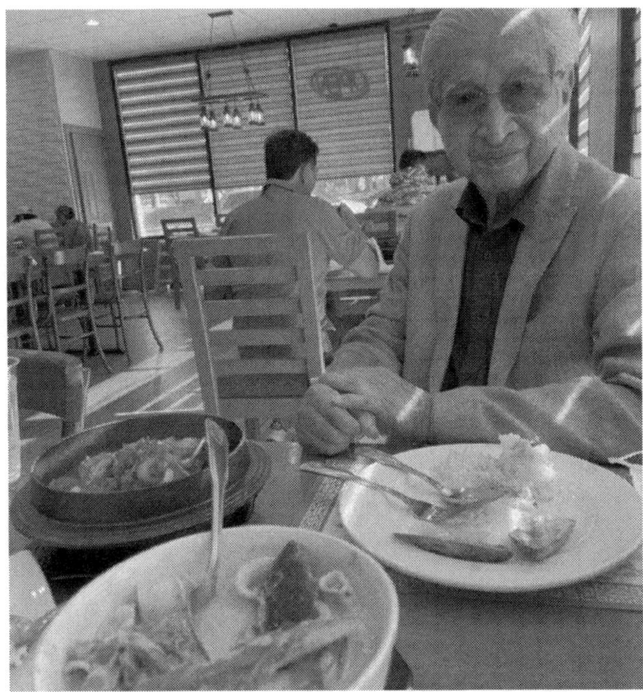

The Author About to Eat His Semi-Plant-Based Meal

Photo Credit: Shutterstock

While Flexitarians eat small portions of meat on certain days of the week, I eat portions of slices or pieces of meat every day, at least in one meal or two meals. Of course, if I eat one egg in the morning with gluten-free whole grains bread, I may eat chicken or pork mixed and small portions of vegetables, small amounts of beans and nuts for lunch or dinner.

My Kidney Disease Journey

I force myself to eat more plant foods than animal foods; that's why my creatinine blood level always remains at about 1 mg/dL, an average number. Remember, plants have no creatine that becomes creatinine, a waste product, upon cooking.

According to Mayo Clinic, the typical ranges for serum creatinine are: For adult men, 0.74 to 1.35 mg/dL (65.4 to 119.3 micromoles/L) For adult women, 0.59 to 1.04 mg/dL (52.2 to 91.9 micromoles/L).

Note: Normal serum creatinine values vary from laboratory to laboratory.

Days to Remember

As mentioned in Chapter 7, my GFR numbers plunged to 35% or (Stage 3b) on Sept, 21, 2016. But the numbers rebounded in 2020 to 73% (Stage 2): Mild decrease in GFR (60-89 mL/min/1.73 m 2), the year that I reversed, stabilized, and put kidney disease into remission. A blood test on July 19, 2022 showed that my GFR was 73%. To this day, my kidney disease is still in remission.

Plant-Based Diets: Good for Diabetes, Kidney Disease, and Heart Disease

As I have said, the kidneys have a harder time processing animal proteins than plant proteins. Plant proteins are suitable for kidney disease because they can lower your blood pressure and saturated fats intake. High blood pressure can damage the kidney more which may lead to end-stage kidney failure.

If you have heart disease, you need to reduce your cholesterol and triglycerides. So by eating more plant foods instead of animal products that contain saturated fats, you'll lower your risk for heart and other cardiovascular diseases.

You Are What You Eat!

The proverbial phrase, "You Are What You Eat," still rings up these days, although the words appeared in a book many, many years ago.

The first mention of the words came from the 1826 work, *Physiologie du Gourt, ou Medetations de Gastronomie Transcendante*, by French author Anthelme Brillat-Savarin, and translated into English, "*Tell me what you eat and I will tell you what you are.*"

Knowing the importance of a plant-based diet may be your key to a long, happy, and prosperous life on Earth. What a wonder!

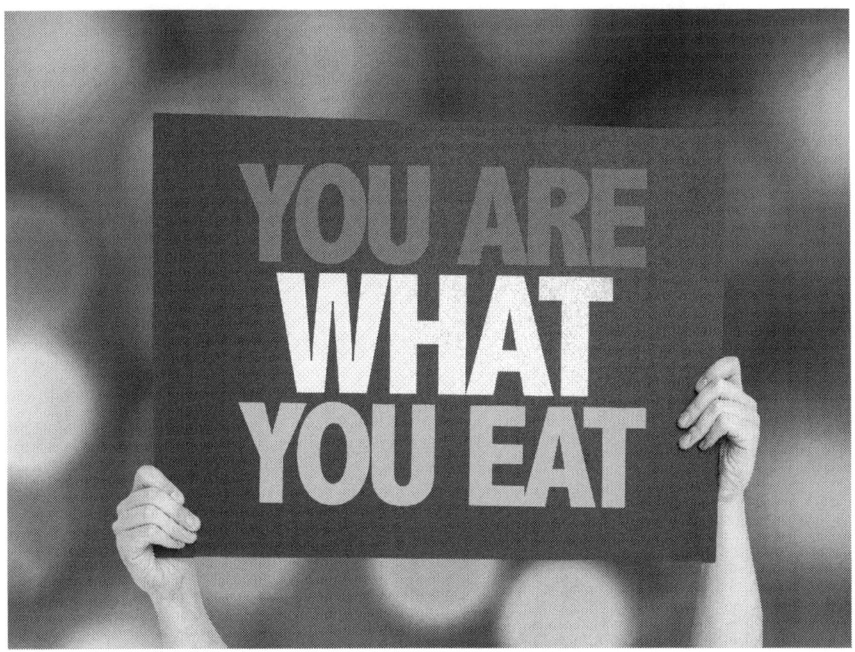

You Are What You Eat Photo Credit: Shutterstock)

Chapter 13

Foods: Eat These, Not Those!

Brief Subject Summary

- What Is the Glycemic Index (GI)?
- What Is the Glycemic Load (GL)?
- The Glycemic Index (GI) Limitations
- The Glycemic Load (GL) Advantage
- Table of Low Glycemic Load Fruits
- Low Glycemic Load of Vegetables and Nuts
- Glycemic Load of Cereal Grains
- Other GI and GL Foods
- Calculation of GL Values
- How to Choose Diabetic Foods
- Where to Find Glycemic Index (GI) and Glycemic Load (GL) Values of Foods?
- Different Kinds of Foods
- Foods with High-Fructose Corn Syrup to Limit or Avoid
- Foods with High Glycemic Index to Limit or Avoid
- Low-Carb Alternatives to White Rice
- Nuts and Seeds

What are the best foods to eat and the worst foods to limit or avoid? It will be a challenge for you if you have diabetes. But you can work on learning the right ways to choose foods to control blood sugar and slow, stabilize, or put your disease into remission.

How? By using the glycemic index (GI) or glycemic load (GL) values of foods. There are two ways to measure the effect of grains, vegetables, and fruits on blood sugar after being eaten: the GI and the GL scales.

In summary, you have to eat low glycemic (GI) and glycemic load (GL) values of foods to be able to stop, reverse, stabilize, and put prediabetes or type 2 diabetes into remission.

I. The Glycemic Index and the Glycemic Load

What Is the Glycemic Index?

The glycemic index (GI) scale indicates how rapidly a carbohydrate digests and gets released as glucose (sugar) into your bloodstream after a meal, based on a scale of 0 to 100.

In other words, the GI measures the blood glucose-raising potential of the carbohydrate content of a food. Foods with high GI raise blood sugar more than foods with low to medium GI.

You can classify carbohydrate-containing foods into the following categories:

- Low GI: 55 or less
- Moderate GI: 56-69
- High GI: >70

Who Created the Glycemic Index?

The glycemic index (GI) was developed in 1981 by Dr. Thomas Wolever and Dr. David Jenkins at the University of Toronto in Canada.

It's a tool for measuring how quickly a food containing 25 or 50 grams of carbohydrate raises blood glucose levels in the bloodstream after a meal.

The Glycemic Index (GI) Limitations

You may use the GI because it has a role in determining the GL of any food. But it has limitations, including:

- The glycemic index only concerns the relative rise of blood glucose after a meal.
- The glycemic index of different foods can vary according to several factors. An example is a particular cooking preparation method used.

- The glycemic response to sugar in certain foods varies among individuals.
- The GI is a relative measure that does not consider the number of carbohydrates in foods. For example, how many grams of carbohydrates per serving of a particular food.

What Is the Glycemic Load?

The glycemic load (GL) is a ranking system for carbohydrate-rich foods that measures the number of carbohydrates in a food serving.

The scale takes cognizance of the planned portion size of foods. The net grams of a carbohydrate content meal are carbohydrates minus the fiber, which the body can not digest and does not affect blood glucose levels, thus decreasing the total carbohydrates.

Typically, some foods have a low carbohydrate content. Because of this fact and the glycemic index concept limitations, Harvard University researchers Liu et al. created the Glycemic Load (GL).

This concept gives cognizance to the number of carbohydrates in a serving of foods to provide useful information.

In other words, the glycemic response to an ingested food is based not only on the GI but also on the total amount of carbohydrates consumed.

The glycemic response can lead to the concept of glycemic load. The glycemic response refers to the effect the food will have on blood glucose after being eaten.

Sydney University in Australia has its international table of GI and GL values of foods in its database on its website:

www.glycemicindex.com.

Glycemic Load System

The glycemic load system is categorized as follows:

- Low GL: 1 to 10
- Medium GL: 11 to 19
- High GL: 20 or more

In simple words, foods with a glycemic load (GL) under 10 are considered low-GL foods and have little impact on your blood sugar.

Those foods whose GL are between 11 and 19 are considered moderate GL foods that impact blood sugar. Those foods above 20 GI cause blood sugar spikes or surges.

With this system, you'll know the carbohydrate content of particular foods. The measurement will be in grams per serving, grams per 1 cup or 1/2 cup per serving, or grams per medium-sized fruit. Thus, GL gives a more real-world value of how a specific food can affect blood sugar levels.

The GI and GL Partnership

It is mentioned in Chapter 10 that there are six essential nutrients for the body's functions, involving macronutrients and micronutrients.

The macronutrients: carbohydrates, proteins, and fats should be included in each meal if you want to have a balanced diet and become healthy.

If you eat high-carb foods, spikes of blood sugar may occur. Proteins have minimal effects on blood glucose, and fats almost do not affect blood sugar.

There are at least four schools of thought on decreasing carb content and successfully managing your diabetes, or they may be a combination of all the following scales:

- 1. The glycemic index (GI)
- 2. Both GI and GL value systems
- 3. Carbohydrate counting
- 4. Fiber counting (to be deducted from total carbs)

The Glycemic Load (GL) Advantage

The GL, a ranking system for carbohydrate-rich foods that measures the net carbohydrates in a food serving, has an advantage over GI.

What advantage? The glycemic load helps determine how different portions of other foods affect blood sugar. The GL scale can not be known without the GI.

The Formula for Determining the GL Value

In calculating the GL value, you must use both the glycemic index and the available carbohydrate content in grams.

Mathematically, GL = GI × available carbohydrate (g) divided by 100.

(Where available carbohydrate = total carbohydrate - dietary fiber = net carbs. A unit of GL approximates the glycemic effect of 1 g of glucose.)

If you want to know a food's glycemic load value, multiply the GI by the number of carbohydrate grams in a serving. Then divide the number by 100 = GL.

As already mentioned, a low GL is between 1 and 10, a moderate GL is 11 to 19, and a high GL is 20 or higher. If you have diabetes, you would want to have a low-glycemic load food to eat.

Here is a classic example of the fruit watermelon, which contains fast-releasing carbohydrates, with a high GI of 72. Yet, a 100-gram serving of watermelon contains only 5 grams of available carbohydrates (because the rest of the fruit is mainly water).

Example: Use a cup per serving of watermelon.

To know the net carbs, search on the internet the net carbs of a serving of watermelon. Here, it is: A 1/2 cup of diced watermelon has 152g and a net carb of 5.5.

Multiply the GI of 72 by the net carbs of 5.5 and divided by 100.

Therefore:

72 x 5.5 = 396 divided by 100 = 3.96 or GL of 4 to round it up.

So watermelon is a low GL food, providing lots of vitamin A, vitamin C, beta-carotene, and lycopene, which reduces the risk of several forms of cancer. If you wish to make it up as a 1 cup serving, you double the figure. In this case, the GL will undoubtedly goes up.

Per servings of food are allowed by the GL system. You can increase or decrease the servings in contrast to the GI system.

You should not avoid some high-GI foods, partnering with low GL food. Why? Because most high-GI foods contain a lot of healthy nutrients for the body.

Though watermelon is a low GL food, your blood glucose will spike if you eat 2 or more servings. So you may think of eliminating watermelon because it's tempting to eat it: it's sweet and refreshing.

As you can see from this example, sometimes, what is considered high glycemic fruit can still be a healthy snack that will barely affect your blood sugar. But it depends on the amount of serving.

This case is not typical, as most foods with a high GI will have a correspondingly high GL.

Lesson: Sometimes, it is best to use the combination of the GI and the net carbs in a particular food. This way, you can have quantity and quality carbohydrate foods to manage your blood sugar successfully.

Advocates of the Use of the Glycemic Load System

Harvard University says, "The glycemic index tells just part of the story. What it does not tell you is how high your blood sugar could go up when you eat the food. To understand a food's effect on blood sugar, you need to know both how quickly it makes glucose enter the bloodstream."

It adds, "A separate measure called the glycemic load does both — which gives you a more accurate picture of a food's real-life impact on your blood sugar."

On the other hand, Krista Wennerstrom, RD, food and nutrition services director at Thorek Memorial Hospital in Chicago, Illinois, has this to say about glycemic load:

"Calculating the glycemic load (GL) can provide an even more accurate picture of what that food will do to your blood sugar."

For its part, www.glycemicindex.com reports that based on the management of diabetes from major diabetes organizations around the world, it advises people with type 1 and type 2 diabetes to use the GI or GL as part of the nutritional management of this condition.

Based on the management of diabetes by several world diabetes organizations, www.glycemicindex.com, for now, advises people with type 1 and type 2 diabetes to use the GI or GL as part of their condition's nutritional management.

Such organizations are the American Diabetes Association, Canadian Diabetes, and Diabetes UK.

The Glycemic Index Website

The www.glycemicndex.com is the official website for the international GI database based at the Boden Institute of Obesity, Nutrition, Exercise and Eating Disorders and Charles Perkins Centre at the University of Sydney in Australia.

The database contains both the glycemic index and the glycemic load of thousands of foods. All those listed have been researched and tested. Of course, thousands of foods have not yet been tested and included in the database: (http://glycemicindex.com/about.php).

Even the World Health Organization (WHO) gives qualified support for the GI-GL concept.

The Combination of GI and GL Scales!

I'm using both the glycemic index (GI) and glycemic load (GL) concepts in creating my meal plan. They are partners. I won't know the GL values without having the GI value. And I can't rely on the GI alone; it has limitations, as cited in the early part of this chapter.

I know that the GL scale is not a perfect system for selecting healthy foods. To reiterate, the GL, for me, is the final judge. I follow its recommendation by experts. It would be best if you did the same.

Of course, it is up to you to follow the GI alone, consuming low glycemic index foods. If you use both scales, you can determine the quantity and quality of healthy foods.

Bottom line: You have to use common sense in selecting quality foods for your health.

How to Choose Diabetic Foods

As mentioned in Chapter 10, there are six essential nutrients for the body's functions involving macronutrients and micronutrients.

If you want to have a balanced diet and become healthy, you should include macronutrients, carbohydrates, proteins, and fats.

If you have prediabetes, type 2 diabetes, or type 1 diabetes, high amounts of carbohydrates will significantly impact sugar or glucose in the bloodstream after a meal.

Spikes in blood sugar may occur if you eat high carbs foods. Proteins have a moderate effect on carbohydrates, and fats almost do not affect blood sugar.

Because of this, you must have a diet plan, select low-carbohydrate foods for diabetes. And, of course, limit or avoid the highly processed foods with too much carb content that causes sugar spikes. It's because carbohydrates turn into glucose when digested.

You can pinpoint the refined carbohydrates that may cause blood glucose spikes after a meal with the GI and GL concepts.

You can increase or decrease GL value by adjusting the carbohydrate content of foods by eliminating most of the meal's carbohydrates.

Moreover, calculating the glycemic load (GL) can provide an even more accurate determination of what a particular food will do to your blood sugar.

Different Bodies, Different Reactions

Different bodies react differently to various foods. We cannot avoid some high carbohydrate foods because sometimes, they are more nutritious and healthy.

You can increase or decrease GL value by adjusting the carbohydrate content of foods per serving or eliminating most of the meal's carbohydrates.

Moreover, calculating the glycemic load (GL) can provide you an even more accurate determination of what a particular food will do to your blood sugar after eating it.

Low-Glycemic Vegetables

- Cabbage
- Bok choy
- Mushrooms
- Lettuce
- Brussels sprouts
- Broccoli
- Cauliflower
- Celery
- Eggplant
- Carrots
- Green peas
- Greens: Green beans, spinach, and kale.
- Hummus
- Different kinds of beans (pinto, black, kidney, and lima beans, plus black-eyed peas

Low-Glycemic Fruits (If Eaten in Small Amounts)

- Cranberries
- Strawberries
- Oranges
- Blueberries
- Apples

Low-Glycemic Grains

- Whole grain pasta
- Sourdough bread
- Wheat tortilla
- Oat bran and rice bran cereals

Low-Glycemic Dairy Products and Dairy-Substitute Products

- Skim, low-fat, and whole milk
- Plain yogurt
- Cheese
- Soy milk and yogurt

Low-Glycemic Legumes

- Tofu
- Hummus
- Lentils
- Edamame
- Split beans

Now, let's compute using both the GL and GI combination system.

Formula to get the glycemic load (GL): Multiply the GI by the net carbs and divide the amount by 100 = GL.

Grains

Here are the GI and GL of 5 varieties of rice:
(Based on 1 cup serving)

GI-GL Values Based on 1 cup serving, 100g, cooked
White Rice: GI 72 x (29g net carbs) = GL 21
Brown Rice: GI 68 x (24g net carbs) = GL 16
Wild Rice: GI 53 x (21g net carbs) = GL 11
Basmati Rice: GI 50-58 x (25g net carbs) = GL 12.5 - GL 14.5

Black Rice: GI 42 x (34g net carbs) = GL 14.28

Calculation of GL Values

White Rice: GI 72 GL 21

Multiply the GI 72 by 29g net carbs = g (2,088) and divide it by 100 = 20.88 GL. So the GL is 20.88 or 21 to round it up.

Brown Rice: GI 68 GL 16

Multiply GI 68 by 24g net carbs = 1,632 and divide the amount by 100 = 16 GL

Wild Rice: GI 53 GL 11

Multiply GI 53 by 21g net carbs = 1,113 and divide the amount by 100 = 11.13 GL or 11 GL to round up

Basmati Rice: GI 50-58 GI = GL 12.54 - GL 14.5

Multiply GI 50g (the lowest GI value among types of basmati rice) by 25 net carbs =1,261 and divide the amount by 100 = 12.5 GL.

Black Rice: GI 42 GL 14

Multiply GI 42 by 34g net carbs = 1,428 and divide the amount by 100 = 14.28 GL or 14 GL to round up.

The figures show that wild rice has the lowest value, GL 11. Thus, wild rice is a moderate or medium value grain.

However, wild rice is not considered true rice; it's a semi-aquatic grass that grows in abundance in North America's Great Lakes region. It has a firm texture and nutty flavor with black-colored grains.

The next lowest GL rice is basmati rice with 12.5 GL. The largest exporter of this rice is India, with Pakistan coming next.

On the other hand, jasmine and regular white rice (including "instant" white rice) are 72-89 GI.

The GL Value

With this system, you will know the glycemic load based on the glycemic index and the net carbohydrates. You will realize a more real-world value of how a specific food can affect blood sugar levels with the GL scale. In other words, the GL concept depends on two factors: the glycemic index (GI) and the serving size.

In other words, the GL concept depends on two factors: the glycemic index (GI) and the serving size.

You can increase or decrease GL value by adjusting the carbohydrate content of foods or eliminating most of the meal's carbohydrates.

Also, calculating the glycemic load (GL) can provide an even more accurate determination of what a particular food will do to your blood sugar levels.

The Usefulness of the GI and GL Values

Even if the glycemic GI scale is not a perfect system, it can help identify lower-glycemic foods with more nutrient-dense content.

Database of Glycemic Index (GI) and Glycemic Load (GL) Values

The lists of foods with their glycemic index and glycemic load values were first published in 2008 in the *Diabetes Care Journal* of the American Diabetes Associatio*n* by the author, Professor Jennie Brand-Miller, of the University of Sydney in Australia

Two websites that contain the glycemic index and glycemic load values of foods to access thousands of laboratory-tested foods worldwide are as follows:

www.mendosa.com/gilist.htm

To look for individual foods, you may visit:

www.glycemicindex.com

The University of Sydney in Australia maintains glycemicindex.com.

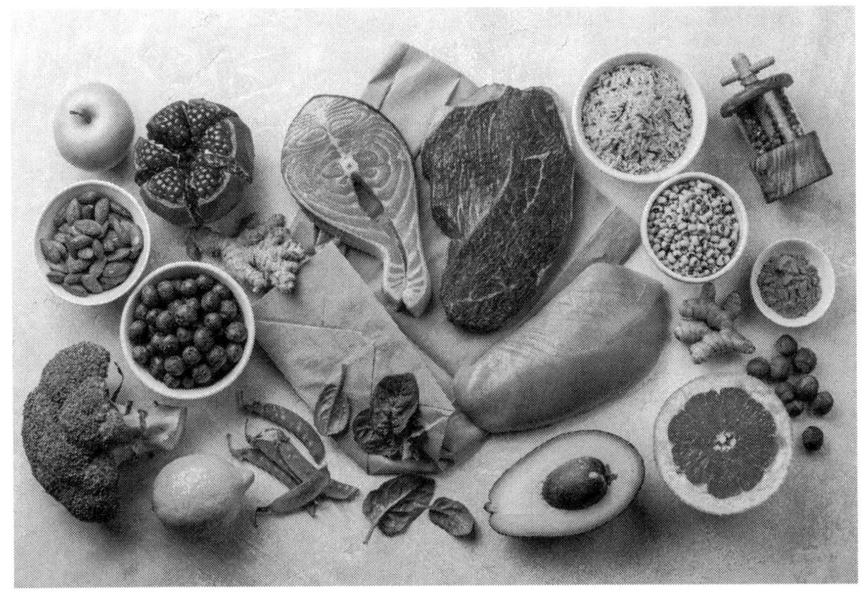

Different Kinds of Foods (Photo Credit: Shutterstock)

II. Different Kinds of Foods

1. Whole Grain Foods

Defining the phrase "whole grains," the Oldways Whole Grains Council says, "All grains start life as whole grains. In their natural state growing in the fields, whole grains are the entire seed of a plant."

Simply put, the seed, called a "kernel" (also called berry), comprises three parts: the bran, germ, and endosperm. An inedible husk covers the kernel, which contains fibers, and B vitamins. It protects the kernel from pests, disease, water, sunlight, and disease.

For a full description of a grain, see chapter 14: *Rice and Whole Grains Feed the World*.

Benefits of Eating Whole Grains

Generally, these are the benefits of eating whole grains:

1. **Fiber:** Whole grains contain a lot of fiber. Government guidelines say that adults need about 25 to 35 grams of daily fiber. Whole grains have two types, soluble and insoluble fibers, which are beneficial to bodily needs.

The fiber content keeps bowel movements regular, and whole grains may prevent diverticulitis that creates little pouches in the sigmoid colon.

2. **Vitamins, minerals, proteins, and antioxidants:** Besides containing vitamins, minerals, and proteins, whole grains also are packed with antioxidants, such as plant compounds of polyphenols, stanols, and sterols (*Trusted Source*).

3. **Lower risk of heart disease and stroke:** Whole grains lower cholesterol, triglycerides, and blood pressure. Whole grains prevent the body from absorbing "bad" or LDL cholesterol.

That's why whole grains reduce your risk of heart disease and stroke. They also regulate the blood sugar of people with diabetes.

4. **Lower risk of diabetes**: Eating whole grains in place of refined grains may lower your risk of type 2 diabetes.

5. **Lower cancer risk:** They may lower the risk of having certain cancers, including breast, colorectal, and pancreatic cancer. (Source: *Healthline).*

6. **Reduce chronic inflammation**: Some studies suggest that whole grains can help reduce inflammation. In one study, women who ate the most whole grains were least likely to die from inflammation-related chronic conditions (*Trusted Source, Healthline.*)

7. **Lower risk of obesity**: Whole grains and their products make your stomach fill up faster than refined grains. That's why research suggests that they may lower the risk of obesity.

Whole Grains Not for Everyone

While whole grains are considered healthy, they are not for everyone. For example, for people with Celiac Disease and gluten sensitivity, and those with Irritable Bowel Syndrome (IBS) and other digestive issues, whole grains can cause a range of symptoms.

Such symptoms include indigestion, bloating, constipation, stomach pain, and diarrhea.

In other words, people with gut issues should adjust or balance their intake of fiber and whole grains in their diet.

How Does Black Rice Stack Up?

Is black rice really a superior grain? Let's look at how it stacks up again other popular rice options.

1/4 Cup Uncooked	**Black Rice**	**White Rice**	**Brown Rice**	**Wild Rice**	**Quinoa**
Calories	160	170	170	**143**	156
Fat	1.5g	**0.5g**	1.3g	**0.5g**	2.6g
Carbs	35g	37g	36g	30.2	**27.3g**
Protein	5g	3g	3.5g	5.6g	**6g**
Fiber	2g	0g	2.7g	2.5g	**3g**
Potassium	**280mg**	53mg	119.9mg	142.8mg	239.3mg
Iron	4%	9%	11%	11%	**25%**
Calcium	**33mg**	13mg	15.3mg	4.2mg	20mg
Lysine	0.286 g	0.1g	0.1g	0.2mg	**0.3g**
Tryptophan	0.096 g	0.0g	0.0g	**0.1g**	**0.1g**
Magnesium	**143mg**	11.6mg	66.8mg	45.2mg	83.7mg
B2 (Riboflavin)	0.043 mg	0.1mg	0.1mg	0.1mg	0.1mg
B1 (Thiamine)	0.413 mg	0.1mg	**0.6mg**	0.1mg	0.2mg
B9 (Folic Acid)	20mcg	3.6mcg	6.1mcg	36.8mcg	**78.2mcg**

Among the types of rice, I like black rice. In fact, it has lower content of carbs than white and brown rice per 1 serving. It also has high magnesium content.

2. Animal Products: Best Sources of Protein

Protein is one of the macronutrients your body needs to form muscles and build and repair tissues. Also, it transports nutrients for the cells of all living things, including you and me. There are two types of protein: complete protein and incomplete protein.

The human body uses about 20 amino acids to build proteins. They are classified either as essential or non-essential.

The body can produce non-essential amino acids. However, it cannot produce essential amino acids; you have to obtain them from your diet.

Meat, fish, poultry, eggs, and dairy, are similar to the protein found in your body. They are all the essential amino acids your body needs to function properly.

On the other hand, plant protein sources, such as beans, lentils, and nuts, are considered incomplete. They don't have one or more of the essential amino acids needed by your body.

Animal foods provide the best sources of complete protein, but generally, plants technically do not give complete proteins, but there are exceptions. You can also combine incomplete plant food proteins to make them have complete proteins.

Many plant foods also can provide complete proteins for vegans, vegetarians, and flexitarians (semi-vegetarians).

There are also non-meat proteins such as fish, eggs, dairy (like milk, yogurt). If you don't eat them, you can also focus on soy products, such as tofu, soy yogurt, and soy milk.

3. Plant Foods (Whole Grains) with Complete or Nearly Complete Sources of Protein

Quinoa: Gluten-free and high in protein, quinoa is one of the most popular health foods. It has complete protein content. A pseudo-grain or pseudocereal, quinoa is a seed of a plant.

It has fiber, iron, potassium, calcium, phosphorus, magnesium, vitamin E, and B vitamins.

Buckwheat: Buckwheat is a plant cultivated for its grain-like seeds. Despite the name, buckwheat has no relation to wheat, as it is not grass.

Instead, buckwheat, a pseudocereal, is related to sorrel, knotweed, and rhubarb. Buckwheat groats (containing complete protein) are the seeds of a flowering plant.

Amaranth: Amaranth, like buckwheat, has been cultivated and eaten since 8,000 years ago.

Considered a staple food in the Inca, Maya, and Aztec civilizations, amaranth grains are classified as a pseudocereal.

What Are Oats?

All oats start as oat groats, meaning whole unbroken grains. After processing, the oats become steel-cut, rolled or old-fashioned, and instant oats, and Scottish oatmeal.

Whole Oat Groats: A whole groat oat has another name: grain kernel. Whole oat groats come from simply harvesting oats, cleaning them, and removing their inedible hull. They take the longest to cook.

These oats: groats, steel-cut, rolled or old-fashioned, and instant oats are whole grains. They come from the same seeds but differ in texture and flavor. Which one do you want? The choice is yours.

Steel-Cut Oats: Often referred to as Irish or Scottish oats, steel-cut oats manufacturers process the whole oat groats by chopping the whole oat groats into several pieces using thin-cutting blades. It looks almost like rice cut into pieces.

Rolled Oats or Old-Fashioned Oats: Made from oat groats with no more husk, manufacturers steam and roll them. Rolled oats are a type of lightly processed whole-grain food.

Instant Oats: Manufacturers fully process instant oats, more processed than old-fashioned and steel-cut oats. Precooked, dried, and then rolled, instant oats are processed thinner than rolled oats. They cook quicker than the rolled oats and steel-cut oats.

4. Soy Products

Soy products are the best sources of plant proteins.

Tofu, Tempeh, and Edamame

There are several plant products with protein made from soybeans. They include:

- Tofu
- Tempeh
- Nato
- Edamame
- Soy yogurt
- Soy milk
- Veggie burgers

Generally, soy products contain complete protein, including food products cited above.

Soybeans have all the nine essential amino acids for human growth and development. Because they contain all the essential amino acids, soybeans are considered complete protein foods.

Because of this, health experts say that by increasing dietary whole soy protein, you can:

- Lower your total level of cholesterol and raise your HDL level
- Reduce your risk of prostate and breast cancer
- Help maintain bone density and decrease fractures in postmenopausal women

5. Other Plants with Proteins

Lentils

Do lentils contain complete proteins? No. According to the Cleveland Clinic, various nuts, seeds, legumes, and whole grains can give you all the essential amino acids from them each day.

While lentils have no complete protein, they can be a complete protein if combined with other foods, such as rice. Put together, and these foods are an equal complete protein.

Spirulina

Spirulina is blue or green algae that have about 8 g of protein per tablespoon. It is rich in various nutrients, such as iron and B vitamins, although they do not have manganese and vitamin B12.

As a supplement, spirulina is available as a powder or a supplement in stores and on the internet.

Mycoprotein

A fungus-based protein, mycoprotein contains about 13g of protein per 1/2 cup of serving. As being advertised, products with mycoproteins are considered suitable meat substitutes.

Seitan

With complete proteins made from mixing wheat gluten with various spices, seitan can be a meat substitute. However, if you have celiac disease or gluten intolerance, you should not eat this product.

Nutritional Yeast

Manufacturers make nutritional yeast into yellow powder or flakes as a deactivated strain of saccharomyces cerevisiae. It has a distinctive flavor that can add a cheese-like flavor to vegan and vegetarian dishes

6. Fruits, Vegetables, Seeds, and Nuts

Fruits

1. **Avocado**: Avocado, a pear-shaped berry, has a single large seed surrounded by buttery pulp and hard skin. Yellowish-green to purple, the avocado flesh is like that of a ripe banana.

Avocado is low in carbohydrates and is jump-packed with fiber, potassium, and folic acid. It also has healthy oils. Avocado's GI is 15, and its GI value is 1.

According to *Healthline*, "The good fats in avocados can help you prevent diabetes complications, like heart attack, stroke, and help your insulin more effectively."

List of low glycemic index and glycemic load per serving of fruits include:

- Plums
- Strawberries
- Raspberries
- Cherries
- Blackberries
- Grapes
- Pears
- Apples

High Glycemic Index Fruits to Limit or Avoid

High glycemic index fruits include:

- Watermelon: 76
- Raisins: 64
- Pineapple: 59
- Banana, ripe: 62

Green Leafy Vegetables

Green leafy vegetables are jam-packed with essential vitamins, minerals, and nutrients. It would help if you ate these leaves because they have minimal impact on blood glucose levels.

Green leafy vegetables include:

- Spinach
- Kale
- Collard greens
- Bok Choy
- Broccoli

Greens like kale and spinach provide potassium, calcium, and vitamin A. Some researchers say that these vegetables help people with diabetes because of their high antioxidant content and starch.

Starchy and Non-Starchy Vegetables

Starch is the primary type of carbohydrate in any diet. Generally, it is often referred to as a complex carb because it consists of joined sugar molecules. Starch is in different foods, including starchy vegetables, cereals, bread, pasta, and noodles.

US health agencies recommend eating 2.5 cups of vegetables each day. Health experts recommend both starchy and non-starchy types, such as:

- Beans: kidney, pinto, black, and starchy vegetables
- Peas, sweet potatoes, taro, and yams
- Parsnips, lentils, and chickpeas
- Corn and butternut squash

Starchy Vegetables

- Corn
- Green potatoes
- Taro
- Beets
- White potatoes

Non-Starchy Vegetables

- Onions, salad greens, and turnips
- Tomatoes, spinach, and peppers
- Mushrooms, cabbage, and cauliflower
- Broccoli, bean sprouts, and asparagus

Both the starchy and non-starchy vegetables have essential vitamins and minerals. Vegetables are some of the richest sources of folate, vitamin K, potassium, and magnesium.

The American Diabetes Association (ADA) recommends that diabetic persons eat more non-starchy vegetables than starchy vegetables.

Healthiest Root Vegetables

Here are the most popular root vegetables that serve as staple ingredients in many cuisines.

Garlic: Garlic is a source of several vital nutrients, including vitamin B6, vitamin C, and manganese.

Onions: Onions are full of antioxidants such as fiber, vitamins, and vitamin C. Research shows that eating onions may be associated with blood sugar control.

One study found that eating 3.5 ounces (100 grams) of raw onions per day significantly reduced blood sugar levels in people with diabetes (*Trusted Source*). They have lots of antioxidants and may help lower blood glucose and your risk of certain cancers.

Sweet Potatoes: They are highly nutritious and loaded with fiber, vitamin A, vitamin C, and manganese. Their glycemic index is lower than that of white potatoes.

Ginger: A flavoring in cuisines, ginger is related to other root vegetables like turmeric. In short, ginger is rich in antioxidants that may help reduce nausea and decrease pain and inflammation in the body.

Turnips: Turnips are rich in vitamin C and may also prevent a lower risk of certain types of cancer.

Carrots: Eating carrots improve antioxidant status and lower cholesterol levels. Low in glycemic index and glycemic load values, carrots are chock-full of antioxidants such as beta-carotene, which reduces risks of eye diseases and certain types of cancers.

Fennel: Fennel is a flowering plant species closely related to carrots. It has vitamin C, fiber, potassium, and manganese. It also reduces blood sugar and stops the growth of bacteria, according to test-tube and animal studies.

Radishes: Radishes, low in calories and carbohydrates, contain fiber and vitamin C. With anti-fungal properties, radishes may protect you against stomach ulcers (*Trusted Source*).

Turmeric: Turmeric, a root vegetable, belongs to the same family as ginger and cardamom.

Celeriac: Also known as celery root, celeriac is a versatile root vegetable. It is a good source of vitamin K, which is for blood clotting and bone health.

7. Nuts and Seeds

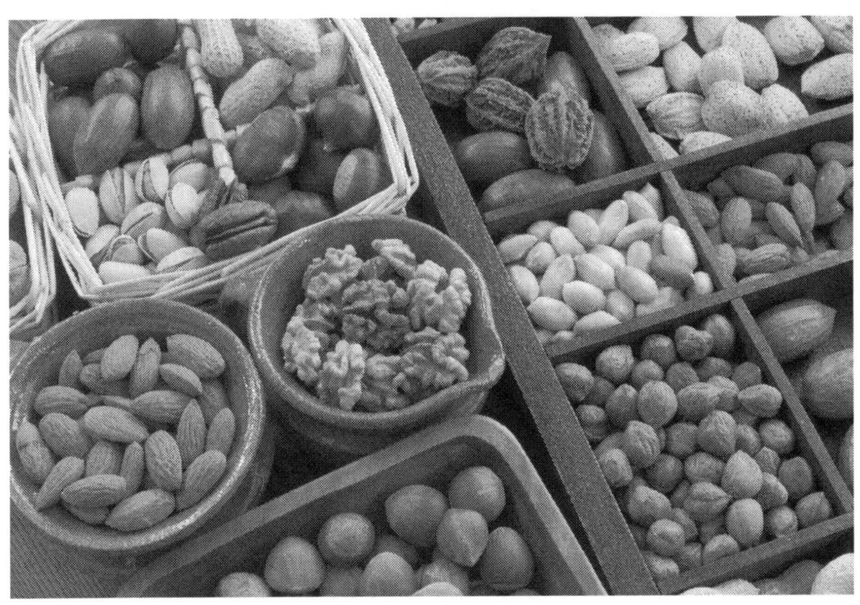

Different Types of Nuts

Photo Source: Shutterstock

Nuts and seeds are healthy snacks for people with diabetes and heart disease. The nutritious nuts and seeds are good sources of fiber, healthy fats, and protein.

Nuts

(Protein in 1 ounce per serving)

- Almonds, protein per 1 oz - 6g
- Walnuts, protein per 1 oz - 4.3g
- Peanuts, protein per 1 oz - 2.4g
- Pistachios, protein per 1 oz - 6g
- Cashews, protein per 1 oz - 4.3g
- Pecans, protein per 1 oz - 2.6g
- Pine Nuts, protein per 1 oz - 2.6g
- Macadamia nuts, protein per 1 oz - 7.9g

Seeds

(Protein in 1 ounce per serving)

- Hemp seeds - 5.2g
- Sunflower seeds - 5.5g
- Chia seeds - 4.7g
- Sesame seeds - 4.8g
- Squash seeds - 8.5g

12 Foods with High-Fructose Corn Syrup to Limit or Avoid

- Ice cream
- Fruit juice
- Canned fruit (Rinse it before eating to reduce salt content.)
- Baked goods
- Bread (see label)
- Soda
- Candy
- Sweetened yogurt
- Breakfast cereal

- Coffee creamer
- Nutritious bars
- Jam and jelly

Source: *Healthline*

7 Foods with High Glycemic Index to Limit or Avoid

- White rice: GI 89
- White bread: GI 75
- Honey: GI 73
- Doughnuts: GI 75
- French fries: GI 76
- Cereals: GI 76
- Instant oatmeal: GI

The American Diabetes Association (ADA) recommends that diabetic persons eat more non-starchy vegetables than starchy vegetables.

Low-Carb Alternatives to White Rice

1. **Cauliflower Rice**: Certainly, cauliflower rice is the most popular choice as a substitute for white rice. Why? Because it's deficient in carbohydrates, which means it doesn't affect blood glucose.

To create it, you should chop heads of cauliflower (called a "curd") into 3 or 4 large chunks in your processor. If you find that hard, you can buy ready-to-cook cauliflower from the nearest grocery in your locality.

Carb-Count: 1 cup contains 4 grams total carbs, 2 grams net carbs.

2. **Edamame/Mung Bean Pasta**: Rice noodles or wheat kinds of pasta are high in carbohydrates. But this bean pasta is a healthy and enticing alternative to regular pasta. You can find edamame pasta in many groceries or buy it from Amazon.com.

3. **Quinoa:** Quinoa is one of the most known health foods in the world; it's chock-full of vitamins and nutrients.

4. **Colored Rice**: Colored rice includes brown rice, red rice, black

Chapter14

Rice and Other Grains Feed the World

Brief Subject Summary

- What Are Grains?
- 2 Types of Grains
- 2 Subgroups of Grains
- What's a Whole Grain?
- What's a Refined Grain?
- What Is Rice?
- What Is Wheat?
- What Is Corn?

What Are Grains?

"Grains, commonly called 'cereals' or 'cereal grains,' are the edible seeds of specific grasses belonging to the Poaceae (also known as Gramineae) family," according to the Grains & Legumes Nutrition Council of Australia.

Grains (or cereal grains) are small and hard, dry seeds that grow on grass-like plants called cereals. So the plants are called cereals as well as the product.

Besides the two types of grains (true cereal grains and pseudocereal grains), grains have two subgroups:

- Whole grains
- Refined grains.

Differences Between Whole Grains and Refined Grains

Whole grains are minimally processed, while refined grains are fully processed.

- Whole grains include brown rice, barley, and sorghum
- Refined grains include white rice, breads, and pasta.
-

I. Types of Grains

The two types of grains are true cereal grains and pseudocereal grains.

1. True Cereal Grains: There are several grains found within the real cereal grains, which are from the botanical family "Poaceae," which include:

- Rice
- Corn (maize)
- Wheat
- Oats
- Barley
- Sorghum
- Rye
- Millet

Within the above groups, there are also several varieties, which include:

- Spelt
- Farro
- Emmer
- Freekeh

2. The Pseudocereal Grains: The "pseudocereal grain" group is not part of the Poaceae botanical family, where the "true or real grains" belong.

This group is considered similar in nutrition and used in ways similar to real cereal grains.

Members of this group include:

- Quinoa
- Buckwheat
- Amaranth

Manufacturers use these pseudocereals as alternatives to rice, pasta, and couscous. They make them into pasta, bread, flatbreads, snacks, crispbreads, and breakfast cereals.

Gluten-Free Grains include**:**

- Amaranth
- Buckwheat
- Corn
- Joe's Tears (or Nato Mugi)
- Millet
- Montina (Indian rice grass)
- Oats
- Quinoa
- Brown rice
- Wild rice
- Black rice
- Red rice
- Sorghum
- Teff
- Oats

Note: Oats (Unless labeled "gluten-free;" some may have gluten, obtained from manufacturing or processing).

II. Whole Grains

What's a Whole Grain?

The Oldways Whole Grains Council reports that "A grain is considered to be a whole grain after being processed as long as all three original parts: the bran, the germ, and the endosperm are still present in the same proportions as when the grain was growing in the fields."

Whole Grain Content

A whole grain contains four layers, which are described as follows:

Husk or Hall: The husk is the outer protective coating of each grain that protects the nutritious grain inside against pests and the weather. The husk is inedible.

When processing the whole grain starts, the husk is stripped away from the entire grain. What will be left will be the grain kernels or berries, which are the edible parts of the entire grain seed with healthy nutrients.

All whole-grain groats or kernels without the husk contain bran, germ, and endosperm. Each section contains health-promoting nutrients.

Bran: The bran is the hard outer layer of cereal grain. The bran. consisting of the combined aleurone and pericarp, is present in cereal grain, including rice, corn (maize), wheat, oats, rye, and millet. The fiber-rich outer layer supplies B vitamins, zinc, iron, copper, magnesium, and antioxidants.

Germ: The germ is the embryo that has the potential to sprout into a new plant. The embryo has large amounts of B vitamins, proteins, healthy fats, and some minerals.

Endosperm: The endosperm serves as the food supply provider that gives growth and vital energy to the new plant.

The endosperm is the largest portion of the seed, called the kernel. It has starchy carbohydrates, proteins, and a small amount of vitamins and minerals.

What Are Groats?

Groats are the whole-grain kernels of various cereal grains, including oat, rye, or wheat. As a whole grain, groats retain the bran, germ, and endosperm after removing the inedible husk, sometimes called the chaff.

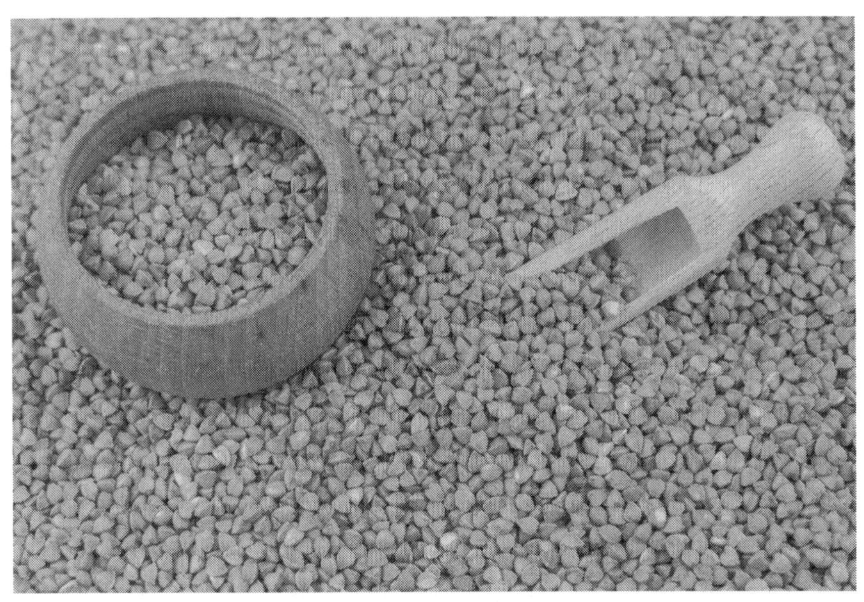

Groats: Whole-Grain Kernels of Buckwheat

Photo Credit: Shutterstock

ANATOMY OF A GRAIN

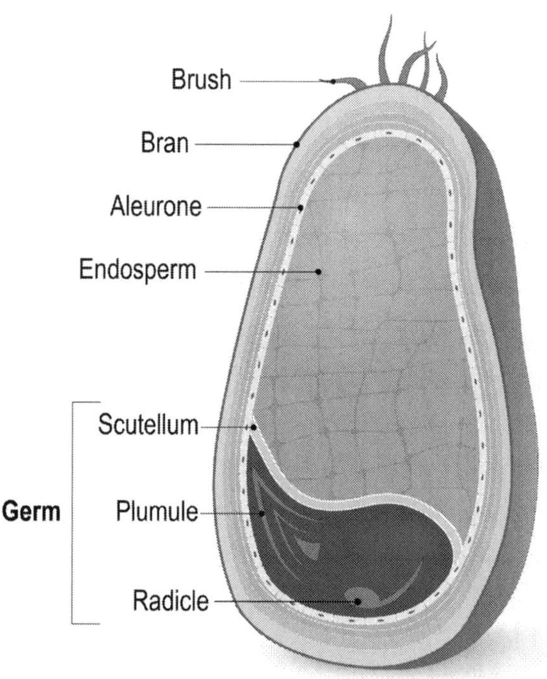

Anatomy of a Whole Grain Seed

Photo Source: Shutterstock

Anatomy of a Whole Grain

Whether they are whole grains of colored rice or whole grains of wheat, all grains start their lives as whole grains. When they are newly harvested, an entire grain consists of four layers: husk or hull, bran, germ, and endosperm. When the husk is removed, the three edible remaining parts become the groats, also called kernels.

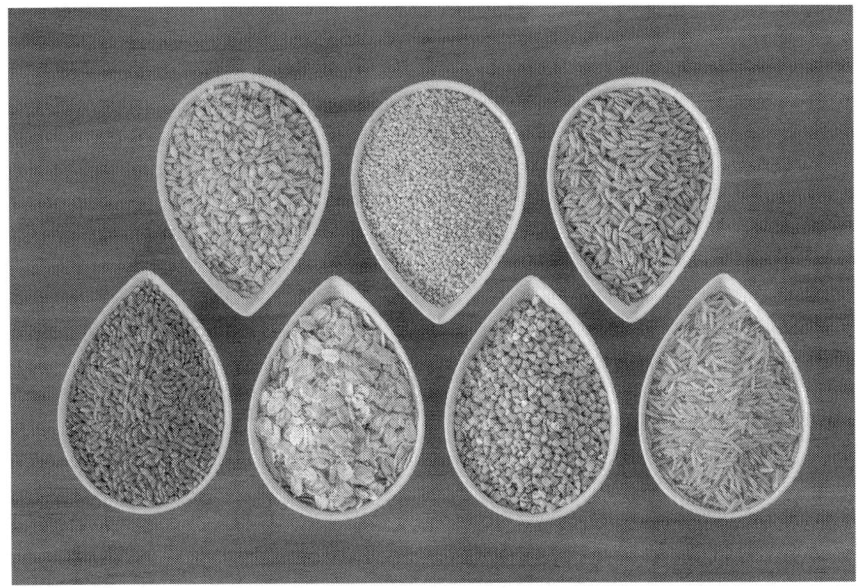

Different Kinds of Whole Grains

Photo Source: Shutterstock

The Old Ways Whole Grains Council.org has identified the whole grains as follows:

Whole Grains A to Z

- Amaranth
- Barley
- Buckwheat
- Bulgar
- Corn (Maize)
- Einkorn
- Farro
- Fonio (see Millet)
- Freekeh
- Kamut Khorasan
- Kaniwa

- Millet
- Oats
- Quinoa
- Rice (Brown rice and other colored rice. White rice is not whole grain.)
- Rye
- Sorghum
- Spelt
- Teff
- Triticale
- Wheat

On the other hand, The Grains & Legumes Nutrition Council of Australia has named the different types of whole grains as follows:

- Rice
- Corn (Maize
- Oats
- Barley
- Sorghum
- Amaranth
- Buckwheat
- Quinoa
- Rye
- Millet
- Triticale
- Quinoa
- Teff

14 Healthiest Whole Grains

1. Whole wheat
2. Whole oats
3. Brown rice
4. Whole rye
5. Freekeh
6. Whole-grain barley

7. Buckwheat
8. Bulgar
9. Quinoa
10. Whole-wheat couscous
11. Corn
12. Amarant
13. Sorghum
14. Farro

Source: *Good House Keeping*

III. Refined Grains

What Is a Refined Grain?

"Refined grain" is a term used to refer to grains that are not whole; it's missing two of their components, the bran and the germ.

During the refining process of grains, manufacturers strip away the bran and the germ, resulting in the loss of several nutrients. The nutrients removed include fiber, vitamins, and minerals.

So manufacturers fortify refined grains with iron, folic acid, and B vitamins to make the refined products nutritious. The nutrients added to the grain are not found in the grain naturally. Then the grain upon fortification becomes an "enriched grain."

Samples of Refined Grains

Refined grains include white flour, white bread, white rice, and white bread.

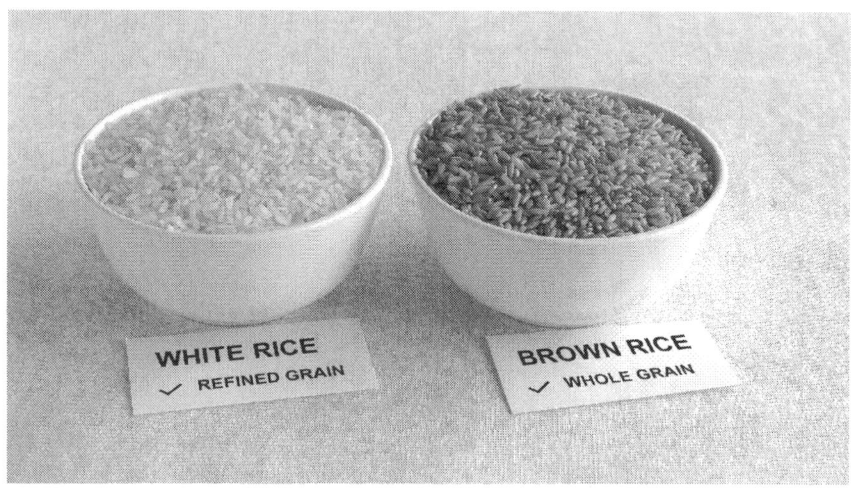

Refined Grain vs. Whole Grain

Photo Credit: Shutterstock

IV. Rice, Wheat, and Corn: Mostly Eaten Food Crops

Leading Food Crops

According to Ricepedia, rice, wheat, and corn (maize) are the world's three leading food crops. These staples directly supply more than 42% of all calories consumed by the entire human population.

In 2009, humans consumed 78% of rice production, compared with 64% for wheat and 14% for corn.

1. What Is Rice?

Rice is the seed of Oryza sativa (Asian rice) or Oryza glaberrima (African rice). As a whole grain, except white rice. Rice is a long, thin seed of grass. It consists of the outermost layer, called the bran, the germ, and the endosperm.

According to Ricepedia, rice is the essential staple food of more than half of the world's population, consisting of more than 3.5 billion people.

Top 10 Rice-Eating Countries in Asia

Asian peoples account for 90% of global rice consumption and rice demand continues yearly.

The rice-eating countries in Asia include, China, Hongkong, Taiwan, Japan, Singapore, the Philippines, India, Thailand, Vietnam, and Indonesia.

Top 10 Rice-Consuming Countries in the World

The 10- top consuming countries globally include China, India, Vietnam, Bangladesh, Indonesia, the Philippines, Thailand, Myanmar (Burma), Japan, and Brazil.

Source: Statista 2020-2021

Types of Rice

Different kinds of rice include:

- White Rice (refined grain)
- Brown Rice
- Wild Rice
- Basmati Rice (white and brown)
- Black Rice
- Red Rice
- And other colored rice

1. White Rice: Among rice varieties, white rice is the most popular staple food consumed worldwide.

In processing white rice, it undergoes depletion of its fiber, vitamins, and minerals.

White rice is considered empty carbs because it has lost its primary sources of nutrition (in the bran and germ). For this reason, countries like the United States enrich it with fiber, vitamins, and minerals to make it healthy.

Health experts have advised people with diabetes to limit or avoid eating white rice due to its high glycemic index values of 72 or more, depending on rice varieties. In addition, it impacts blood sugar immediately after a meal.

Instead, they suggest brown rice or any other rice type, like wild rice, Basmati rice, or black rice.

2. Brown Rice: Rice millers only strip the brown rice of its husk because it is not edible. So the nutrients remain in the seed: the bran, germ, and endosperm that consist of the kernel. That's why it's called healthy rice.

In other words, brown rice is a whole grain., unlike the white rice. Doctors and dietitians recommend brown rice for diabetes patients.

It has 52 grams of carbs per 1 cup per serving of cooked brown rice.

Brown rice has long, medium, and short varieties. It is 100% whole grain and is widely considered healthier than white rice. It has a slightly chewy texture and nutty flavor.

Besides the fiber, the seed contains magnesium and selenium, making it a better staple for people with diabetes. Brown rice is also nutty or sweet.

3. Wild Rice: Technically, wild rice is not rice but is the grain of four different grass species. It has a chewy and earthy, nutty flavor. Each serving of cooked one cup of wild rice contains 35 grams of carbohydrates.

4. Basmati Rice: **(White and Brown)**: Basmati rice, a long grain aromatic rice, has been an international rice in many parts of the world. The grain is about 6.61 to 7.5 mm.

The rice is available in two colors: white and brown. Of course, the white Basmati is similar to the standard white rice, fully processed, and lacks nutrients found in brown rice. On the other hand, manufacturers minimally process brown rice to make it whole grain.

Basmati white rice is not a whole grain because it has no bran and germ stripped away during the processing. Hence, it's not a whole grain. On the other hand, the Basmati brown rice is a whole grain since it has the bran, germ, and endosperm.

Basmati rice is traditionally grown in a specific geographical area, at the Himalayan foothills of the Indian sub-continent. Many countries, including the United States, cultivate Basmati rice.

Rice is widely grown in India and Pakistan. It is known for its extra-long slender grain that elongates at least twice its original size when cooked. The rice has a delicious taste, superior aroma, and distinct flavor upon cooking.

Basmati, a non-sticky rice, contains a high amylose content of 25%-30% and has a lower GI value of 50% to 58%.

Amylose is a long, straight starch molecule that does not gelatinize upon cooking, so it tends to cook firm and dry; grains don't stick together, making the rice ideal for making curries and pilafs. Its grains cook up soft fluffy, and the aroma is reminiscent of pandan leaves containing aromatic compounds.

India exports 2/3 of the global demand for Basmati, followed by Pakistan.

Many health professionals and dietitians consider Basmati rice an ideal staple for diabetes because of its low GI, especially brown rice, considered a whole grain. There are about 29 varieties of Basmati in India.

A variety of Basmati known as Texmati is grown in the United States.

5. **Black Rice**: Black rice is jump-packed with fiber, iron, protein, and antioxidants such as anthocyanin.

During the ancient times in China, black rice, tasty and nutritious, was so rare that authorities declared it for the emperors only and banned ordinary people from eating it. Hence, the name, the Forbidden Rice.

Rice producers partially mill black rice. They remove only the outer, inedible layer ('husked' rice). Like brown rice, black rice is a whole grain.

It has a distinct texture. It looks black with white spots, and emits purple color when soaked in water and cooked. It tastes nutty and a little bit sweet in some types of this rice.

Black rice, when cooked, has a total of 34 grams of carbohydrates per one-cup serving cooked.

6. **Red Rice**: Red rice is a whole grain food that includes germ, bran, and endosperm, the nutrients which white rice does not have.

Like black rice, red rice is also a proven fiber source and consists of many nutritional elements. It is grown explicitly in the Himalayan Mountains, southern Tibet, India, and Bhutan.

2. What Is Wheat?

Cultivated for its seed, wheat is a cereal grain eaten as staple food worldwide. The most widely grown wheat is the common wheat, called, Tuber aestivum.

Wheat Products

More than one-third of the world's population depends on wheat as the main staple of its diet. When milled into flour, the grain accounts for nearly 20% of humans' calories and proteins, more than any other single food source. China is the leading wheat-producing country in the world.

Wheat Grain Products with Gluten

Wheat berries and other wheat products with gluten include:

- Spelt
- Kamut
- Farro
- Durum
- Bulgar
- Semolina
- Barley
- Rye (closely related to wheat and barley)
- Triticale (a hybrid of wheat)

1. **Wheat Berries:** Wheat berries are the edible part of the wheat kernel (seed) that includes the bran, germ, and endosperm. Only the husk is removed before being turned into wheat products for different foods.

2. **Spelt:** According to *Medical News Today,* "Spelt is an ancient grain that is a subspecies of wheat. Spelt and wheat are similar in terms of appearance, but spelt has a stronger husk and slightly different nutritional content."

From spelt, you can get carbohydrates and dietary fiber. It is rich in zinc, niacin (Vitamin B3), iron, phosphorous, and magnesium.

3. **Kamut**: Kamut, an ancient form of wheat whose name originated from the Egyptian word for "wheat," has a nutty flavor with kernels measuring two to three times the wheat size.

Even if kamut is related to wheat, most people with gluten allergies can eat it.

4. **Farro**: A protein and fiber-packed whole grain, farro is rich in nutrients, minerals, and antioxidants. Chewy, the grain of farro looks and tastes like a bowl of lighter brown rice. Originally from Italy, farro is used in soups, desserts, and salads.

5. **Durum:** Durum or Triticum turgidum, a type of wheat, is the second most cultivated species of wheat after bread wheat, also called common wheat. Durum has bearded ears and is made into flour to make pasta.

A hard wheat grain, durum can be ground into semolina, a coarse flour typically used in pasta, including couscous.

6. Bulgar: Made from the cracked whole grains of different wheat species, Bulgar is parboiled. That merely means it's partially boiled and dried before packing it.

Bulgar's flavor is light and nutty. Like other whole grains, it has a chewy texture when cooked.

7. Einkorn: Centuries ago, the einkorn wheat grew wild worldwide. But later, farmers cultivated it for human consumption. The plant is produced mainly in Turkey, France, Morocco, and the former Soviet Union republics.

8. Semolina: Semolina is a flour made from durum wheat. It has a more earthy aroma than ordinary wheat flour. People mainly use it in making upma (a South Indian traditional breakfast dish), pasta, and couscous.

9. Barley: Barley is one of the oldest cultivated grains in the world. It is a highly adopted crop, growing north of the Arctic circle and south of Ethiopia.

Containing a rigid hull, which is hard to remove without losing some of the bran, hulled barley is available at health food stores and amazon.com.

10. Rye: Rye, made into flour, is cultivated widely on the France-Germany border and north of Hungary. Rye bread, including pumpernickel, is made of rye flour.

Rye flour is high in gliadin (a protein class in wheat) but low in glutenin than wheat flour. Still, it has gluten.

11. Triticale: A hybrid of wheat and rye, triticale resembles wheat in size, shape, and color.

However, the triticale cultivators have improved the grain that matches the grains' yield for the past few years. It contains less gluten than wheat.

Chapter 15

Fatty Fish: Are They Good for You or Not?

Brief Subject Summary

- Should You Eat Fatty Fish?
- Fish with Highest Proteins and Creatine
- Fatty Fish: Bad for Kidney Disease
- Omega 3 Acids: Good for Diabetes, Heart, and Brain

Should You Eat Fatty Fish?

It is beneficial to eat species of fatty fish, whether or not you have diabetes or not. Why? Because by eating them, you will get omega-3 fatty acids which are considered to be healthy.

In a report, The American Diabetes Association (ADA) says healthy fats enhance blood sugar control and blood lipids in people with diabetes. Such healthy fats are polyunsaturated and monounsaturated fats of fish.

Fish that have healthy fats include:

- Salmon
- Tuna
- Herring
- Mackerel
- Sardines
- Trout

Because I have kidney disease, I limit or avoid eating the above fish species because of the high protein and creaatine contents. It's just common sense that when you eat a lot of protein and creatine, you produce a big amount of blood urea nitrogen (BUN), the waste product of protein and creatinine (the toxin of creatine) in your bloodstream.

And this is bad for the diseased kidney because it will have a hard time filtering the toxic wastes. And this can lead to worsening your renal disease, progressing it instead of reversing it.

14 Fish With Highest Proteins and Creatine

Persons with kidney disease should limit or avoid these fish species so that their creatinine and BUN won't skyrocket.

1. **Anchovy** (Canned in oil): A 4-oz serving delivers 52g of protein
2 **Sardines**: You can get 50g of protein from a 6-oz serving.
3. **Trout**: A serving of 6 oz delivers 40g of protein.
4. **Salmon**: A 6-oz serving gives 38g of protein.
5. **Yellowtail**: A 4-oz serving has 34 grams of protein.
6. **Haddock** (Wild): Has 34g of protein from a 6-oz serving.
7. **Mackerel**: A 6 oz serving gives 32g of protein.
8. **Perch** (Wild): A 6-oz serving delivers 32g of protein.
9. **Cod**: A 6-oz serving gives 30g of protein.
10. **Bluefish**: A 4-oz serving delivers 29 grams of protein.
11. **Grouper**: It has 28 grams of protein per 4-oz serving.
12. **Pollock**: A 4-oz serving has 29 grams of protein.
13. **Tilapia**: A 4-oz serving gives 23 grams of protein.
14. **Flounder** (Wild): You can get 22g of protein per 6 oz serving.

Source: *Men's Magazine.*

Fatty Fish: Bad for Kidney Disease

To simply put it, it's too hard for the diseased kidneys to handle the creatinine, more so with the BUN. The two kidneys maintain the blood creatinine in a normal range. Creatinine level is a relatively reliable indicator of kidney function.

It's okay for the normal kidney to process and secrete the creatinine. However, if the creatinine amount is already too much, the damaged kidney may not be able to clear it out. Both BUN and creatinine are poison to the body.

Omega 3 Acids: Good for Diabetes, Heart, and Brain

While fatty acids are not good for the diseased kidney, Omega-3 acids in fish strengthen blood sugar control and promote heart and brain health.

In a report, The American Diabetes Association (ADA0 says healthy fats enhance blood sugar control and blood lipids in people with diabetes. The healthy fats are polyunsaturated and monounsaturated.

These fats are considered healthy fats. Fish that are healthy in fats include:

- Salmon
- Tuna
- Herring
- Mackerel
- Sardines
- Trout

While fish with high protein and creatine are detrimental to kidney disease, fatty fish are beneficial for diabetes, heart disease, or the brain.

I take 4,000 grams of Omega-3 Acid daily, a generic of Lovaza, the first fish oil approved by the FDA. The medication is available only prescription.

Supposing you have kidney and heart disease, would you eat fatty fish? Me? Having kidney disease and heart disease, I limit or sometimes totally avoid consuming fatty fish.

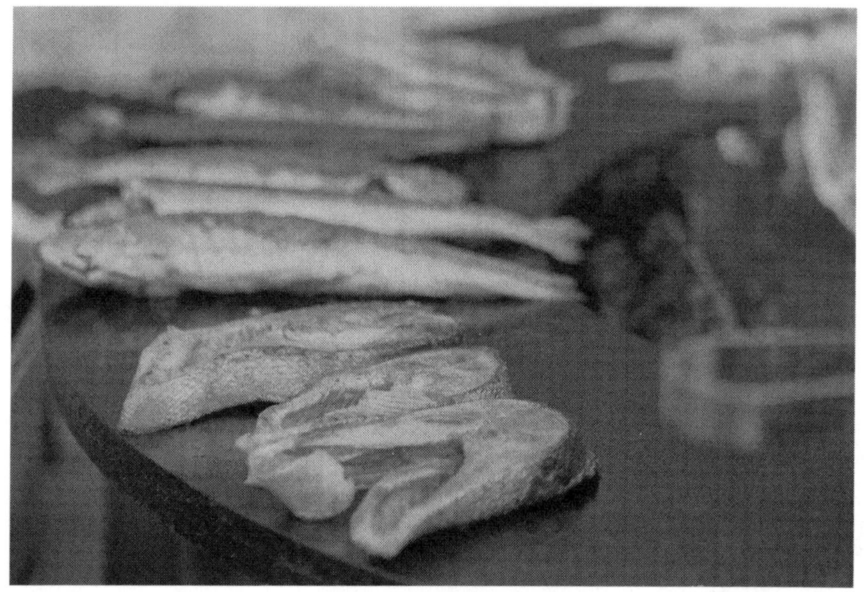

Species of Fatty Fish

Photo Credit: Shutterstock

Chapter 16

Which Bread Is Good for You?

Brief Subject Summary

- What Is White Bread?
- What Is Brown Bread?
- What Are Whole Grain Breads?
- Types of Sprouted Grain Breads and Other Whole Grain Breads
- Breads from Around the World

Generally, people in different countries worldwide eat bread with coffee, tea, chocolate, or any other drinks in the morning.

For you, which types of bread do you eat? Do you ingest bread made of different kinds of flour from whole grains, whole wheat, or sprouted grains?

People bake regular whole-wheat bread or whole white wheat from the whole grains with the bran, germ, and endosperm intact. The difference between the two whole wheat bread lies in the grain used.

I. White, Brown, Whole Grain, & Whole Wheat Breads

What Is White Bread?

White bread is made from Maida flour or refined wheat flour from the wheat grains. Of the three parts of the seed, the bran and the germ are removed, leaving only the endosperm.

.(Maida is a white flour from the Indian subcontinent, made from wheat.)

The endosperm contains only starch and has minimal vitamins, and minerals. It's because white bread is highly processed. So what manufacturers do is add nutrients, except fiber, to the bread, which is called enriched bread. White bread is not a whole grain bread.

What Is Brown Bread?

Brown bread is usually a mixture of refined flour and whole wheat flour, with added ingredients, for instance, caramel, molasses, or coffee, to make its color brown.

In some parts of the United States, brown bread is called wheat bread.

What Are Whole Grain Breads?

Like whole wheat bread, whole grain bread is made up of the main components of a seed, the bran, germ, and endosperm. The entire grain brain can also include other whole grains, such as brown rice, whole grain oats, rye, barley, quinoa, amaranth, and millet.

Whole Grain Sourdough (origin: unknown)

Sourdough, a whole grain bread, is made from flour's natural yeast and bacteria. There are four ingredients: sourdough starter, flour, water, and salt.

In making this bread, the three ingredients used are the sourdough starter, salt, and flour in the traditional way of making sourdough bread.

The sourdough startter consists of flour and water. The sourdough bread is considered exceptional. Why? Because of its signature tartness. The tartness comes from the same bacteria that gives yogurt and sour cream their different taste.

What Is the Whole-Wheat Bread?

Wikipedia says, "Whole wheat bread or wholemeal bread is a type of bread made using flour that is partly or entirely milled from whole or almost-whole wheat grains."

Whole wheat bread has more fiber than brown bread made with a large amount of refined wheat flour. It has no artificial color.

Whole wheat bread, made from red wheat, has more nutrition than brown bread.

Whole White Wheat Bread

White wheat is a different type of wheat with no major genes for bran color, unlike traditional red wheat, which has one to three ban color genes.

The whole white wheat bread and the traditional whole wheat bread have the same nutrition because they both have the flour's bran, germ, and endosperm.

But while the whole red wheat bread has the strongly-flavored phenolic compounds found in red wheat, the white wheat bread has a milder flavor.

II. Types of Sprouted Grain Bread and Other Whole Grain Breads

Sprouted Grain Breads

Bakers use sprouted grains from different plants to make foods, like sprouted bread. While there's no regulated definition of a "sprouted grain, the Whole Grains Council in Boston, Massachusetts, describes it as "a whole grain seed that has just begun to sprout."

Manny dietitians recommend sprouted bread because of its nutritional health benefits.

Benefits of Sprouted Grain Breads

- High protein and vitamins, including Vitamins B and C, folate, and lysine, an essential amino acid in protein
- More fiber than other types of bread
- Low glycemic index
- More antioxidants

Samples of Sprouted Grain Breads

1. Food For Life Ezekiel 4:9 Bread and Other Breads: Ezekiel bread 4:9 bread is a sprouted whole grains bread whose name was an inspiration from the Bible verse Ezekiel 4:9. It offers a unique blend of nutrients, like folic acid and amino acids.

Ezekiel 4:9 bread is made from whole grains and legumes that are organically sprouted, including soybeans, barley, wheat, lentils, millet, corn, and spelt.

Containing a complete protein, Ezekiel 4:9 is considered a good alternative for low glycemic bread for people with diabetes. Its glycemic index (GI) is 36. It doesn't contain sugar.

Note: I'm familiar with Ezekiel Sprouted Bread because it's the one I eat every breakfast. In restaurants, I eat sourdough bread, if available.

2. **Angelic Bakehouse 7-Grain Sprouted Bread:** No-salt added bread

3. **Silver Hills 100% Sprouted Power Bread Low-Fat Multi-Grain Spouted Bread**

4. Angelic Bakehouse Sprouted Bread

5. **Alvarado Street Bakery Sprouted** .No-Salt Added Bread Loaf

Samples of Other Grain Breads

Chia Bread

This bread has a total carb amount of 24 grams and 5 grams of fiber per slice. (Baker: Udi's Gluten-Free Millet-Chia Bread.)

Spelt Bread

Boasting a light, fluffy texture, manufacturers make this bread with stone-milled, whole grain spelt flour. One slice contains 16 grams of carbs and 2 grams of fiber. (Baker: Berlin Bakery Whole Grain Spelt Bread.)

Flax Bread

This bread contains 7 grams of carbs and 7 grams of fiber, which decreases the carb count to zero. Wow! How nice! (Baker: Thin Slim Zero Carb Bread.)

Pumpernickel Bread: Country of Origin - Germany

This bread contains 8 net carbs and 7 grams of fiber. (Baker: Great Low Carb Bread Company.)

7 Healthiest Types of Breads

According to *Healthline,* the healthiest types of breads are:

- Sprouted whole grain bread
- Sourdough.
- 100% whole wheat
- Oat bread
- Flaxseed bread
- 100% sprouted rye bread
- Healthy gluten-free bread

III. Breads From Around the World

Bagel: Country of Origin - Poland

Bagel is a ring-shaped bread made from flour and similar to a doughnut. Usually, the bread is eaten in the morning as a sandwich with cream cheese serving and sometimes with a fillet of brined or smoked salmon. This bread originated in Jewish communities in Poland in 1610. They have a crisp, shiny crust.

Pita: Region of Origin - Middle East

Pita, a slightly leavened flatbread, has a pocket inside, stuffed with fillings. It is traditionally associated with Greek and Middle Eastern foods.

Pumpernickel: Country of Origin - Germany

Pumpernickel is a heavy and dark type of rye bread. After serving it to German soldiers during the Thirty Years War, the bread began being called pumpernickel.

The traditional pumpernickel bread is made from coarsely ground rye flour and fermented with a dough starter.

Tortilla: Country of Origin - Mexico

Tortilla is a thin, unleavened flatbread made from ground corn (maize), flour, or whole wheat. Usually, it is used as a wrap to stuff it with different fillings, like baked beans, meat, chicken, and veggies.

Rye Bread: Region of Origin - Europe

People make rye bread in different types, including flat rye bread and multi-grain bread. The bread can vary in taste, texture, and color. It all depends on its ingredients.

Pretzel: Country of Origin - Germany

A pretzel is made from dough commonly shaped into a knot. The traditional pretzel shape is a distinctive symmetrical form.

Chapter 17

Drinking Water, Coffee, and Tea: Their Benefits and Risks

Brief Subject Summary

- What Are the Best Drinks for Diabetics?
- Water: The Best Drink of Them All
- Different Types of Water
- Is Coffee Safe for Diabetics or Not?
- Benefits of Consuming Caffeine
- Side Effects of Caffeine
- How Much Caffeine Is Enough?
- Different Types of Tea

What Are the Best Drinks for Diabetics?

What do you drink when you eat your breakfast to avoid raising your blood sugar levels?

According to *Healthline,* the best drinks for people with diabetes include:

- Water
- Seltzer water
- Herbal tea
- Hot or cold unsweetened tea
- Unsweetened coffee
- Vegetable juice
- Sugar-free diet beverages
- Sugar-free home-made lemonade
- Milk alternatives (low-sugar soy milk, low-sugar almond milk)

I. Water: The Best Drink of Them All

Water is an essential nutrient since your body relies on water to function. Sure, whether you have diabetes or not, you need enough water because it's vital for maintaining overall health.

Generally, health professionals recommend drinking 8-12 cups or glasses of 8 ounces each of water.

Among the drinks above, water is the best drink for nondiabetics and diabetics, as well.

Different Types of Water

There are different types of water which include:

1. Tap Water
2. Ionized Water
3. Alkaline Bottled Water
4. Purified Water
5. Distilled Water
6. Spring or Glacier Water
7. Sparkling Water
8. Artesian Well Water

In many parts of the world, people drink and use water from many sources for home use. But the question is, is the water safe for consumption?

The U.S. Centers for Disease Control and Prevention (CDC) reports that "In many parts of the world the water is not safe to drink, so filtration if you use this water, (referring to tap water), is one option to protect your health with the use of water filters."

1. Tap Water

Tap water, coming from household faucets, is the cheapest water you can buy. Such water may come from the surface or underground sources of water.

It is supplied to the household in every community by city, town, or municipal water systems.

Water Filtration

Filtration is a separation process in which a filter medium is used to remove contaminants from an aqueous solution by passage through a porous membrane. The size of the pores in the membranes determines which particles are removed. Particles that are larger than the pores in the membranes are removed while smaller particles pass through.

Filtration Filters

Microfiltration Filter: A microfiltration filter has a pore size of approximately 0.1 microns to 5 microns. They are permeable to fluids but remove particles, such as bacteria and suspended solids.

Ultrafiltration Filter: An ultrafiltration filter has a pore size of approximately 0.001 microns to 0.01 microns which are permeable to fluids but remove particles, such as bacteria, suspended solids, and viruses.

Nanofiltration Filter: A nanofiltration filter has a pore size of approximately 0.001 microns (the smallest) to 0.01 microns which are permeable to fluids but remove particles, such as bacteria, suspended solids, viruses, and multivalent ions.

Reverse Osmosis (RO) Filtration Filter: Reverse osmosis has a pore size ranging from 0.0001 (the smallest among microns) to 0.001 microns. It is the only water filtration procedure to remove all elements; nothing is left except pure water. And it has no nutrients like magnesium.

Types of Water Filters

There are two household water purifying systems, which are:

Point of Entry (POE) or Whole House System: The POE system, connected directly to your main water line, filters all the water to your house. This whole house system has a high water flow rate. It also removes odors and chlorine taste.

Kitchen Point Of Use System: POU filters are installed at a single water connection, typically under the kitchen or bathroom sink counter.

Depending on the size of the unit, a POU filter typically lasts only three to six months.

Other Kinds of Filters

- Faucet Filters
- Counter top Filters
- Under the Counter Filters
- Reverse Osmosis Filters
- Alkaline Water Pitcher Filters

Faucet Filters: The faucet filter attached to the end of the kitchen or bathroom faucet uses a diverter for filtered water.

Countertop Pitchers. This filter sits on the counter top next to the kitchen or bathroom sink. And it is connected with a small hose to the faucet.

Under the Counter Filters: In a plumbed-in system, a counter filter is connected to your cold water line under the sink and dispenses filtered water using a second small faucet. You may install the filter at the main kitchen sink or a secondary sink.

Reverse Osmosis Systems: A reverse osmosis system uses a process that reverses water flow in a natural osmosis process.

In this process, the water passes from a more concentrated solution to a more dilute solution through a semi-permeable membrane. The filter has a pore size of approximately 0.0001 microns, the smallest among microns.

What Is pH?

The pH of water measures the acidity of water. Based on pure water ion concentration, the pH scale ranges from 0 to 14, neutral—pH 7.

A pH below 7 is considered acidic, and above a pH of 7 is referred to as basic. Alkaline water typically has a pH of 8 or 9.

The pH measures the relative amount of free hydrogen and hydroxyl ions in the water.

A simple alkaline pitcher water filter, on average, can make the filtration of water with pH between 8 and 9.5, depending on the ability of the ionized pitcher filter.

pH Test Drops

According to some sources, using quality test drops is one of the most efficient and straightforward methods to do an alkaline pH test. Just be sure that you'll be using the right ratio of pH test-drops-to water and allow enough time to go by the water to alkalize properly.

What pH Is Safe for Drinking?

The U.S. Environmental Protection Agency (EPA) requires municipal drinking water suppliers to keep their water supply at a pH of 6.5 to 8.5. EPA is in charge of monitoring public drinking water quality in the country.

If the pH is higher than 8.5 (but not exceeding 9), it probably is safe to drink, but you may want to acidify the water if you notice any skin problems (not due to diabetes).

Common Water pH Levels

- Tap water: varies, typically above 7.0
- Distilled Reverse Osmosis Water: 5 to 7
- Common bottled waters: 6.5 to 7.5
- Bottled water labeled as alkaline: 8 to 9
- Ocean Water: Above 8
- Acid rain: 5 to 5.5 (Source: *Healthline*)

Generally, a pH of less than 6.5 is considered more likely to be contaminated with pollutants. The optimal pH for water is between 8.0 and 9.5.

An “alkaline” is described as a solution (or water) with a pH above 7. A pH below that means it’s acidic.

2. Ionized Water

What Is Ionized Water?

Ionized water is tap water that has gone through water ionizing, either by non-electric or electric ionizers. The ionizers use bicarbonate and mineral ions to convert tap water to alkaline water by having more OH-ions than H+ ions increase its pH level.

The mineral ions come from tap water minerals, such as calcium, magnesium, and potassium, and became ionized when they gained or lost electrons. Tap water, which contains equal numbers of OH-ions and H+, becomes neutral.

Regular tap water contains a mixture of these two kinds of ions: minerals and bicarbonate ions. That’s why it’s the ideal water to turn into alkaline water.

Tap water is a mixture of bicarbonate and mineral ions. When CO2 dissolves, it becomes bicarbonate. CO2 (carbon dioxide) is an odorless, colorless gas.

Non-Electric and Electric Alkaline Water Ionizers

There are two types of water ionizer devices that you can use to make healthy alkaline water: Non-electric and electric water Ionizers.

1. Non-Electric Water Ionizers: Non-electric water ionizers are composed of several internal filters combinations, such as zinc, calcium, magnesium, and potassium, which give the water a mild electrical charge.

The filters purify the water and remove harmful contaminants from the water without using electricity.

Non-electric water ionizers work by using minerals infused into the water to adjust or raise the pH level. They do it this way, instead of using electricity.

The pitcher water filter is the cheapest non-electric water alkaline device. But there are also simple home water machine ionizers.

What Do the Pitcher Filters Create?

- The pitcher filter adds beneficial minerals into the water, such as magnesium, bicarbonate, and calcium, which the body needs appropriately to function.
- It incorporates a push-down lid, which makes it easier to fill up. Usually, people put it on the counter top in the kitchen. Also, one or more alkaline water devices can be in the kitchen.
- Good non-electric water filters can also provide hydrogen water, wherein hydrogen gas is added to regular water, as electric water ionizers do.

2. Electric Water Ionizers: These machines are connected to the household plumbing and located on the countertop or below it. They increase drinking water quality by using electricity to adjust the water pH through electrolysis.

Inside the water ionizer, an electric current is run, and it causes the water to be ionized as it flows through the ionizer.

Compared to regular water, ionized water is steeped in antioxidants. Antioxidants reduce the risk of heart disease, certain cancers, and other diseases because they help neutralize the damaging effects of free radicals in our bodies.

3. Alkaline Bottled Water and Other Types of Bottled Water: As concerns about the nation's municipal tap water safety have increased, many people turn to bottled alkaline water and other types of bottled water.

As a result, sales of bottled water have soared! Bottled water has become the country's top-selling bottled beverage.

Alkaline water is ionized (through electrolysis) and bottled. The water has a pH of 8 to 9.5.

CDC Guidelines

According to the CDC, the filter can hold any bigger than 1 micron or smaller contaminants and not go with the filtered water.

A thing to remember: the smaller the pores, the better because they can remove many, if not all, of the contaminants and pollutants.

4. Purified Water

The U.S. Food and Drug Administration (FDA) and the Environmental Protection Agency (EPA) take responsibility for drinking water safety. The FDA oversees bottled drinking water, while EPA regulates public drinking water (tap water).

According to the FDA, "Purified water is produced by distillation, deionization, reverse osmosis or other suitable processes." It may also be called "demineralized water, deionized water, distilled water, or reverse osmosis water."

5. Distilled Water

Distilling water is a process used to boil water to remove contaminants, such as metals and inorganic minerals. Those impurities have a much higher boiling point than water's boiling point of 212 degrees Fahrenheit.

The steam that comes from the boiling water is captured and cooled. And the water that results from the condensation is known as distilled water. Many steamed water compounds boil off first because they have a lower boiling point than water.

6. Spring Water or Glacier Water: Mineral Water

The FDA describes spring water as "derived from an underground formation from which water flows naturally to the surface of the earth, at an identified location and may be collected at the spring or through a borehole, tapping the underground formation that feeds the spring."

Spring water, the least processed, goes through very little distillation since the purpose is to keep the minerals that naturally occur in the water.

Many people consider spring water as natural alkaline water because it contains minerals that make it more alkaline or is ionized to make it that way.

Mineral water is water from a mineral spring that contains various minerals, such as salts, calcium, magnesium, and sulfur compounds.

7. Sparkling (Carbonated) Water

Sparkling water, also known as carbonated water, is mostly drunk in European countries, particularly Germany. But it has been gaining popularity in the United States and other nations.

Manufacturers infuse water with carbon dioxide gas under pressure to make sparkling water. That's why it produces a bubbly drink. Sparkling water names include soda water, club soda, fizzy water, and seltzer water.

Is It Safe to Drink?

"The bottom line is that these sparkling waters do not cause any type of harm," says Anne Linge, a registered dietitian nutritionist and certified diabetes educator at the Nutrition Clinic at the University of Washington Medical Center-Roosevelt.

"They're fine to drink as long as they don't contain added sugar," she adds.

One of the biggest concerns about carbonated water is its effect on teeth. Too much acid that the water contains may destroy the enamel.

8. Well Water

Know the alkalinity or acidity of your well water. If you use well water for drinking, make it safe, with an ideal pH.

Water from wells is usually hard. That means hardness is the amount of dissolved calcium and magnesium. Solid calcium carbonate deposits can form when you heat the hard water, such as in a water heater.

II. Coffee: Is It Safe for Diabetics or Not?

What Is Caffeine?

Caffeine is a nitrogenous organic compound that acts as a stimulant in the central nervous system, heart, blood vessels, and kidneys. It blocks adenosine, a molecule that inhibits neural activity and causes drowsiness, from binding to its receptors.

It does this by attaching itself to these same receptors that adenosine usually binds to. Hence, it prevents drowsiness caused by adenosine.

Caffeine, a bitter stimulant substance, occurs naturally in many plants, including:

- Coffee beans
- Tea beans
- Kola nuts for flavoring soft drink colas
- Cacao pods used to make chocolate products

How Does Caffeine Affect the Human Body?

The U.S. Institute of Health, in its online newsletter, *MedlinePlus,* assesses how caffeine affects the human body for certain functions:

- It increases blood pressure.
- It interferes with the body's absorption of calcium.
- It stimulates the central nervous system, increasing mental focus and alertness and boosting energy.
- Since it is a diuretic, it helps your body get rid of extra salt and water by causing you to urinate more.
- It increases acid release in our stomach and can trigger an upset stomach or heartburn.

According to the U.S. National Institute of Health (NIH)), the caffeine contents in coffee and other drinks generally are as follows:

- An 8-ounce cup of coffee: 95-200 mg
- A 12-ounce can of cola: 35-45 mg

- An 8-ounce can or bottle of energy drink: 70-100 mg
- An 8-ounce cup of tea: 14-60 mg

What Is Coffee?

Coffee is a drink brewed from the roasted and ground seeds of the tropical coffee plant. Along with water and tea, it is one of the three most popular drinks globally.

Brewing Techniques

People use several types of brewing techniques to cause a different amount of caffeine each time. These are:

- Variations in the coffee blend
- The amount of ground coffee used
- The brewing technique

What Are Flavored Coffees?

Flavored coffee is made by adding flavoring oils – natural or synthetic – to coffee beans. The natural flavoring oils come from vanilla, cocoa beans (chocolate!), nuts, and berries.

3 to 5 Cups of Coffee Per Day

The Food and Drug Administration (FDA) has recommended up to 400 mg of caffeine, roughly 3 to 5 cups of coffee daily. In other words, the maximum limit is about 400 mg of caffeine per day for healthy people.

The FDA estimates that a typical 8-ounce (oz) coffee cup contains around 80–100 mg of caffeine.

Coffee: Good for What?

A new research, funded by the American Diabetes Association (ADA), indicates that coffee is suitable for:

- Cardiovascular disease
- Cancer (prostate, breast, etc.
- Type 2 diabetes

WHO Endorses U.S. Guidelines

For its part, the World Health Organization (WHO) has released the Guidelines for *Dietary Recommendation for Americans for 2015-2020*, indicating its endorsement of the quantity of caffeine consumption, as per the Guide for Dietary Recommendation for Americans.

According to WHO, 3-5 cups of coffee per day or up to 400 mg of caffeine benefit people. They include those with type 2 diabetes.

What's the Amount of Coffee Ideal for Diabetics?

There has not been any fixed amount of caffeine intake for people with diabetes, whether prediabetic, type 2 diabetic, or type 1 diabetic.

There's no "one-size-fits-all" caffeine quota for anyone. The appropriate amount depends on many factors; a particular diabetic's body reaction to the effect of caffeine or "sensitivity,"

But research indicates that 1 or 2 cups of coffee per day is safe for people with diabetes. Two cups of coffee may have 200 mg or less caffeine, which should be the maximum for people with diabetes.

How About Kidney Disease, In Case You Have It?

The (U.S.) National Kidney Foundation, commenting on the effect of caffeine on kidney disease, says, "Caffeine causes a short but sudden increase in blood pressure. Research has not shown that drinking 3-4 cups of coffee a day increases the risk of kidney disease or increases the rate of decline of kidney function."

Side Effects and Risks of Caffeine

The common side effects of drinking too much coffee, even for healthy individuals, may include:

- Fast heart rate (palpitations)
- Headaches
- Nausea
- Anxiousness
- Jitters

The risks may include:

- Caffeine stimulation of the central nervous system
- Elevated blood glucose levels after a meal
- An increased risk of heartburn
- An increase in cholesterol with unfiltered or espresso-type coffees

Who Should Limit or Avoid Caffeine?

You should talk to your doctor about whether you should limit or avoid consuming caffeine if you:

- Have GERD or ulcer
- Have high blood pressure
- Have anxiety or nervousness

The FDA has not set any amount of caffeine for adolescents and teens. However, the American College of Pediatrics discourages drinking coffee and other stimulants by children and adolescents.

Caffeine Content of Beverages

Starbucks Hot Beverage Caffeine

Beverage	Short (8 fl oz)	Tall (12 oz)	Grande (16 oz)	Venti (20 oz)
Pike Place Brewed Coffee	155mg	235mg	310mg	410mg
Blonde Roast	180mg	270mg	360mg	475mg
Featured Dark Roast	130mg	195mg	260mg	340mg
Clover® Brewed Coffees	–	–	–	–
Reserve Roasts	190mg	280mg	380mg	470mg
Blonde Roasts	155mg	255mg	340mg	425mg
Medium Roasts	170mg	280mg	375mg	445mg
Dark Roasts	190mg	280mg	380mg	470mg
Brewed Decaf Coffee	15mg	20mg	25mg	30mg
Caffe Americano	75mg	150mg	225mg	300mg

USA UK/Europe (Sample only)

Source: CaffeineInformer.com: For a complete guide, Starbucks drink caffeine, go to: https://www.caffeineinformer.com/the-complete-guide-to-starbucks-caffeine.

For all brands of the caffeine content of beverages, go to: https://www.caffeineinformer.com/the-caffeine-database

McCafe Coffee and Tea Caffeine Content

Beverage	Small (12 oz)	Medium (16 oz)	Large (21-24 oz)	X-Large (32 oz)
Coffee (Brewed)	109mg	145mg	180mg	–
Decaf Coffee (Brewed)	8mg	11mg	14mg	–
Espresso	71mg (single)	142mg (double)	–	–
Americano	71mg	142mg	178mg	–
Latte	71mg	142mg	178mg	–
Cinnamon Cookie Latte	71mg	142mg	178mg	–
Caramel Latte	71mg	142mg	178mg	–
French Vanilla Latte	71mg	142mg	178mg	–
Cappuccino	71mg	142mg	178mg	–
Caramel Cappuccino	71mg	142mg	178mg	–
Mocha	86mg	167mg	200mg	–
Iced Sweet Tea	38mg	50mg	66mg	
Hot Tea	42mg	42mg	42mg	–
Hot Chocolate	7mg	10mg	12mg	

Source: *https://*www.caffeineinformer.com/mccafe-coffee-caffeine-content

Dunkin' Donuts Coffee and Tea Caffeine Content

Beverage	Small (10 fl oz)	Medium (14 oz)	Large (20 oz)	Extra-Large (24 oz)
Coffee (Brewed)	150mg	210mg	300mg	359mg
Decaf Coffee (Brewed)	7mg	10mg	15mg	18mg
Brewed Dark Roast	117mg	164mg	235mg	282mg
Espresso	118mg (single)	–	–	–
Americano	237mg	284mg	371mg	
Latte	118mg	166mg	252mg	n/a
Decaf Latte	<5mg	<5mg	7mg	n/a
Cappuccino	118mg	166mg	252mg	n/a
Macchiato	237mg	284mg	371mg	

Hot Green Tea	70mg	70mg	140mg	n/a
Hot Tea	90mg	90mg	180mg	N/a
Hot Chocolate	9mg	13mg	18mg	19mg

Source: CaffeineInformer.com. For a complete guide, go to:
https://www.caffeineinformer.com/complete-guide-to-dunkin-donuts-caffeine-content

Caribou Caffeine Content in Drinks

Source: Caffeineinformer.com: For a complete guide, go to:

Beverage	**Small**	**Medium**	**Large**
Brewed Coffee	230mg	305mg	385mg
Coffee with Steamed Milk	153mg	192mg	230mg
Brewed Decaf Coffee	4mg	5mg	6mg
Hot Press Coffee	230mg	305mg	385mg
Crafted Press Hot	130mg	205mg	235mg
Cold Press Latte	115mg	155mg	190mg
Caffè Latte & Lite	180mg	180mg	270mg
Caffè Mocha	190mg	195mg	290mg
Spicy Mocha	190mg	195mg	290mg
Caffè Americano	180mg	270mg	360mg
Cappuccino	180mg	270mg	360mg

https://www.caffeineinformer.com/caribou-coffee-the-complete-caffeine-guide

(Note: LibroCasa published caffeine content of different brands of coffee shown above with permission from caffeineiformer.com)

Caffeine Calculator

Wanna know how much caffeine you can consume in different coffee brands without endangering your health?

Then, go to the Caffeine Calculator:
https://www.caffeineinformer.com/death-by-caffeine

III. Tea

What Is Tea?

Tea is a beverage made by adding hot water to a teapot containing dried leaves or small tea bugs with semi-powdered leaves, putting the water temperature into the nearly boiling point at 100° C (212° F). But many people boil the water, which may be a mistake, as explained in the latter part of this chapter.

Tea comes from the buds and leaves of the plant's upper area. The plant grows up to 4 feet tall, so the uppermost leaves are easily accessible.

5 Types of True Teas

The five main types of true teas are black, oolong, green, white, and pu-erh tea. They all come from the plant *camellia sinensis.*

There are five significant components found in all tea from the plant *Camellia sinensis,* which include:

- **Essential Oils:** They are a source of tea's delicious flavor and aroma
- **Polyphenols:** Antioxidants that provide the tea's brisk flavor and many of its potential health benefits.
- **Phytonutrients:** There are small amounts of vitamins, minerals, and amino acids, including L-theanine (a rare molecule found in only three sources, including *camellia sinensis.*).
- **Enzymes:** Macromolecular biological catalysts accelerate chemical reactions in the body.
- **Methylxanthines:** They are a family of alkaloids that include caffeine.

  Source: Arbor Teas

Caffeine Content of Teas Per 8 oz Serving

- Herbal: 0mg
- White: 10-15mg
- Arabica: 10-20mg

- Green: 15-30mg
- Oolong: 30-45mg
- Black: 60-75mg
- Matcha: 60-80mg
- Mate: 70-85mg
- Coffee: 125-150mg
  (Estimates only.)

Source: Adagio Teas

What Are Tannins?

The chemical compounds in teas include tannins and antioxidants belonging to polyphenols groups. Tannins are natural compounds found in plants, such as fruits, tree bark, roots, and leaves.

However, although serving as antioxidants themselves, these tannins block the absorption of iron in the body, resulting in a deficiency of this mineral that may lead to anemia.

Description of 5 True Teas

1. **Black Tea**: Black tea is one of the most widely known worldwide. It is also known as red tea in China with a darker shade.

Black tea contains the most amounts of caffeine and tannins. But it has more theaflavins (antioxidant polyphenols) than any other tea type. Black tea's taste is something rich and bold.

Black tea is fully oxidized through manufacturing processes, including sun-drying. Later, it undergoes natural fermentation when bacteria and fungi break down tea and make chemical changes. During the oxidation the tea develops its flavor and coloring during the oxidation, depending on how it's oxidized, whether fully or lightly.

Benefits of Black Tea

- Lowers blood sugar levels and blood pressure
- Improves immune system function
- Reduces inflammation
- Lowers bad LDL cholesterol

- Reduces risk of cancer
- Improves gut health

2. Oolong Tea: In China, Oolong tea, known as Black Dragon Oolong tea, falls somewhere between the black and green tea varieties.

Oolong tea is semi-oxidized (30-70% oxidized). It has a more complex flavor than green and white teas. It has smooth, soft astringency (slight acidity or bitterness of taste or smell) and has a floral or fruity flavor.

Benefits of Oolong Tea

- Lowers bad LDL cholesterol and triglycerides
- Serves as the natural defense from the sun's ultraviolet rays
- Makes bones stronger
- Reduces blood sugar levels and blood pressure
- Boasts heart health
- Promotes tooth and bone strength

3. Green Tea: Like other teas, green tea has different types, including the well-known *Sencha* and *Matcha*. Green tea has lots of antioxidants and other nutrients. The flavor profiles of green tea are mellow, grassy, and nutty.

Benefits of Green Tea

Green tea benefits include:

- Offers a lot of antioxidants, almost the same as those of white tea
- Promotes heart health
- Reduces blood sugar levels
- Lowers blood pressure due to its polyphenols and polysaccharides
- Minimizes the risk of some cancers
- Reduces inflammation

However, green tea is rich in tannins, a group of bitter and astringent compounds considered antinutrients like any other true tea.

4. White Tea: This tea is the simplest form of tea. It undergoes the least processing, so it has a delicate taste and aroma. This tea comes from the soft buds of the plant *Camellia Sinensis*. White tea has the lowest content of caffeine and tannins and is known for being the lightest of the teas.

White tea has the lowest amount of tannins, also an oxidant, but should not be consumed in high amounts because it hinders iron absorption in the body. It has a very delicate, calming, and slightly sweet.

Benefits of White Tea

- Acts as a natural supplement for cleansing and detoxing
- Protects the immune system
- Promotes cardiovascular health
- Promotes dental health due to its fluoride content
- Lowers blood sugar levels and blood pressure

5. Pu-erh Tea: Pu-erh or pu'er is a variety of fermented tea traditionally produced in Yunnan province, China. It is also grown in Taiwan and other parts of the globe. The taste of pu-erh tea varies; it depends on how long it's aged. It can stay fresh for up to 50 years and ages like a good-tasting wine because of its fermentation.

Pu-erh undergoes a process similar to green tea's sun-drying of the leaves. However, after the enzymatic oxidation of the leaves, pu-erh tea undergoes its fermentation through the aid of fungi and bacteria and then ages from a few months to several years.

The pu-erh tea has an earthy aroma and rich, smooth taste when aged like wine.

Benefits of Pu-erh Tea

- Promotes heart health
- Aids weight loss
- Increases energy
- Boasts cognitive health
- Improves metabolic syndrome

Types of Herbal Teas

The exceptions to the above teas are the so-called herbal teas or tisanes. These herbal teas have no caffeine. Why? Because these herbal teas come from the seeds, roots, stems, leaves, and flowers of different kinds of plants.

Examples of herbal teas include moringa tea, chamomile tea, peppermint tea, and ginger tea.

Moringa Oleifera Tea

The moringa tea comes from the leaves of the moringa tree. It is widely grown in India and subtropical regions of Africa, Asia, including the Philippines, and Latin America. However, it is a new tea globally,

This herbal tea is made by steeping moringa leaves or tea bags in hot water. It is naturally caffeine-free, and the tea's tannins and antinutrients are negligible. It has a delightful taste, flavor, and aroma.

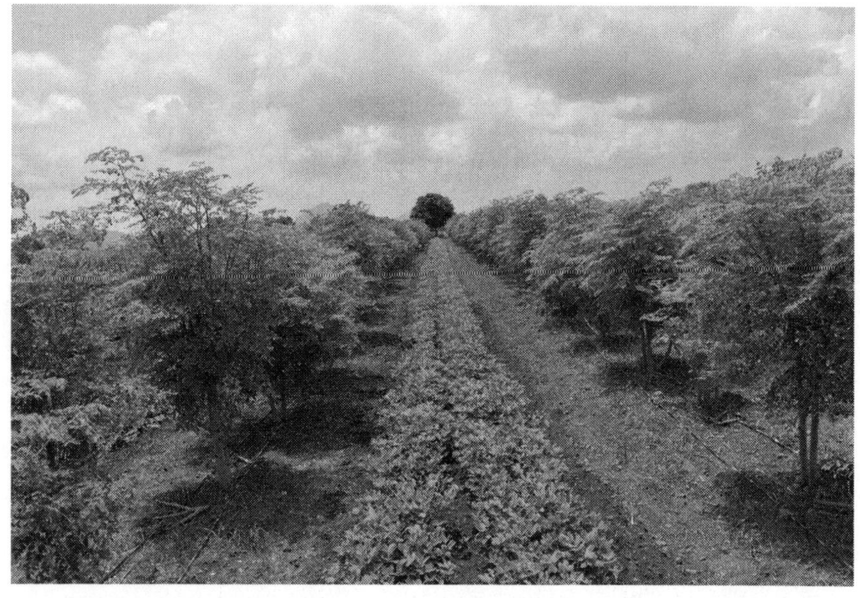

Moringa Tree Plantation

Photo Credit: Shutterstock

Benefits of Moringa Tea

Nutritional benefits of moringa tea include:

- Lowers blood sugar, helping in reducing the amount of sugar in the blood, as well as glucose and protein in the urine
- Reduces high blood pressure because its compounds isothiocyanate and niaziminin help in stopping arteries from thickening, which causes blood pressure to rise
- Protects the cardiovascular system because the powerful antioxidants in moringa extract might help prevent any cardiac damage, maintaining a healthy heart
- Fights inflammation because it has anti-inflammation properties
- Protects kidney disorders by preventing the development of kidney stones

Side Effects

- May interact with your diabetes and blood pressure medicines, resulting in very low blood sugar and blood pressure.
- May interact with some other medications.
- May be dangerous for pregnant women because of its anti-fertility qualities.
- May cause some stomach problems, like diarrhea, for some people.

Other herbal teas: Although containing antioxidants beneficial to health, true teas, and some other herbal teas may interact with medicines and other conditions. Before you drink any tea, you may consult with your physician.

The Correct Ways to Steep or Brew Tea

The true teas, white tea, green tea, oolong tea, and black te4a all come from the *camellia sinensis* plant. These teas contain many chemical compounds that give flavor and nutritional content to the tea.

To get enough nutritional compounds, you have to extract the compounds from the teas though the correct ways of steeping or brewing.

Generally, you have to submerge the dried tea leaves or tea bags in a cup or mug with hot water (but not boiling water).

Then the tea's compounds leach into the liquid through *osmosis diffusion*, which happens when there's fluid on both sides of a selectively permeable membrane, the tea leaves or tea bag. The teabags contain the leftover, broken tea leaves, called the "dust and fanning." done in selecting quality tea leaves.

In other words, when you heat water for tea steeping, wait for the water to simmer, during which a few bubbles break into the surface.

Yes, small bubbles from the bottom pop up in a liquid form, creating a simmering boil, not a rolling boil.

The temperature should not reach or exceed the boiling point at 212°F (100°C). To put it simply, don't heat the water at a rolling boil, which means a kind of churning, active motion coming from a high amount of heat.

Water that is too hot can destroy, degrade, or lose some of the chemical compounds such as vitamins, nutrients, and antioxidants extracted by hot water from the tea bag.

Stages of Chemical Compounds Release from Tea

Bioactive compounds, a type of substances found in small amounts in plants and certain foods, give good health to the body.

When you submerge tea leaves or tea bags in hot water, bioactive compounds released in succession from the tea are:

- Substances that give the tea's aroma, taste, and nutritional content
- Micronutrients, flavanols, polyphenols, and caffeine
- The heavier micronutrients
- Bitter tannins, which are considered antinutrients

Timing of steeping tea is of importance: If you soak or brew tea leaves or tea bags long enough, you'll miss some of the bioactive compounds. If you submerge it in hot water too long, the more tannins and caffeine you'll get; let the osmosis diffusion work. Be patient.

Hot Tea Steeping Time

Guidelines for the best steeping time and temperature for various teas follow:

Tea	Time	Temperature
White tea	4–5 minutes	175°F (79°C)
Green tea	3–4 minutes	175°F (79°C)
Oolong tea	3–5 minutes	195°F (91°C)
Black tea	3–4 minutes	195°F (91°C)
Dried herbal tea (e.g., dried chamomile, peppermint, hibiscus, lemon balm)	Up to 15 minutes or according to the manufacturer's instructions	212°F (100°C)
Fresh herbal tea (e.g., fresh herbs, ginger, turmeric)	5–15 minutes for tender herbs, 15–30 minutes for chopped or grated roots	212°F (100°C)e

Source: Healthline

Several Don'ts

- Don't use tap water; instead, use filtered (not distilled) water.
- Don't boil water. That's too hot that it may destroy or degrade some chemical compounds.
- Under normal atmospheric pressure, the temperature should be below the boiling point of pure water at 100°C (212°F). Or heat water in a pot; if you see enough bubbles at the bottom, that's a sign that the water is about to boil.
- Don't poke or jiggle the tea bag; don't move it around.
- Don't squeeze it before putting out the tea bag from the cup or mug.
- Don't drink tea with meals because tannins, being antinutrients, interfere with iron absorption by the body.
- Consume the tea at least one hour after a meal; at that time, the body should have already absorbed the iron.

Chapter 18

Sweeteners: Are They Good for Diabetics?

Brief Subject Summary

- What Are High-Intensity Sweeteners?
- Advantages of Using Sugar Substitutes
- Requirements for Approval of Sweeteners
- What Is GRAS?
- Sweeteners Approved by the FDA as Food Additives
- What Is Stevia?
- What Are Stevia Sweeteners?
- What Are Highly-Purity Steviol Glycosides?
- Most Popular Sweeteners
- What Are Some Other Sugar Substitutes?
- Other Food Additives

I. The Sweeteners: Food Additives

As we know, people with diabetes can't eat or should omit table sugar in their diet because it will cause blood sugar spikes in the bloodstream. That's why many people with diabetes are forced to use sugar substitutes or sweeteners in their diet.

But are these sweeteners good for you and me? Or bad for the body? Let's find out.

High-intensity sweeteners are commonly used as sugar substitutes or sugar alternatives because they are sweeter than regular table sugar, called sucrose.

What Are High-Intensity Sweeteners

FDA says, "High-intensity sweeteners are commonly used as sugar substitutes or sugar alternatives because they are many times sweeter than sugar but contribute only a few to no calories when added to foods."

And it adds, "High-intensity sweeteners, like all other ingredients added to food in the United States, must be safe for consumption."

Simply put, high-intensity sweeteners are ingredients used to sweeten and enhance the flavor of foods.

Because they are often sweeter than table sugar (sucrose), only smaller amounts of high-intensity sweeteners are needed to achieve the same sweetness level as the regular table sugar.

Advantages in Using These Sugar Substitutes

- High-intensity sweeteners contribute only a few to no calories when added to foods
- They are many times' sweeter than regular table sugar, so it needs only small amounts of these sugar substitutes to achieve the same sweetness level as the regular sugar in foods

What Is Generally Recognized as Safe (GRAS)?

According to the International Food Information Council Foundation (IFICF), food ingredients permitted for use in the United States, fall into one of two categories:

- Food additives (which require review before approval from the FDA) or;
- Generally Recognized as Safe (GRAS) ingredients

8 Sweeteners Approved by the FDA as Food Additives

The FDA had earlier approved six high-intensity sweeteners: aspartame, advantame, acesulfame potassium, neotame, saccharin, and sucralose, used in the United States as food sugar alternatives to enhance flavor in foods. But they are subject to strict scrutiny to be safe for human consumption.

They underwent premarket review, scrutiny, and approval by the FDA, basing its decision on premarket reviews and studies made by the manufacturers of these food additives.

The FDA then approved two more sugar substitutes: Luo han guo (Monk fruit extract) and Stevia Sweeteners.

The total 8 nonnutritive sweeteners approved by the U.S. Food and Drug Administration (FDA) are as follows:

- Aspartame (Equal® or NutraSweet®)
- Advantame
- Acesulfame potassium (Sunett® and Sweet One®)
- Neotame
- Saccharin (Sweet 'N Low®, Sweet Twin®, and Sugar Twin®)
- Sucralose (Splenda® and Equal Sucralose)
- Luo han guo (Monk fruit extract) (Monk Fruit in the Raw ®)
- Stevia (Truvia®, Stevia in the Raw®, SweetLeaf® Stevia, Sweet Drops™, Sun Crystals®, and PureVia®)

1. **Aspartame:** With about 200 times sweeter than table sugar, the FDA approved aspartame as a nutritive sweetener. Aspartame has been one of the most exhaustively studied substances in the human food supply.

Aspartame brand names include NutraSweet®, Equal®, and *S*ugar Twin®.

Upon reviewing scientific data, FDA scientists have concluded that aspartame is safe for the general population under certain conditions.

2. **Advantame:** The FDA approved advantame for use in food as a nonnutritive sweetener. Advantame is about 20,000 times sweeter than table sugar.

3. **Acesulfame Potassium**: The FDA approved acesulfame potassium as a nonnutritive sweetener. It's about 200 times sweeter than table sugar. Brand names of this sweetener include Sunette and Sweet One.

4. **Neotame:** About 7,000 to 13,000 sweeter than table sugar, the FDA approved neotame for foods as a nonnutritive sweetener.

In 2002, the FDA approved it as a general-purpose sweetener and flavor enhancer in foods (except meat and poultry) under certain conditions. Stores sell Neotame's brand name, *Newtame.*

5. **Saccharin**: This sugar substitute is 200 to 700 times sweeter than table sugar (sucrose.). The FDA approved saccharin for use in food as a nonnutritive sweetener. One example of a saccharin sweetener is Sweet'N Low®.

6. **Sucralose:** The FDA approved sucralose, sold under Splenda's name for food use as a nonnutritive sweetener. It is 600 times sweeter than regular sugar.

In 1998, the FDA approved sucralose for use in 15 food categories. Then in 1999, it was approved by the FDA as a general-purpose sugar substitute.

7. **Luo han guo (monk fruit extract)**: (Monk Fruit in the Raw ®): Monk fruit, or lou han guo, is a small green melon native to southern China and named after the monks who first cultivated it centuries ago.

8. **Stevia Sweeteners:** Brand Names -- SweetLeaf®, Truvia®, Stevia in the Raw®, Sweet Drops™, Sun Crystals®, and PureVia®)

II. What Are Stevia Sweeteners?

Generally, Stevia sweeteners were approved as sugar substitutes by the US FDA and declared safe for food and drink additives, as long as they have achieved the GRAS status.

The International Food Information Council Foundation, representing leading global health agencies, has found purified stevia sweeteners to be safe.

The agencies include:

- European Food Safety Authority (EFSA)
- Joint FAO/WHO Expert Committee on Food Additives (JECFA)
- Japan Ministry of Health and Welfare
- Food Standards of Australia, New Zealand, and Health Canada

According to *Medical News Today*, "Stevia is an intensely sweet-tasting plant that has been used to sweeten beverages and make tea since the 16th century."

Originally native to Paraguay and Brazil, stevia is also grown in Japan and China. A nonnutritive sweetener, Stevia contains few or no calories and zero glycemic indexes. It does not affect blood sugar levels.

Is Stevia Safe?

In 1991, the FDA banned stevia products as a food additive in the United States, saying it had questions about its safety. Early studies suggested it may cause cancer. Subsequent studies refuted these earlier studies, and the FDA later ruled stevia as GRAS for use in general food production.

Endorsed with Condition

According to Dr. Ben Brown, the Ornish Lifestyle Medicine medical director, taking stevia is safe. However, he recommends that you use stevia in smaller quantities because some case reports suggest that it may cause some side effects for some people. When taken in large amounts, these conditions include stomach upset, muscle pain, and allergies.

Dr. Brown says, "Stevia has been around for a long time in Latin America. Most research on stevia shows that it appears to be safe and has some potential benefits, including possibly lowering blood pressure and blood sugar."

What Are Highly-Purity Steviol Glycosides?

Steviol glycosides are natural constituents of highly-purity (95%) minimum purity) that make the leaves of Stevia rebaudiana taste sweet. The plant is native to Paraguay and Brazil in South America and is commonly known as stevia in South America.

The glycosides, as nonnutritive sweeteners, are considered 200 to 400 times sweeter than table sugar.

The US FDA has received many GRAS notices for using these high-purity steviol glycosides.

They include Rebaudioside A (also known as Reb A); Stevioside; Rebaudioside D; steviol glycoside mixture preparations with Rebaudioside A; and Stevioside being the predominant components.

The FDA has not questioned the notifiers' GRAS determination for these high-purity stevia-derived sweeteners under the intended conditions of use identified in the GRAS notices submitted to the FDA.

The process of approving a Stevia sweetener by the FDA is quite simple. If the FDA does not question the submitted Notifiers' Gras status or determination, the sweetener has already gained approval for use as a sweetener.

However, stevia leaf and crude stevia extracts (instead of purified steviol glycosides) are not considered GRAS by the FDA. Thus, it's illegal to import them to the U.S. as sweeteners.

8 Glycosides

Stevia contains 8 glycosides, which are the sweet components isolated and purified from the leaves of stevia. These include:

- Stevioside
- Rebaudioside A
- Rebaudioside C
- Rebaudioside D
- Rebaudioside E
- Rebaudioside F
- Steviolbioside
- Dulioside A

Beverages with Stevia Sweeteners

Frequently, foods and drinks made with stevia sweeteners are recommended for people with diabetes, whether prediabetes, type 2 diabetes, or type 1 diabetes.

According to the International Food Information Council Foundation, "Extensive research shows that stevia sweeteners do not raise blood sugar levels in humans (Nichol 2018, Romo-Romo 2017, Maki 2008), and recognized in a recent consensus statement by experts in nutrition, medicine, and physical activity."

The legality of stevia as a food additive or sweetener differs from nation to nation. In the United States, a stevia product is approved as a sugar substitute so long as it has achieved GRAS status.

In 2011, the European Union approved stevia products as food additives or a table sugar substitute. In Japan, people have widely used stevia for the past many years.

The Most Popular Sweeteners?

At present, for some people, the most popular sugar substitutes used by people with diabetes (cited not in order of popularity) are Splenda (Sucralose), Equal (aspartame), Sweet and Low (Saccharin), and SweetLeaf Stevia and Truvia.

Splenda, Equal, and Sweet and Low have been approved as food additives by the FDA (that underwent premarket review, scrutiny, and approval by the FDA).

The FDA has approved SweetLeaf Stevia and Truvia as sweeteners for having GRAS status or determination.

Descriptions

Splenda: Splenda, sucralose, isn't broken down in the body, so it has zero calories and is about 400-700 times sweeter than table sugar.

Sweet and Low: It is one of the first available artificial sugar substitutes used in foods, toothpaste, and medicine.

Equal (Aspartame): Typically found in diet soda, puddings, chewing gum, and other "sugar-free" snacks, aspartame is about 200 sweeter than sugar. It does have some calories, and it also loses its sweetness when heated.

SweetLeaf Stevia: SweetLeaf Stevia is a highly refined stevia called *rebaudioside* A (marketed as *Rebiana*). It is approved as a sweetener by the FDA, having the status of GRAS.

Truvia: A product created by The Coca-Cola Company and Cargill, a chemical company, is made from Stevia leaves and other ingredients. Truvia has also gained the status of GRAS.

Sweetleaf Stevia Sweetener Processing

SweetLeaf Stevia Sweetener on its website says it uses high-grade stevia leaves in extracting sweeteners in a proprietary cool and purified water filtration process.

The company adds that it doesn't use alcohol or chemicals in the processing.

Ingredients of SweetLeaf Stevia Sweetener

The main ingredients of SweetLeaf Stevia Sweetener are:

- Stevia leaf extract
- Purified water

What Is Truvia?

Truvia, which sounds like Stevia, is a sweetener created by The Coca-Cola Company and Cargill, a food and chemical company.

A competitor of SweetLeaf Stevia Sweetener and other sweet manufacturers, Truvia also uses stevia plant leaves.

Stevia and Truvia have almost similar names, but they are different; stevia is a plant while Truvia is a commercial product.

Truvia uses stevia leaves as ingredients in whatever amounts of food additives in manufacturing, like all other sweeteners

Ingredients of Truvia

Truvia Natural Sweetener has three components:

- Stevia leaf extract
- Erythritol
- Natural flavors

The first step in making the sugar substitute is to take the sweetest part of the stevia leaf and extract its natural sweetness. A raw sugar alcohol called erythritol and a particular amount of natural flavors are included in the ingredients to create a good-tasting, zero-calorie sweetness.

What Are Some of the Other Sugar Substitutes?

They include PureVia, Eliten, Rebiana, Steviacane, and Stevia Extract In the Raw.

III. Other Food Additives

What Are Other Food Additives?

While high-intensity sweeteners are considered food additives, other food additives also give eaters a good taste, flavor, and appearance. They include:

- **Sodium Glutamate (MSG):** A common food additive used to enhance the flavor of foods
- **Sodium Benzoate:** Sodium benzoate acts as a preservative for carbonated drinks and acidic foods
- **Artificial food coloring**: Brightens the appearance of candies, condiments, and other foods
- **Sodium nitrite:** Sodium nitrate acting as a preservative and adding a salty flavor and reddish-pink color to foods
- **High-fructose corn syrup:** A sweetener made from corn and found in soda, juice, candy, and breakfast cereals

Source: *Healthline*

Part II: Book 2

Exposing Longevity & Old Age Secrets to Living into Your 90s

Chapter 19

The Quest for Healthy Aging & Longevity

Brief Subject Summary

- Where's the Fountain of Youth?
- What Is Aging?
- What's Healthy Living?
- Differences Between Longevity, Lifespan, and Life Expectancy
- Average World Life Expectancy
- What Are You Called Based on Your Age?
- Can You Lengthen Your Life?
- Estimated Long Life Expectancy

Where's the Fountain of Youth?

Since time immemorial, the human race has been seeking the Fountain of Youth. Scientists worldwide have been making studies to discover the secrets to slowing down aging and lengthening human longevity. It is their belief that aging can be slowed down through healthy living.

What Is Aging, By the Way?

"Aging is associated with changes in dynamic biological, physiological, environmental, behavioral, and social processes," says the National Institute on Aging (NIA) of the National Institute of Health (NIH).

Simply put, such age-related changes result in declines in body and mental functions, causing the advancing age to become the risk factor for many human chronic diseases.

What's the Meaning of Healthy Living?

The World Health Organization (WHO) defines healthy living "as the process of developing and maintaining the functional ability that enables well-being in older age."

Other Definitions of Terms

Before we proceed further, let us discuss first the terms: longevity, lifespan, life expectancy, and health span which may often be used in this second part of this book.

Differences Between Longevity, Lifespan, and Life Expectancy

The terms, longevity, lifespan, and life expectancy are sometimes used interchangeably. But they are different from each other, with specific definition.

- **Longevity**: Longevity which means "long" refers to the duration of life, particularly of exceptionally long-lived persons. In other words, longevity has the ability to last for a long time. In fact, the word longevity has been in existence since the 1600s. The word, longevity, is often used to define the length of an individual's life but it may also mean a long duration, such as a person living into the 90s and beyond. Put simply, longevity may mean how long you actually live past averages. For example, the average life expectancy for both men and women worldwide is 72 to 73. If you reach the age 72 or 73, you have a little bit of longevity. It means it's not impressive.
- **Lifespan:** Lifespan is the duration of life of a person, while longevity typically describes a particularly long lifespan. To clarify, human lifespan is the maximum number of years an individual from the human species can live based on observed examples.
- **Life Expectancy:** Although the words lifespan and life expectancy both refer to the number of living years, they actually describe different concepts. The term lifespan refers to the maximum years a person can live while life expectancy defines an estimate or average number of years an individual can expect to live. Simply put, life expectancy is described by a scientific calculation of an individual's estimate number of years of existence. Such calculation, of course, may depend on several factors, including genetics, diet, lifestyle, and environment.

Health Span: Health span may be described as the period of life spent by an individual in good health, without having suffered from chronic diseases and aging disabilities. (Aging is a process of growing older and showing bad effects of increasing age, such as wrinkles and diminishing body of humans.)

A Look at Life Expectancy

Demographic research indicates that at the turn of the 19th century no country had achieved the life expectancy of people of more than 40 years.

However, in 1950, the life expectancy of newborns was already more than 60 years in some progressive nations, such as people living in Europe, North America, Japan, Oceania, and some places of South America. For instance, at that time, Norway had a life expectancy (for males and females), of 60 years.

Of course, in some poor countries, people could only expect to have a life expectancy of 30 years. So therefore, there was no equality in life expectancy. The higher life expectancy in progressive countries had been attributed to advancement in health and technology, including the discoveries of new medicines.

As countries progressed, bolstered by improved economy and education, life expectancy continued to rise.

Average World Life Expectancy

- **75 years**: For female at birth
- **70 years:** For male at birth

Latest US Average Life Expectancy at Birth for Both Sexes

- **80 years:** (for both sexes) - Central Intelligence Agency (CIA)
- **78.6 years** ((or both sexes) - Centers for Disease Control and Prevention (CDC)
- **78.5 years (for both sexes)** - Organization for Economic Co-operation and Development (OECD)

US Gender Specific Figures

- **81.1 years:** Average life expectancy for females
- **76.1 years:** Average life expectancy for males

Life Expectancy for Females and Males Over 65 years

- **20.6 Years:** Average life expectancy for females over 65
- 1 **8.1 years**: Average life expectancy for males over 65

U.S. Latest Life Expectancy From 2019 to 2022

- **79.05 years:** Life expectancy in 2022
- **78.99 years**: Life expectancy in 2021
- **78.87 years:** Life expectancy in 2020
- **78.93 years:** Life expectancy in 2019

Note: All 2020 and later figures are projections of the United Nations and DO NOT include impacts of COVID-19 virus.

How Does U.S. Rank in Life Expectancy Worldwide?

The United States currently ranks 43rd in life expectancy among countries globally.

Countries with Highest Global Life Expectancy

- **Monaco:** 89.4 years
- **Japan:** 85.3 years
- **Singapore:** 85.3 years

How Old Are You Now?

At whatever age you're right now, you have the chance of a life-time in lengthening your longevity, provided you adhere to the factors that determine your longevity.

What Are You Called Based on Your Age?

Are you a sexagenarian or an oldest old? Yes, you can extend your life, barring accidents or the dreaded disease, cancer. Well, you may be able to survive cancer, if it's discovered in its early stages.

For me, being 90 years old, I'm called a nonagenarian or an oldest old.

Age by Decade

There are different group names for people in each decade of age which are:

10 to 19 - denarian
20 to 29 - vicenarian.
30-to 39 - tricenarian
40 to 49 - quadragenarian
50 to 59 - quinquagenarian
60 to 69 - sexgenarian
70 to 79 - septuagenarian
80 to 89 - octogenarian
90 to 99 - nonagenarian
100 to 109 - centenarian

Classification of Elderly Based on Age Groups:

The elderly is classified into these age groups:

65 to 74 - youngest old
75 to 84 - middle old
85 and over - oldest old

For me, being 90 years old, (I'm more than 90 now) is called a nonagenarian or an oldest old.

Can You Lengthen Your Life?

Today, newly-born babies in the United States can be expected to have a life expectancy of about 80 years. In retrospect, a century ago, the life expectancy throughout the world was closer to 54 years only.

"We've had a significant increase in lifespan over the last century," says Dr. Marie Bernard, deputy director of National Institute on Aging of the US National Institute of Health (NIH)

She adds, "Now if you make it to age 65, the likelihood that you'll make it to 85 is very high. And if you make it to 85, the likelihood that you'll make it to 92 is very high. So people are living longer on average than most Americans. and it's happening across the globe."

"If I had to rank behaviors in terms of priority, I'd say that exercise is the most important thing associated with living longer and healthier," says Dr. Luigi Ferrucci, an NIH geriatrician who oversees research on aging and health.

"Exercise is especially important for lengthening active life expectancy, which is life without disease and without physical and mental/ thinking disability," adds Ferrucci.

For exercise, review Chapter 9: *Walking: The Best Exercise for Reversing Type 2 Diabetes, Kidney Disease, and Heart Disease.*

Estimated Life Long Expectancy

Generally, it is a widely accepted fact that the maximum long life expectancy could be up to 125. So far, the long life expectancy was established by a French woman, named Jeanne Calment, who died at the age of 122.

The Gerontology Research Group validates current longevity records based on modern standards. It maintains a list of super-centenarians and other invalidated longevity claims.

The list of supercentenarians include:

Jean Calment (a French woman (1875-1997, 122 years, 164 days): The oldest human being who ever lived, whose record was verified through modern standard verifications.

Sarah Knauss (1880-1999, 119 years, 97 days): The second oldest documented person in the world and the oldest American.

Christian Mortensen (1882-1998, 115 years, 252 days): The oldest man who ever lived.

Super-Centinarian

Kane Tanaka, a Japanese woman (Jane 2, 1903), was 119 years old and 107 days when she died on April 19, 2022.

Chapter 20

How to Live into Your 90s and Beyond

Brief Subject Summary

- Setting Goals Is Required
- A Massive Heart Attack
- Is Longevity Determined by Genetics?
- Can You Do Some Changes in Lifestyle?
- The 90+ Study
- Factors That Influence Human Longevity
- Overall Tips for Having a Long Life

At the age of 63, I had survived a massive heart attack, resulting in about 40% damage to my body machine and that ended in having heart failure with an ejection fraction of only 27%.

Also, I have no family history of a long life, no clan members that had reached the age 90 or more. My mother passed away when I was two years old and my father died at the age of 45. My grandfather, on my mother's side, passed away at age 75, which is still not impressive.

Yet, this year, I reached age 90 and now I'm already in my 90s. What a way to live!

Over the years, I have reversed my type 2 diabetes and kidney disease into remission and reversed my heart disease gravity and put it in a better condition up to 47% fraction from 15%.

Not to brag, but at this age now, living in the 90s, I can still do moderate-intensity walk, covering 3 to 4 miles daily, in a 3-session-20-minute exercise, month after month.

Wow! Yes, it's incredible; it's satisfying and enjoyable! I almost could not believe it, but it's true.

This is just to prove that your dream of living into your 90s can be achieved, too, if you are really determined to accomplish it.

Setting Goals Is Required

Having a long life does not happen just like that. You have to work for it. It's only you who can do it barring accidents and the dreaded disease, cancer; you have the power and ability to slow down aging and achieve longevity.

Is Longevity Determined by Genetics?

MedlinePlus, a reliable government website, commenting on longevity reports, "The duration of human life (longevity) is influenced by genetics, the environment, and lifestyle. Environmental improvements beginning in the 1900s extended the average lifespan dramatically with significant improvements in the availability of food and clean water, better housing and living conditions, reduced exposure to infectious diseases, and access to medical care."

It adds, "Most significant were public health advances that reduced premature death by decreasing the risk of infant mortality, increasing the chances of surviving childhood, and avoiding infection and communicable diseases. Now, people in the United States live about 80 years on average, but some individuals survive for much longer."

Can You Do Some Changes in Lifestyles?

True, we cannot change our genes, but we can alter our diet, form of exercise, lifestyle, and environment. Of course, if you have a family whose members who lived into their 90s, you have the edge over other human beings.

Also, other factors can be changed, like changing your overall lifestyle, involving behaviors, like smoking, drinking alcohol, and not having enough sleep. If you are eating bad foods for your body, you can minimize or eliminate them.

If you are living in a city with lots of pollutions, including poisonous chemicals, you may move to another place to change your environment to avoid being afflicted with cancer. The list goes on and on.

The 90+ Study

The 90+ Study was started in 1981 as an investigation of the oldest old, regarding their diet, medical history, lifestyle, behaviors, and other factors.

The initial healthy male participants, about 1,600, were once members of the Leisure World, (a community in Orange County, California, now known as the City of Laguna Woods, California).

Later, men about 600 participants, with average age 70 or more, were enrolled in the study. So all in all, the number totalled about 2,200, which may be considered as the largest study of the oldest old in the world.

All the men were given yearly surveys about aging and lifestyle. They were visited by researchers or investigators every six months, undergoing neurological and and other tests.

What Happened?

By the end of the study, sixteen years later, 970 men (41 percent of the surviving participants of the 90+ study) had lived into their 90s.

Specifically, the study discovered that:

- None-smokers are twice as likely to reach 90 and beyond as smokers.
- Over 40% of individuals aged 90 and more suffer from dementia and almost 80% are disabled.
- People aged 90 and over with an APOE2 gene are less likely to have Alzheimer's dementia. However, they are likely to have Alzheimer's neuropathology in their brains to explain their cognitive loss.
- Diabetes increases the risk of dying before the age of 90 by 86 percent.
- High blood pressure increases the risk of dying before 90 by 28 percent..
- Overweight people have a 44 percent risk of dying before age 90.
- People who exercise regularly reduce their risk of death before 90 by 20 percent to 30 percent.
- About half of people afflicted with dementia over 90 didn't have sufficient neuropathology in their brain, indicating cognitive loss.

What Do the 90+Study Results Indicate?

It's loud and clear! The results suggested that in order to reach age 90 and beyond, you have to do he following:

- Stop smoking, if you are addicted to it.
- Prevent the occurrence of type 2 diabetes, kidney disease, and heart disease by eating semi-plant based foods (more plant foods than animal foods.)
- Reduce weight to lower the risk of diabetes.
- Exercise regularly, doing moderate-intensity walking or any aerobic exercises that reduce blood sugar, creatinine, and blood urea nitrogen (BUN), if you have diabetes, or kidney disease.
- Normalize your high blood pressure to prevent the risk of diabetes stroke, heart attack, and kidney disease.

Factors That Influence Human Longevity

Besides genetics (it's inherited, and you can not change it), you must know the factors that may affect your lifespan, which are within your reach.

The major factors that may determine your being able to reach the age of 90 and beyond are:

- Genetics
- Lifestyle
- Environment

1. Genetics

Having a family history of people who had lived a long life, is a plus. Yes, you may think that you should have good genes to be able to have a long life. But it's a fact that genetics has only 20 to 30 percent influence in determining your longevity.

So don't worry, if you don't have the genes of a family of people who have reached the age of 90 or more, you can improve other factors that you have.

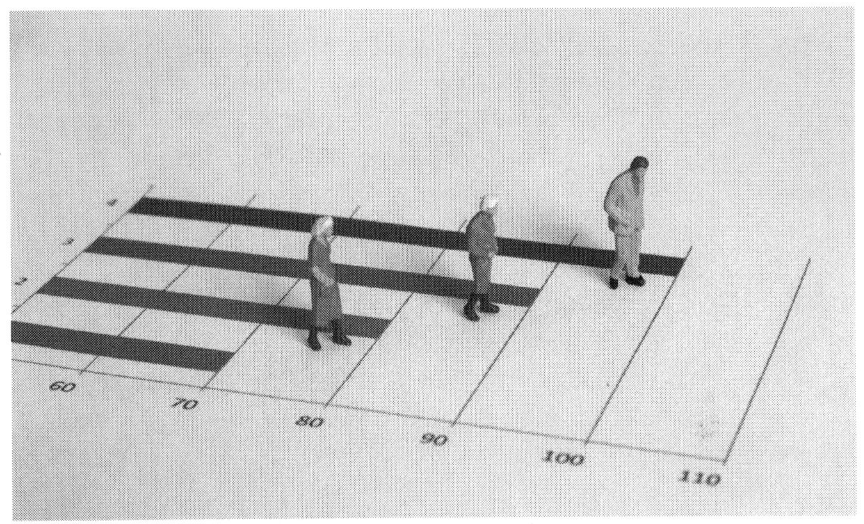

Miniature People and the Concept of an Aging Society

Photo Source: Shutterstock

2. Lifestyle

Generally, lifestyle involves many factors, including your habits, behaviors, interactions with family members, friends, and other members of society, as a whole.

Smoking: For example, if you're a chain smoker, you are susceptible to several diseases, including chronic obstructive pulmonary disease (COPD), kidney disease, and lung cancer. What to do if you're a smoker? Well, you have to stop doing it.

Drinking alcohol. If you have the habit of drinking too much alcohol, then you are bound to having mouth cancer, liver cirrhosis, and cardiovascular diseases. In other words, drinking alcohol should be in moderation.

Lack of Enough Sleep: The recommended number of hours of sleep is from 7 to 9 hours. But most people sleep only for about 4 to 6 hours. Sleep deprivation causes bad effects, including health issues such as chronic diseases or conditions, like heat attack, and other cardiovascular diseases, high blood pressure, irregular heart beat, kidney diseases, diabetes, and obesity.

Needless to say, you have to stop or minimize doing bad habits turning them into good ones. In that way, you can extend your lifespan.

Diet: Your overall diet plays a major role in aspiring to have a long life. Your health good condition will depend on what you eat, whether you are following a particular diet, for instance, the Mediterranean diet, the MIND diet, vegetarian diet, or the flexible diet, or any plant-based diet. The general recommendation is to eat more plant foods such as whole grains, vegetables, and fruits. (Review chapter 11: *Best Diets for 2023* for discussion of different diets.)

Exercise, Leisure Time, and Other Activities: Doing physical activities such as aerobic exercises, including moderate-intensity walking (or brisk walking), can help your body become healthy. It can enhance your heart pumping enough blood to all parts of the body. (Review chapter 9: *Walking System: Why Is It Works for Diabetes, Kidney Disease, and Heart Disease.)*

Also, many studies suggest that the elderly should engage in leisure time for good physical condition and mental alertness

For good health, the Centers for Disease and Prevention (CDC), recommends to do an exercise 3 to 5 times a week, at least for 30 minutes per session.

Being Obese: Being overweight is an established risk factor for several diseases, such as diabetes, kidney disease, and heart disease that can cause stroke or heart attack.

So what's the solution? Lessen your body weight by at least 5 to 10%, depending on your body mass index (BMI). In other words, you should have a healthy BMI.

Social Networking: According to several studies, senior social networking has been established to influence mortality. However, the problem is how can a senior, especially the oldest old, interact with members of society, since they cannot drive anymore and they are stuck in their homes alone.

What can you do, if you're already an oldest old, is to let your close family members, and some friends visit you. If they can't do it, talking to them by phone is an option.

Stress: A stressful lifestyle has a strong influence on your longevity and health. A Yale University research indicates that chronic stress due to diseases, such as diabetes, kidney disease, heart disease, and other cardiovascular diseases, can shorten an individual's lifespan.

"A lot of people have felt on a gut level that stress makes us age faster, and our study shows that is true," says Zach Harvanek, a resident psychiatrist at Yale University and one of the researchers who made the study.

"

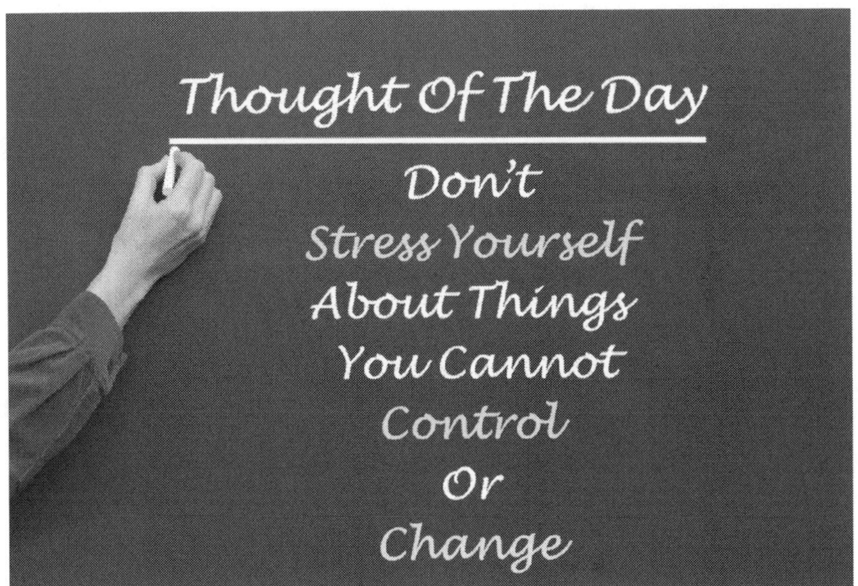

Image Credit: Shutterstock

Depression: According to the American Psychiatric Association, in defining depression, says, "Depression (major depressive disorder) is a common and serious medical illness that negatively affects how you feel, the way you think and how you act."

3. Environment

The environment plays a major role in seeking one's longevity. Environmental factors may affect an individual's health.

While stress is a natural part of life, it should be minimized for the elderly. Stress can make chemical changes in the brain, involving memory and leading to developing Alzheimer's or related dementia. Research shows the conditions are aggravated by isolation, depression, and loneliness. As an older adults, you should avoid deep sadness, lack of sleep, and lack of appetite, because they will have a big impact on your health.

Toxins and Other Pollutants: If you live in a modern city, you will ingest toxins, such as poisonous smoke and polluted air that can wreck havoc on your body. They are bad for the body's organs, such as the lungs, that may cause you have cancer.

For instance, ingestion of metals can cause cardiometabolic conditions and breast cancer. Persistent pesticides (such as DDT and DDE) can result in lactation impairments.

Traffic jams may cause you stress, and due to many vehicles, you may meet an accident, especially if you're already an elderly. Factories, of course, use chemicals that emit poisonous smoke, as they process and pack manufactured goods.

Several studies have shown that unhealthy environmental quality, such as poor air quality, can cause increased mortality in urban areas due to air pollution.

Change of Environment: So, if possible, if you're already retired, you may move to the suburbs with less pollution, or to the rural areas with lots of fresh air. In other words, you may change your environment.

Overall Tips for Having a Long Life

1. Having a Healthy Diet: If possible select a plant-based diet, a semi-plant based diet (more plant foods than animal foods). To select a particularly diet, go to Chapter 11: *Best Diets for 2023*, as sponsored by *U.S. News & World Report* on page 239.

You may select the Mediterranean Diet or any vegetarian diet, such as the Flexitarian Diet or any other flexible diet. Or select a semi-plant-based diet that advocates more plant foods than animal foods, and other plant-based proteins that can lead to healthy aging.

2. Exercising: Regular aerobic exercises, such as moderate-intensity walking for 30 minutes daily, 3 to 5 times a week, is recommended by the centers for Disease Control and Prevention (CDC). Regarding my exercising, I do walking and different workout every day.

3. **Stopping smoking**: Smoking, as described in this chapter, results in having many diseases. So it's but wise to stop smoking,

4. **Limiting or avoiding alcohol:** Ingestion of alcohol, like smoking, causes many diseases that will damage your body, making your

lifespan shorter. Drink alcohol moderately, if you can't totally ignore it.

If you have more goals to achieve, then those can be your inspiration to continue living with your family, especially your grand kids, for a much longer time, and to pursue some more work that you enjoy doing.

5. Practicing Healthy Lifestyle: Changing bad habits to good habits can greatly influence healthy aging.

6. Drinking Enough Water: Make the habit of drinking enough water, probably 8 to 10 measuring cups or glasses with 8-ounce fluid is recommended by health professionals. The kidneys and other body organs need enough water, the best drink, to have a healthy body; for instance, preventing the formations of kidney stones, and making the kidneys healthy. Water, as already mentioned, dilute blood sugar, creatinine and BUN (blood sugar urea), the waste product of protein),

7. Getting Enough Sleep: Health professionals recommend that you sleep for 7 to 9 hours per day in order to have a healthy body. They say that if you sleep only for 6 hours, you'll increase the risk of developing diseases, such as type 2 diabetes, kidney disease, and heart disease.

8. Improving Cognitive Health: What is cognitive health? The Centers for Diseases Control and Prevention (CDC) describes cognitive health as "a healthy brain that is one that can perform all the mental processes that are collectively known as cognition, including the ability to learn new things, intuition, judgment, language, and remembering."

9. Being Socially Active: Although you may not have the ability and capacity to fully interact with other people in a society in general, because of your physical health, at least you may be active in interacting with your family members and friends.

Chapter 21

Overcoming 8 Grand Challenges of Aging

Brief Subject Summary

- Key Facts and Figures
- 8 Challenges of Aging

Key Facts and Figures

Problems facing all countries for their growing populations are the following:

- All countries face major challenges to ensure that their health and social systems are ready to make the most of this demographic shift.
- In 2050, 80% of older people will be living in low- and middle-income countries.
- The pace of population aging is much faster than in the past.
- In 2020, the number of people age 60 years and older outnumbered children younger than 5 years.
- Between 2015 and 2050, the proportion of the world's population over 60 years will nearly double from 12% to 22%.

Source: World Health Organization (WHO)

8 Challenges of Aging

The 8 major challenges of getting old are as defined by the Aging 2.0 Alliance, a network of senior specialists in the United States and experts are as follows:

1. Engagement & Purpose
2. Financial Wellness
3. Mobility & Movement
4. Daily Living & Lifestyle

5. Caregiving
6. Care Coordination
7. Brain Health
8. End of Life

These challenges of aging can be applied to older adults in any place worldwide. Whether you are an American, Canadian, Japanese, British, Filipino, Australian, or Brazilian, the problems of old age are similar, wherever you may go.

1. Engagement & Purpose

As an elderly, especially if you belong to the group of oldest adult, you are faced with the major challenges of old age. You need to maintain your social contact, especially with your family members, and friends, not necessarily the society as a whole.

And of course, you need a purpose to continue living. If you have no more purpose in life or whatever work you still want to do, you continue to set goals, to have a purpose to continue living. Have new hobbies and attend social functions. If not, you get stuck in your room most of the day, suffering from loneliness and depression. Simply put, have a purpose in life.

2. Financial Wellness

In the United States, many of the growing older adults live in poverty. A generation ago, the country's oldest populations had he highest risk of living in poverty.

Of course, in some countries, many local, city, provincial, and national governments have some kind of programs for senior citizens. But those programs are not enough. Among those benefits for older adults are discounts for food, transportation, or entertainment and more.

In the Philippines, for instance, senior citizens are given a certain allowance each per month, and they have discount cards for food or services.

Not only that, if you are a Filipino and you live into your 100, you'll be given a lump sum of P100,000 for being a centenarian. That's big money in the Philippines.

Wow! That's why senior citizens are trying to reach age 100,. Yes, that's an incentive to live longer!

3. Mobility & Movement

Being an elderly, you lose your independence. Before, if you have a car, you used to drive anywhere. But not now; therefore, your family members are worried about your safety.

In general, particularly if you're frail and old; you little by little, depending on your age, lose your balance and increase your risks of falls, during which you may break your bones. That may result in your being disabled and you'll get stuck at home. (For improving balance, see Chapter 23).

In the house, if you already have balance problems, you need to have bars on walls and rubber mats on the tub for safety reasons. You should also use a walking can or walker, depending on your physical conditions.

Outdoor, you may use, if needed, a walking can for safety reasons while doing walking as an exercise. Some people are ashamed doing this, as a denial of getting old. "I don't need it," some seniors say, even if they are walking unsteadily.

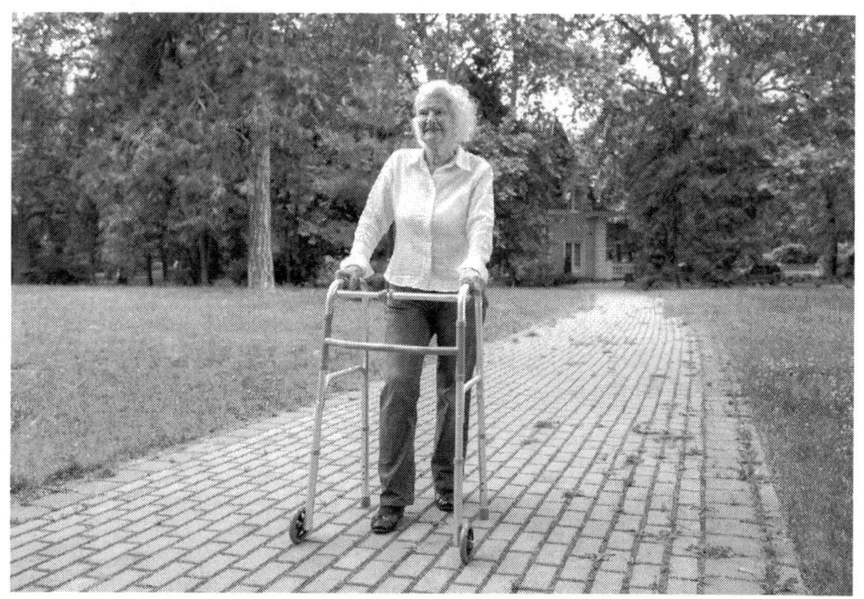

Elderly Woman Uses a Walker as She Strolls Through the Park

Photo Credit: Shutterstock

4. Daily Living and Lifestyle

Almost all seniors want to get old in place, (meaning in their own homes), some seniors who can afford it, prefer to live in an independent living facility. Other old adults, those living alone in their own abodes, depending on their physical fitness, need assistance in daily living,

For instance, seniors who no longer drive, need someone to buy them groceries. If you are a senior living alone, you may check if there are any local government or private assistance programs, providing assistance, buying foods, or companies that make home deliveries.

5. Caregiving

There are two types of caregivers: professional caregivers and family member or relative caregivers. If you are an elderly and you have the financial capacity, you may hire a professional caregiver who can provide you assistance, if you need it.

There are agencies in the care-taking business that provide caregivers. Or you may get the services of an independent parttime caregiver, if you want.

6. Care Coordination

Care coordination simplifies the care of the elderly. For example, many old people save money by using a care coordinator such as a registered nurse or a certified nursing assistant (CNA). He or she can help you work directly with your health care providers.

7. Brain Health

Make your body healthy as well as the brain. It's because cognitive conditions such as Alzheimer's and Parkinson's disease, occur as we age, if we don't take care of our brain.

For instance, you must eat healthy balanced meals for brain health, and you must use your brain to have mental alertness by reading, doing crossword puzzles, and computing figures, or playing cards and games.

Regarding the brain, there's a saying that, "If you don't use it, you'll lose it!"

8. End of Life

We cannot escape death; we all die. This is the most difficult challenge that face the older adults. You and I have to prepare for it, for the benefit of your love ones who will be left behind.

You have to prepare for these documents:

- Will
- Living will
- Durable power of attorney for health care
- Durable power of attorney for finances
- Do not resuscitate (DNR) order
- Living trust

Will: A Will or Last Will and Testament is a legal document that stipulates your wishes for the distribution of your assets and wealth and the care of minor child or children, after your death.

Living will: A living will is a legal document that states medical treatments you would want and would not want to keep you alive. It is also a legal document that states your preferences for other medical decisions.

Durable power of attorney for health care: It is a legal document that grants a person to make medical decisions for another individual, like a relative, or a friend. The provisions of the document remains in effect until the person who gave it dies or cancels it.

Durable power of attorney for finances: It is a document that gives a person the legal authority to manage your finances while you are alive.

Do not resuscitate (DNR) order: This is an order of a doctor to the medical staff that stipulates not to do any cardiopulmonary resuscitation (CPR) to a diseased person for various reasons The document is a simple form, signed by a person authorized to sign such an instruction. It is included in a sick person's medical records.

Living trust: A living trust, also known as a revocable living trust, is a legal document that establishes a trust for any assets you want to transfer to it. You are the grantor of the trust, and you can designate a person who will distribute the assets to heirs, after your death.

Chapter 22

Aging in Place: Home Alone or Elsewhere?

Brief Subject Summary

•2 Options for Retirement
- What Is Independent Living?
- What Is Aging in Place?
- Aging Changes
- Aging Concerns
- What Do Surveys Show

2 Options for Retirement

If you are an older adult, you have two options for your retirement. Of course, it depends on your physical and mental conditions, and where you want to live for the rest of your life.

The two options for you for retirement are:

- **Aging in Place**, Alone or with a spouse or a caregiver. That means you have to continue living in your original home or family home.
- **Living Independently** in a senior housing, or staying in an assisted living facility.

What Is Independent Living?

Independent living simply means, you'll be living independently in your home, condo unit or apartment, or in a senior living community.

If you continue to live, alone or with a spouse, in your original place of abode, that is called aging in place.

What Is Aging in Place?

The Centers for Disease Control and Prevention (CDC) defines aging in place, "as the ability to live in one's own home and community safely, independently, and comfortably, regardless of age, income, or ability level."

Simply put, aging in place is a term used to describe older adults' living in the residence of their choice. For instance, they expect to live in a place where services and supports are available, which are needed as they continue to grow old.

Aging in place is a good alternative, but if you live in your own house, you may face some unique challenges and problems.

Aging Changes

As you age, your needs change. Whether you are 65, 75, 85 or in the 90s, you have to plan and learn how to manage your finances, diet, and physical activities.

Where you can live: at home, in an independent living community or an assisted living facility, or in a nursing home, depending on financial status and your physical ability.

Some of the changes you will face include the following:

- How to care for yourself with the help of a relative or a part-time or a professional caregiver.
- Which type of assistance you need, depending on your age and physical ability.
- How you will socialize whether you stay in your own home or in a living facility

Aging Concerns

Aging concerns may include the following:

- Reduced vision
- Decreased mental processing capabilities
- Hearing impairment
- Managing your disease or diseases if you already have them
- Managing your health
- Reduced muscle strength
- Risk of falls due to balance problems while standing still or walking
- Cooking and home upkeep if you are living in your own home
- Driving safely if you are still driving
- Transportation if you have no car

I. Home Alone Living

According to the AARP, about 90% of older adults who are over 65 want to live in their own homes as they age. They don't want to stay in a nursing home, or in an independent, or assisted living facility.

Of course, it would be better if you could stay in an independent living facility where you can get services you need. But that cost too much money. If you didn't save enough money, then that's a problem.

According to statistics seniors aged 65 and older are living either with a spouse or alone in their own home. If you are living with a spouse, then it would be much easier for doing some household chores and other activities. And you would have someone to talk to.

Where I'm Staying Right Now

As an older adult, at present, I'm living with my son, Melvin, and Faith, my daughter-in-law, their teen-aged son, in Michigan. I don't know yet about my future plans, whether I would like to go back, to the Philippines, or not, in the final years of my life. As I said, I'm now in my 90s.

Aging in Place

Majority of seniors in the U.S. age in place (or own home), instead of staying in communities of elders, for better or worse. Yes, staying in place, is the norm among older adults.

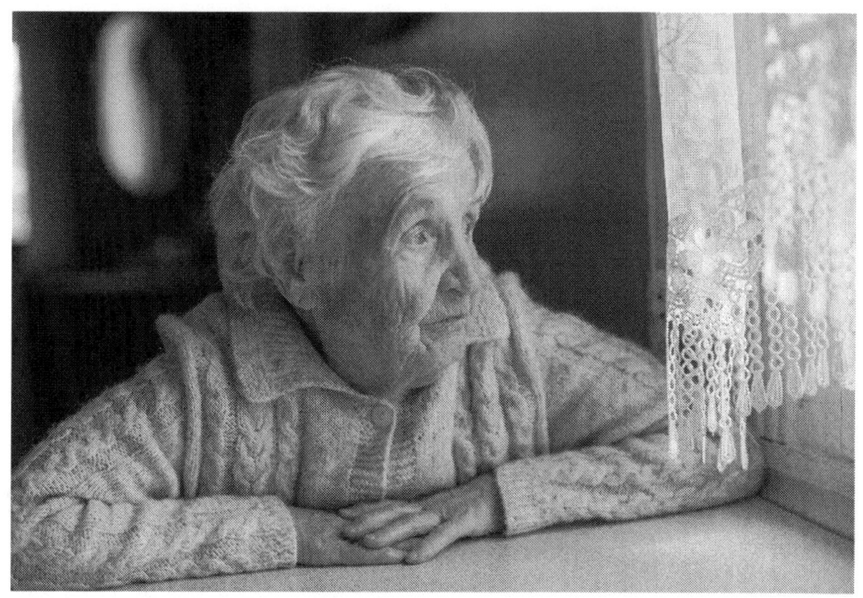

An Elderly Woman Looks Sadly Out the Window

Photo Credit: Shutterstock.

What Do Surveys Show?

Survey after survey shows that older adults would want to live in their homes, rather than move to senior communities or a nursing home, or an assisted living center.

Prediction

By 2000, the majority of 35 million Americans seniors were over the age of 65. Now, the U.S. Bureau of Census predicts that by 2030, there will be about 71.5 million Americans who will be 65 and over.

If you are a senior who has a wife or husband living with you, you may be lucky. Why? Because you can assist each other, in any undertakings in the house. You can still enjoy life because you talk to each other, may even set new goals in life, and know where to travel, if you can still do it. If you're already a widower or a widow, then that's another story.

In the United States, the Pew Research says, "27 percent of adults ages 60 and older live alone, compared with 16 percent in the 130 countries and territories."

What's Happening?

In the U.S., Americans value independence, more than anything else.. That's why the elderly prefer to live alone. in their homes or in condos or apartments.

On the other hand, people in many countries, like the Philippines, usually stay with their families, with a daughter's or a son's family. No wonder, they have close relationships.

In other words, grown children, usually take care of their aging parents.

Of course, there are instances, when an aging parent or parents live separately from their children, either in an assisted living facility or a nursing home.

Want Another Place? No Problem

If you don't want to live alone, you may stay in a senior community where you can interact with other residents.

Apartment living is a an option to have a companion like a relative or a friend to share with expenses and do their activities together. If you're a widow or a widower, you can get a companion for companionship or marriage. In that way, you can take care of each other. It's your choice!

Advantages of Living Alone in Your Own Home or Apartment

- You're free like a solo flying bird! You are your own boss; therefore, you can do what you want and when try painting or writing. Who knows? You can be a famous painter, creating your artistic masterpieces, or a prolific author, who can write books to be read worldwide through the Internet at Amazon.com.
- You can stay connected with families and friends through your i-phone, laptop, or computer.

- You can explore yourself, planning your activities and pursuing other dreams in life.
- You can travel in your country, or any other places that interest you, worldwide, like Korea, Indonesia, or Africa, depending on your physical ability to travel.

Disadvantages of Being Home Alone

- You'll experience isolation, loneliness, and depression.
- You'll have no one to talk with you, day in and day out in your own world, except if you want to talk to yourself in front of a mirror. Of course, you can communicate with a pet: a cat or a dog. Why not? It may talk with you, a cat just looking at you, and meowing at you, or a dog barking at you.
- If you are home alone, you'll have lack of safety. Burglars may make forced entry into your home, whether you are in your house or apartment, and ransack your home, exposing yourself to be hurt and even killed, if you shout for help.
- There is no one to take care of you when you get sick or incapacitated.
- It may cost you more money to live alone without someone who can share household expenses with you.

II. 55+ Retirement Communities With Independent Living Facilities

Retirement communities are restricted areas that are ideal for people whose ages range from 55 years old and beyond. They are also called senior communities.

In many ways, the seniors living there share the same needs, interests, and lifestyle. Some of them need some kind of special assistance. But many of them live on their own: cooking, doing household chores, and no need of assistance in taking medications, if they have certain illnesses.

In other words, these communities cater to people like you, to be with residents around your age.

- 3Independent Living
- Assisted Living

- Memory Care
- Nursing Home Facilities
- Hospice Care

Benefits of Age-Restricted Communities

- **Independence**: You live in a place, where you can reminisce your failures and successes in life and set goals for the coming months and years to come with people your age. What a joy to reminisce the memories of your youth!
- **Home, without maintenance**: No more fixing up home issues. No more mowing or no more snow shoveling during winter time.
- **Availability of accessible features:** If you live in a retirement place, you don't have to manage, for example, long staircases, and small doorways or hallways.
- **On-site services:** Many senior communities provide on-site services, like beauty salons, laundry services, dining, and more, without going outside to have these services.
- **Social and entertainment opportunities:** In this kind of community, you can socialize with other people of your age.
- **Supportive services:** In senior living, there are supportive services to help you age. There are also friends or neighbors, who will comfort you when you're down and depressed.

III. Assisted Living Facilities

You can live in an assisted living facility. However, community living is expensive, too. To live in community of older adults, you have to spend maybe $4,000 to $8,000 per month, depending on location.

Naturally, community living maybe more affordable in communities in Florida, than in other states. In California, it may cost you to pay $6,000 to $8,000 per month. What, if you didn't save enough money for retirement? That's a big problem!

Eligible seniors who have some disabilities are qualified for a place in independent living facilities, and get services, such as cooking, eating, bathing, assistance in taking medications, and others.

Assisted Living Facilities

Assisted living facilities may include the following:

- Memory Care
- Nursing Home Facilities
- Hospice Care

Memory Care: Usually, some assisted living communities have their own memory care wings within the building complex. Those who live here, are people afflicted with Alzheimer's disease, Parkinson's disease, or any form of dementia with reduced cognitive functions, involving memory.

In this kind of facility, there are teams of caregivers, including nursing assistants, who take care of a number of residents. These nursing assistances, give services, such as feeding, giving medications, or bathing or showering.

Nursing Home Facilities: These facilities, similar to hospitals, offer more assistance to residence. A skilled nursing facility offers the highest level of care, among these assisted living facilities. The patients assigned here are either recuperating after a stroke or surgery.

These patients need around-the clock medical care. Medical professionals, such as doctors, registered nurses, and therapists are always available in the premises for any medical situation. Yes, it's expensive to stay in a nursing home.

Hospice Care: The stay of a patient is only temporary in this facility. Often, when you are already not in need of medical treatment for your disease, you may be brought there by your relatives, for a peaceful end of your life.

That is, you'll be given only pain killers for the inflammation in your body, causing you so much pain. That is, you have to have comfort and tranquility in the face of death, and die peacefully.

Chapter 23

11 Senior Common Diseases & Disorders

Brief Subject Summary

- Cognitive Impairment and Dementia
- Type 2 Diabetes
- Kidney Disease
- Heart Disease
- Respiratory Diseases & Condition
- Cancer
- Falls
- Overactive bladder
- Osteoarthritis
- Osteoporosis
- Tinnitus (Ringing in the Ear), Symptoms, & Treatments

More than ever before, humans can expect to live longer now due to modern technology, medicine, and healthful lifestyles. In fact, it won't be surprising, if you live into your 80s or 90s and beyond.

However, you must know how to deal with the 11 common diseases and other disorders that older adults, including the oldest old. In this case, you have to face them as you grow old, like what I do. Purpose: To prevent or treat any of these diseases, as you continue on your life journey, towards your goal of living into your 90s and beyond.

I. Cognitive Impairment and Dementia

What is cognitive impairment? The term cognitive impairment refers to the decline of the brain's ability to function effectively, in remembering, focusing, making decisions, and learning new things.

When you have cognitive impairment, it means you may have been afflicted with dementia, a disease that affects memory and thinking skills.

Types of Dementia

According to Cleveland Clinic, dementias may be divided into three groups:

- Primary: Diseases and conditions in which dementia is the main illness.
- Secondary: It means the dementia is due to another disease or disorder.
- Reversible demantia-like symptoms: These are caused by other conditions, like taking certain medications or sleeping pills.

Dementia is an umbrella category or disorders.of Alzheimer's Disease and Related Dementias (ADRDs)

In other words, AD is only one of diseases that are caused by cognitive impairment. Simply defined, Alzheimer's disease is a form of dementia.

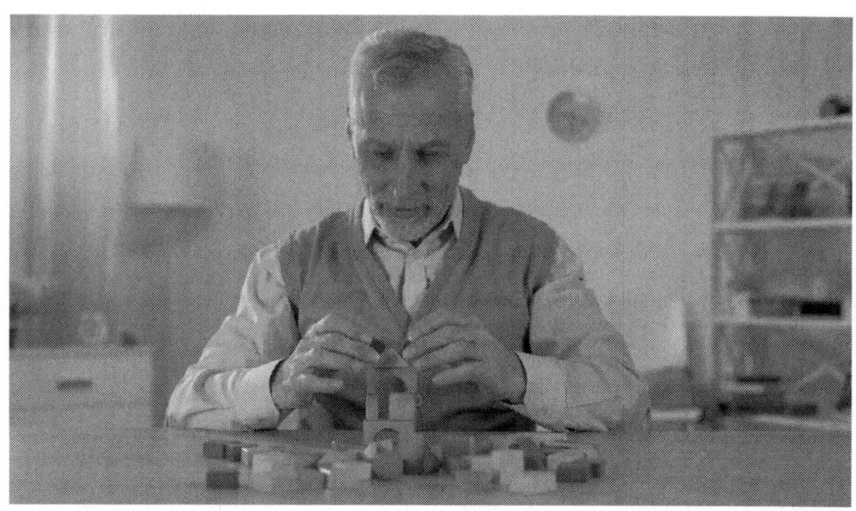

Positive Old Man Playing with Wooden Cubes, Cognitive Training in Alzheimer's Disease

Photo Credit: Shutterstock

Symptoms of Dementia

- Memory loss
- Difficulty communicating or finding words to say
- Taking hard time in handling simple and complex tasks
- Difficulty with planning or organizing
- Having trouble with visual and spatial abilities
- Seeing things that they are not there (visual hallucinations)
- Having lack of concentration and attention
- Having uncoordinated or slow movement, and sometimes, tremor

Causes of Dementia

1. Alzheimer's Disease and Other Dementia Disorders: According to current estimates, Alzheimer's disease comprises 70% to 80% of all dementias.

2. **Other types of dementias.** Alzheimer's include the most disorders in people 60 and below. They affect the frontal and temporal lobes of the brain that control the changes in brain functions.

Like Alzheimer's disease, other dementias are all progressive and irreversible. Besides Alzheimer's disease, dementias include the following:

- **Vascular dementia:** Vascular dementia, the second most common type of dementia, involves the damage of the vessels that supply blood to your brain.
- **Frontotemporal dementia:** They affect the frontal and temporal lobes of the brain that control the changes in brain functions.
- **Lew body dementia:** An abnormal balloon-like clumps of protein. They have been located in the brains of people with Alzheimer's disease and Parkinson's disease.
- **Mixed dementia:** Brains of people in the age of 80 and above. In a study, for instance, they have a mixture of Alzheimer's disease, vascular dementia, and Lewy body dementia.

Other Dementia Conditions

There are also other disorders linked to dementia, which include:

- **Parkinson's disease:** Many people who have Parkinson's disease develop dementia in the later stages of their disease
- **Huntington's disease:** A single defective gene may cause this brain condition, due to breakdown in your brain's nerve cells.
- **Creutzfeldt-Jakob disease:** According to CDC, Creutzfeldt-Jakob disease (CJD) is a rapidly progressive, invariably fatal neurodegenerative disorder believed to be caused by an abnormal isoform of a cellular glycoprotein known as the prion protein.
- **Wernicke-Korsakoff syndrome:** This brain condition is caused by too much of thiamine (Vitamin B1)
- **Traumatic brain injury (TBI)**

Prevention and Treatment of Dementia

The treatment of dementia may include:

- Doing mental stimulating activities such as moderate-intensity walking and doing reading, solving word puzzles, playing word games, and memory training. Purpose: To avoid the onset of Alzheimer's disease, (AD) or to delay the progression of a current AD or any other forms of dementia.
- Reducing blood sugar level, if you have diabetes, that joins the plaques in arteries and veins, tha cause blockages that may lead to stroke or heart attack.
- Quiting smoking to avoid depositing nicotine in the body that damages arteries and veins, and blocking the flow of blood throughout the body
- Lowering LDL (bad cholesterol) and increasing HDL (good) cholesterol, and reducing triglycerides
- Reducing elevated blood pressure level, to avoid the occurrence of kidney disease, and minimize the risk of developing dementia
- Managing cardiovascular diseases, such as heart disease
- Eating a healthy diet, for instance, following a semi-plant-based diet, meaning more plant foods, than animal foods
- Getting enough sleep, at least 7 to 9 hours per night

- Drinking enough water, at least 7 to 10 glasses or cups of water, a measurement of 8 ounces per glass or cup, depending on your body's size, height, and weight

II. Type 2 Diabetes

Research shows that 25% of adults age 65 and older have type 2 diabetes. If you have type 2 diabetes, it means you have elevated blood sugar or glucose in your bloodstream.

To know whether you have type 2 diabetes, or at risk of having diabetes, you have to monitor your blood sugar and try not to eat too many carbohydrates that turn into glucose when you consume them.

Controlling blood sugar levels is important because, if not treated or controlled, your disease may lead to kidney and heart disease and other diseases. (Review Chapter 4, *Type 2 Diabetes)*.

Diabetes affects 27% of older adults in the US.

My Type 2 Diabetes Journey

Here's my latest results of my Hemoglobin A1C details:

Veltisezar Bautista

HEMOGLOBIN A1C - Details

Study Results

Component Results

Component	Your Value	Standard Range	Flag
Hemoglobin A1C	5.6 %	4.0 to 5.6 %4.0 - 5.6 %	
Estimated Average Glucose	114 mg/dL	mg/dLmg/dL	

Collected on 12/10/2022 7:36 AM from Blood, Venous (Blood)

III. Kidney Disease

According to current statistics, chronic kidney disease (CKD) affects 18% of seniors in the United States. CKD causes a slow decline of kidney function over time.

Of course, the kidneys play a significant role in normal kidney functions, you must be aware of the consequences that may occur, if you don't control and slow down your disease, if you have it. (See Chapter 7 *How to Reverse, Stabilize, & Put Kidney Disease into Remission,) on page 83.* My GFR for the past years: 35%, September 21, 2016, page 123, Chapter 7, increasing to 73% on July 7, 2022. (See page 126, Chapter 7.) On December 9, 2023, my GFR was 72%.

IV. Heart Disease

Heart and blood vessel disease (also called heart disease) includes numerous problems, many of which are related to a process called atherosclerosis," says the American Heart Association.

Heart and blood vessel disease (also called heart disease) includes numerous problems, many of which are related to a process called atherosclerosis," says the American Heart Association.

(For more information, review Chapter 8: *Can You Reverse Your Heart Disease Severity & Put into Better Condition*?)

Heart disease is the No. 1 killer in the United States. If you don't want to have a heart disease that can lead to heart attacks and strokes, you may take steps to prevent them. You should lower your levels of glucose, cholesterol, triglycerides, and blood pressure.

Coronary heart disease, research shows, affects 29% of older adults and oldest old.

(For more information, review Chapter 8: *Can You Reverse Your Heart Disease Severity & Put into Better Condition*?)

My Heart Disease Journey: Ejection Fraction

Through my rehabilitation efforts, I have reversed my heart disease severity, proven by the fact that I had increased my ejection fraction (percentage of the heart's blood pumping power) from 15% on September 21, 2018 to August 27, 2022.

The next two pages show the test results of an echocardiogram doppler report, taken on August 27, 2022 (latest.GFR 44%).

[redacted]
Diplomate, American Board of Internal Medicine
[redacted]
[redacted]

[redacted] [redacted]

ECHOCARDIOGRAM/DOPPLER REPORT

Patient Name: Veltisezar Bautista **Date of Service:** 8-27-22
Ordering Physician: Raad P. Kasmikha **Date of Birth:** 10-31-33
Daianoses/IN

Left Ventricular Dimension		Mitral Valve		Tricuspid Valve	
Diastole (3.5-5.7)	6.37	Peak Velocity (0.6-1.3/sec)		Peak Velocity (0.3-0.7m/sec)	
Systole (less than 4 cm)	4.96	Regurgitation		Regurgitation	
Septal wall (0.6-1.1 cm)	.92	Pressure ½ time		RVSP	
Posterior wall (0.6-1.1 cm)	1.34	Mean Gradient			
%FS (>50%)	44	Mitral Valve Area			
EF (>50%)					

Aortic Valve		Aortic valve		Pulmonary Valve	
Aortic Root (2.0-3.7 cm)	3.48	Peak Velocity (1-1.7m/sec)		Peak Velocity (0.6-0.9/sec)	
Cusp Separation (1.5-2.6 cm)	1.68	Regurgitation		Regurgitation	
		Peak Gradient			
LAD (1.9-4.0 cm)	4.53	Mean Gradient		RVD (0.7-2.6)	1.11
		A1 Pressure ½			
		Aortic Valve Area			

Summary and Interpretations:

1) Left Ventricle dilated, normal Contractility
2) Right Ventricle normal.
3) Left Atrium dilated
4) Right Atrium Dilated
5) Aortic Root normal
6) Aortic Valve Calcified with normal opening
7) Mitral Valve prolapse
8) Tricuspid Valve normal
9) Pulmonic Valve normal
10) Pericardial Effusion none

Doppler Study Reveals:

mild pulmonic & Tricuspid Regurg.
mild to mod. MR

Ordering physician

Summary of My Ejection Fraction Numbers (Leading to heart failure reversal)

September 21, 2016 - 15%
March 28, 2017 - 23%
March 16, 2018 - 30%
August 22, 2020 - 47%
August 27, 2022 - 44%
August 26, 2023 - 43%

V. Respiratory Diseases and Conditions

The top 8 respiratory diseases are as follows:

- Chronic Obstructive Pulmonary Disease (COPD)
- Asthma
- Chronic Bronchitis
- Emphysema
- Lung Cancer
- Cystic Fibrosis
- Pneumonia
- Pleural Effusion

1. Constructive pulmonary disease (COPD): It involves a reduction of airflow into and out of the lungs, caused by inflammation in the airways. This thickens the lining of the lungs, resulting in the over production of mucus in the air tubes. Hence, this results in hard breathing for the individual who has this condition.

2. Asthma: Defining asthma, the American Lung Association says, "Asthma is a chronic disease that makes it harder to move air in and out of your lungs."

Why does this happen? It's because when there's an inflammation in the airways (tubes), they cause them to be extra sensitive to viruses and irritants. Next. more mucus is produced, making the airways tighten, resulting in hard breathing for the person who has the disease.

3. Chronic Bronchitis: Chronic bronchitis is a long-term inflammation of the air passageway, called bronchi, which is common among chain smokers.

When the airways (trachea and bronchi), leading to your lungs become damaged, inflamed, and filled with mucus, you'll have persistent coughing which may last two or more weeks, to get rid of the mucus.

And when the persistent coughing lasts too long, that may mean that you already have an acute bronchitis. This may mean too, that the condition is caused by virus and it will go away on its own.

Actually, chronic bronchitis never goes away, but you can manage it.

4. Emphysema: Emphysema is a lung disorder that involves the air sacs in the lungs, called alveoli. When the air sacs become damaged, that may result in the weakening and rupturing of the alveoli. When this happens, the air spaces become larger, instead of many small ones.

MedicinePlus, in describing emphysema says, "In emphysema, the walls between many of the air sacs in the lungs are damaged. This causes the air sacs to lose their shape and become floppy. The damage also can destroy the walls of the air sacs, leading to fewer and larger air sacs instead of many tiny ones. This makes it harder for your lungs to move oxygen in and carbon dioxide out of your body."

5. Lung cancer: What is lung cancer? Lung cancer is one of the most frequently diagnosed cancers worldwide. That is, more people die from it than colon, breast, and prostate cancer combined.

The two main types of lung cancer are:

- Non-small cell lung cancer
- Small cell lung cancer

6. Cystic Fibrosis/Bronchiectasis: What is cystic fibrosis and what is bronchiectasis? Cystic fibrosis, the most common inherited life-shortening disorder in the Caucasian population, is caused by the body's production of thick and sticky mucus produced by glands of the mucous membrane that clogs the lungs. The mucus is also called mucosa. When this happens, lung infections occur, leading to the dilation and destruction of airways, called bronchiectasis, an abnormal widening of the bronchi or their branches that causes a risk of infection.

Simply put, bronchiectasis, a part of cystic fibrosis lung disease, can also appear for other reasons. It is defined as the permanent dilation and obstruction of the airway wall.

Thus, due to the airway damage, the condition obstructs the the pancreas and stops the natural enzymes from aiding the body to break down and absorb nutrients.

7. Pneumonia: *MedicinePlus,* a website of the National Library of Medicine of the National Institutes of Health, defines pneumonia as, "an infection in one or both of the lungs. It causes the air sacs of the lungs to fill up with fluid or pus. It can range from mild to severe, depending on the type of germ causing the infection, your age, and your overall health."

What causes pneumonia? Bacterial, viral, and fungal infections can cause this condition. The main treatment for pneumonia, a serious condition, is antibiotics. Doctors advise people with pneumonia to drink plenty of water and other liquids.

This disorder is common among older adults, especially the oldest old with alzheimer's disease.

8. Pleural effusion: Pleural effusion involves the buildup of fluid between the layers of tissue that line the chest cavity and the lungs. In other words, smoking and drinking alcohol, cause heart, lung and liver disease, which can lead to pleural effusion.

To further explain, pleura is a two-layer membrane that covers the lungs and lines the chest cavity. The fluid inside the fluid inside the pleura is called pleural fluid, produced by the body.

Put simply, pleural effusion is an excessive collection of this fluid. in the lungs. Such accumulation of fluid is medically termed as pulmonary edema or pleural effusion. Normally, the lungs contain fluid for lubrication of their membranes.

But if the fluid is excessive, the lungs can start to swell and deteriorate. Such swelling can cause too much pressure on the blood vessels, making fluids leak into the lungs' tiny air sac units, called alveoli.

If you have this abnormality, you'll experience chest pain and a lot of coughing, causing you shortness of breath. The condition can be treated in the hospital.

VI. Cancer

"Cancer starts when gene changes make one cell or a few cells begin to grow and multiply too much. This may cause a growth called a tumour,".according to the Cancer Research UK.

Is Cancer Hereditary?

Answering his question, the National Cancer Institute of the National Institute of Health says, "Cancer itself can't be passed down from parents to children. And genetic changes in tumor cells can't be passed down. But a genetic change that increases the risk of cancer can be passed down (inherited) if it is present in a parent's egg or sperm cells."

Cancer Groups

Cancers are divided into groups, according to the type of cell they start from. They include

- Carcinomas
- Lymphomas
- Leukemias
- Brain tumors
- Sarcomas

Many cancers can be cured, especially if they are discovered in the early stages. In other words, they can be put into remission, but some can come back.

The American Cancer Society says, "77% of all cancers are diagnosed in people over the age of 55."

The most common cancers of seniors include:

- Lung cancer
- Breast
- Cervical
- Colorectal
- Prostate
- Bladder
- Non-Hodgkin's lymphoma

- Stomach
- Brain tumors

1. Lung cancer: What is lung cancer? Lung cancer is one of the most frequently diagnosed cancers worldwide. Lung cancer is also considered as one of the eight respiratory diseases.

The two main types of lung cancer are:

- Non-small cell lung cancer
- Small cell lung cancer

2. Breast cancer: Breast cancer occurs when cells in the breast grow and divide in an uncontrolled way. Breast cancer is most often found in women, but men can have breast cancer, too. About 1 out of every 100 breast cancers diagnosed in the United States is discovered in a man.

3. Cervical cancer: As already mentioned, cancer is a disease that causes cells in the body grow uncontrollably. When the disease starts in the cervix, that is called cervical cancer. The cervix is the lower, narrow end of the uterus (or womb).

4. Colorectal cancer: Colorectal cancer, also known as bowel cancer, develops in the inner lining of the bowel. Usually, it is preceded by growths, known as polyps. If not detected early, the polyps become the so-called invasive cancer. Depending on where it starts, the bowel cancer may be called rectal or colon cancer.

5. Prostate cancer: This disease is the most non-skin cancer in the United States. In fact, according to estimates, 1 in 8 men is diagnosed with prostate cancer.

6. Bladder cancer: Bladder cancer develops when cells that make up the urinary bladder begin to grow out of control. As more cancer cells develop, they form a tumor. Later, the tumor spreads to other parts of the body.

The bladder is a hollow organ in the lower pelvis whose main function is to store urine and to move it out. For instance, when you urinate, the bladder pushes out the urine through a tube called the urethra.

7. Non-Hodgkin's lymphoma: Non-Hodgkin's lymphoma is a type of cancer that develops in your lymphatic systems, a part of the body's germ-fighting immune system. In this disease, white blood cells, known as lymphocytes, grow abnormally, forming growths or tumors in the whole body.

8. Stomach cancer: Stomach cancer occurs when cancerous cells grow within the lining of the stomach. This type of cancer is also called gastric cancer, and it can be difficult to diagnose because most people typically don't show symptoms in the earlier stages," says *Healthline.*

9. Brain tumors: Usually, brain tumors develop in brain tissue itself, but sometimes, though, they spread in the brain from other parts of the body, according to the Mayo Clinic.

VII. Falls (Balance Issue)

(See the next chapter.)

VIII. Overactive Bladder (OAB) Incontinence

What is overactive bladder? Overactive bladder or incontinence is a health condition involving the frequent, urgent need to urinate.

The disorder is described as urinary symptoms, rather than a disease. The condition causes different types of diseases and other health issues.

Symptoms

Symptoms of overactive bladder (OB) differ from person to person, a condition that older adults suffer from. Women are more susceptible, than men, to this condition.

The symptoms may include:

- Sudden, urgent need to urinate
- Waking up more than four, five, or more, at night to urinate
- Sudden, urgent need to urinate, often occurring 8 or more within 24 hours
- Unintentional loss of urine with urgent need to urinate (urgency incontinence)

Overactive bladder causes the bladder muscle to contract, even when the bladder is nearly empty. Because of this contraction, there can be a sudden and strong urge to pee, which may lead to incontinence. Usually the doctor orders several tests to diagnose this condition.

Causes of Frequent Urination

- Diabetes
- Nerve related problems
- Enlarged prostate in middle-aged and older men
- Swelling and infection of the urethra
- Vaginitis (swelling or discharge of the vulva and vagina in women)
- Caffeine intake
- Urinary tract infection (UTI)

Types of Incontinence

Mayo Clinic categorizes different types of incontinence that may include the following:

1. Stress incontinence: When you exert pressure on your bladder you may have some leaks of urine due to exerting pressure on your bladder caused by:

- Laughing
- Exercising
- Coughing
- Lifting heavy objects

Then, suddenly you feel the urge to pee.

2.Overflow incontinence: This condition involves frequent dribbling of urine. Why? It's because the bladder may not empty completely, in one instant. In fact, you may do double urination to empty fully you bladder.

3. Functional incontinence: A physical or mental impairment that may keep you from making it to the toilet in time.

4. Mixed incontinence: Sometimes, you may experience more than one type of urinary incontinence. Most often, this incontinence involves a combination of stress incontinence and urge incontinence.

Medicine Treatments and Behavioral Therapies

1. Medicines: The medicines for overactive bladder may include:

- Mirabegron (Myrbetriq)
- Fesoterodine (Toviaz)
- Tolterodine (Detrol)
- Oxybutynin
- Solifenacin (Vesicare)

The mentioned medications can relax the bladder to help in relieving symptoms of overactive bladder and in reducing episodes of urge incontinence.

2. Behavioral Therapies: Behavioral therapies include.

- Doing Kegel exercise or Pelvic floor muscle exercise
- Wearing absorbent pads and undergarments
- Bladder training by scheduling urination

Kegel exercise or pelvic floor exercise: The exercise strengthens your pelvic floor muscles and urinary sphincter. The strong muscles thus stop the bladder's involuntary contractions that give you the urge to urinate instantly.

Therefore, you should exercise the muscles that are part of the pelvic floor. In performing the Kegel exercise, you can make the muscles stronger, so that they can have the power to control any urgent emergency urination or leaking.

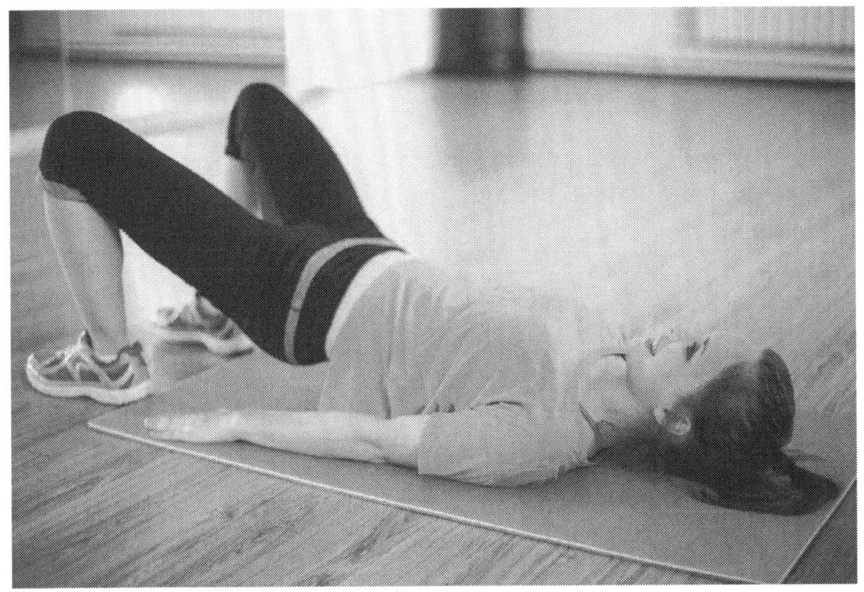

A Young Woman Does the Kegel or Pelvic Floor Exercise

Photo Source: Shutterstock

I practice this Kegel or pelvic floor exercise as soon as I wake up in the morning, after practicing some stretching and balancing xercises.

You can do the pelvic floor exercise while lying on the floor, facing the ceiling, by putting your two hands downward on the floor, and then pushing your thighs and half body upward, and then pulling them downward, in sequence. You can do this regimen anytime during the day, but more preferably in the early morning after you wake up, as you do your warm-up, like stretching or practicing tai chi, a Chinese exercise or doing other workouts, to strengthen your lower body.

You may limit the time duration for your exercises to about 15 to 20 minutes.

To know fully how to do the pelvic floor exercise, or any other exercises, you may also talk to your doctor or a therapist to get advice on kegel exercise or pelvic floor muscle exercise.

Wearing absorbent pads and/or undergarments: If you have overactive bladder you should wear, either one or both of them. Wearing either one or both of them can protect your clothing from being wet. You can also avoid embarrassing incidents in front of other people.

Training the bladder: Bladder training involves your bladder and mind, to delay an urge to urinate. You can gradually work your way up to urinating every one or two hours or more. In short, try to limit your toilet trips.

However, your accomplishing this feat depends on how you can tighten (contract) successfully your pelvic floor muscles.

Where Is the Pelvic Floor?

The pelvic floor is a group of muscles, a bit like a small muscle hammock that runs between the pubic bone in the front, and the so-called tailbone at the back.

Woman's pelvic floor muscles: A woman's floor muscles support her womb (uterus), bladder, and bowel (colon). The urine tube (urethra), the vagina, and the anus and urine tube (urethra) pass through it. Kegel exercises help strengthen your pelvic floor muscles.

Your pelvic floor muscles support organs in your pelvis, like your bladder, bowel, and vagina. Your pelvic floor muscles hold your organs in place while also assisting with bodily functions like peeing, pooping and sex.

My Journey: Overactive Bladder

I must confess, as an oldest old, I'm a victim of incontinence. I usually wake up, four or five times at night. I'm managing my incontinence by wearing pampers all the time, training my bladder to release urine at least once after more than 2 hours. Before, I could only schedule my urination up to one hour only.

As an oldest old, I have tried several medicines for an overactive bladder. If you have incontinence, you may ask your doctor about taking any medications, but you must know that all medicines cause unwanted side effects. If you can tolerate the side effects of any medication, then you may try taking it, if it is giving you some relief.

I tried to take different incontinence medications, but all of them gave me some side effects, I had headaches, groin pain, and other bad things. Yes, they didn't all work for me. And, I don't know if any of the medicines can work for you.

The last medication that I tried was called Oxybutynin. But this tablet made my mouth swollen and my lip crack.

In summary, I have lessened my trips to the bathroom, as a result of my exercises for this condition. Well, that's a big improvement. I did it, without taking any medications. It's very seldom that I get sometimes, unlike before, when they were in volumes.. What a relief!

Pelvic Floor Exercise

With my practice of doing the pelvic exercise and the scheduling of my urination to train my bladder not to do it, too. Yes, I can delay my urination in a certain time. In other words, I did some improvements.

When traveling, I can delay my urination for an extended period of time, especially when I know the next rest area is still far. With that thought in my mind, I can delay my going to the restroom.

Of course, once in a while I still have some little leaks, not like before when I had urine discharge in volume. Imagine, when I would wake up, and walk to the restroom, sometimes I would think it's coming. Most of the times, I would reach the toilet without any accidents.

In summary, I have lessened my trips to the bathroom, day or night. Well, that's a big improvement. I did it, without taking any medications.

Drinking Less Fluid, Especially Water?

Oh no! I can't do it. I may have a kidney failure, if I do that. While my kidney disease is in remission, I can't take the risk having kidney failure. It's because the kidneys need enough water to survive.

It's because insufficient water or liquid can make damages in the kidney and you can have kidney failure.

The more I drink water, the more my GFR increases, making it to 47% percent in 2020. Before, my GFR was in the 30s; but now, it's hovering from 44% to 47%, which are in the normal range for a senior. Generally, the whole body, including the brain, needs a lot of water, about 8 to 10 glasses of water every day, unless you have heart failure that may limit your taking of water. Of course, it's based on your heart condition, too.

Although, I have heart failure, (which gives no symptoms to me), I manage to drink 8 to 10 cups or glasses of water, containing 8 ounces of water or fluids, without a problem.

And I have had only one incidence of cardiovascular event; that is, the intake of too much water, causing me lung congestion. But I have learned many things on my own. My cardiologist told me that I have no problems with my heart's ejection fraction right now, because it ranges from 44 to 47%, near the normal range of 50% to 70%. So that's good news for me.

IX. Osteoarthritis

Osteoarthritis, also known as osteogenesis (brittle bone disease)," is a degenerative joint disease and a common form of arthritis worldwide. As people age, this appears and anatomical factors may cause osteoarthritis.

In short, osteoarthritis involves the swelling and pain in the joints.

Why is this condition usually occurs in older adults, especially in women? Aging changes in the musculoskeletal system naturally increase the risk of having osteoarthritis.

Hormonal differences between men and women may play a role in the development of osteoarthritis. Postmenopausal women, in particular, have an increased risk of developing osteoarthritis. This has been linked to the decrease in estrogen during this period.

Postmenopausal women means having undergone menopause or occurring after menopause. It is estimated that half of all women over the age of 50 break a bone because of hip fractures.

If you have osteoporosis, you may ask your doctor about the proper medications for this disorder.

The treatments of osteoarthritis may depend on the severity of the condition.

X. Osteoporosis

Osteoporosis involves bone mass loss, characterized by the thinning and weakening of bones. Simply put, the disorder may be treated to prevent fractures.

Most people at risk of having osteoporosis are Caucasian and Asian women.

According to Mayo Clinic, in people with osteoporosis, bone tissue breaks down faster than it is replaced. The bones become thinner and brittle; hence, they are more likely to break with pressure or after a fall. Bones are made up of calcium and other minerals are being broken down and rebuilt.

The National Osteoporosis Foundation reports that as many as half of all women over the age of 50 can break a bone because of osteoporosis. On the other hand, 27% of men over 50 may develop osteoporosis.

Osteoporosis-related fractures commonly occur in the wrist, hip, or spine.

If you're an older adult, you should reduce weight if you are overweight, and eat foods that are rich in calcium and Vitamin D. Or you may take Vitamin D3 if you have deficiency in this vitamin.

XI. Tinnitus

Defining tinnitus or ringing in the ear the Johns Hopkins Medicine, says, "Tinnitus is the sound of ringing in the ear. It may also be described as roaring, buzzing, hissing or clicking inside of the head. The sounds may come and go. Or they may be ongoing."

Besides the above, some sources also describe the noisy sounds in the ears, that can occur in one or both ears as:

- Humming
- Buzzing
- Whining
- Clicking
- Chirping
- Whistling
- Roaring
- Other insect sounds or voices

To put it simply, tinnitus causes the sensation of hearing, either a continuous or an intermittent noise that is not coming from the outside.

Tinnitus is a common problem of older adults, affecting more than 50 million people in the United States.

According to Cleveland Clinic, tinnitus is a symptom of more than 75% of all disorders that affect the ears.

If you have tinnitus, you may suffer from irritability, loss of concentration on whatever you do, and not being able to get enough sleep because of certain sounds that keep you awake, most of the time.

Having tinnitus can make you feel angry, frustrated, and depressed. In fact, a CEO of a well-known chain restaurant, was reported to have committed suicide because he could not sleep, night and day. Yes, you can go crazy if your ringing in the ear is so serious.

In reality, even doctors say that there is no cure for this condition, and you have to live with it, the rest of your life. Even one of my doctors has told me that there is no cure for my tinnitus, and no medicine can cure it. But, I didn't surrender, I continued my search for a solution to tinnitus, and at last, I did defeat it! Yes, you can take some steps to be able to cope with it, in whatever ways. (See *Treatments of Tinnitus* on the next page.)

Signs or Symptoms of Tinnitus

The causes of ringing in the ears include the following:

- Age-related hearing loss
- An ear injury or a problem with the circulatory system
- Misplacement of the white crystals in the ears
- Too much accumulation of wax in the inner ears
- Damage to the tiny hairs on auditory cells within the inner ear that changes the signal they send to the brain.

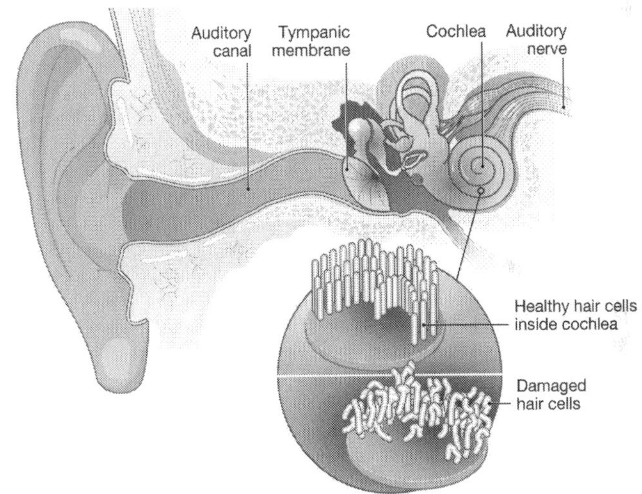

Illustration Shows the Way of Sound to the Brain, Labeled

Image Source: Shutterstock

Treatments of Tinnitus

Treatments may include:

- **Earwax removal:** Removing the earwax that accumulated in your ears
- **Blood vessel condition:** Treating any blood vessel disorder that may require surgery, or medications, such as anti-depressants, to reduce the noises
- **Simple Tinnitus Exercises:** Massaging involving the head, neck and pulling down the ear lobes can make a difference in alleviating sounds seems to be coming from the ear. (I did stop it, successfully.)
- **Lying on body's left or right side:** Lying on the body's side, (whether left or right) opposite the ear that's creating the noise
- If the sound is occurring in the right ear, you should lie on your left side. (I did this technique, which I found to be effective, too, especially when you are about to sleep.)
- **Correct positioning of the head:** Doing the right positioning of the head, when you are ready to sleep. This works for me, too.
- **Simple tinnitus exercises, called massage therapy:** The water massaging therapy involves the head, neck, and pulling the ear in different ways. Such practice can make a difference in stopping sounds in the ear. (I did stop them, successfully.)

Massage Therapy: Exercises for Ears, Neck and Jaw Muscles to Get Rid of Tinnitus. This is the message therapy that I got rid of my tinnitus.

Did you know that simple exercises can end your tinnitus sufferings? Yes, with simple exercises, you can get rid of tinnitus, which is not a disease, but merely symptoms .

The Simple Exercises

The exercising procedure involves massaging of the whole head, the neck (especially the back at the base of your head, the boundary between the head and the neck), and the jaw and facial muscles. Put a little pressure on your skin and afterwards, pump your ears with air with the palms of your hands, covering your ears, at the same time opening your mouth as wide as possible.

With these several simple exercises, called message therapy, you can reverse the condition that makes your life miserable.

This is based on what I do, and I'm still doing, to be free from tinnitus attacks. The exercises include:

1. **Pumping the Ear with Air**: With this method, hold your head with both hands, with your fingers toward your back, you pump your ears with air, with both thumbs of your hands, holding your head, at the time opening your mouth as wide as possible.

2. **The massage therapy for the ear:** It pertains to the gentle pulling of parts of the ears in different directions, including the ear lobes, up and down, and side to side pulling of the ear parts.

3. **Messaging the muscles at the base of the head:** The base of the head is located in the boundary between the head and the neck.

The purpose for doing these simple exercises is to make the different muscles reduce tension, improve blood circulation, and give more flexibility to the muscles, as they move to do their tasks.

If you are bothered by tinnitus, and want to learn the secrets to tinnitus solution, you may watch videos about it on Youtube.com.

Almost all people who do these exercises, can make tinnitus go away.

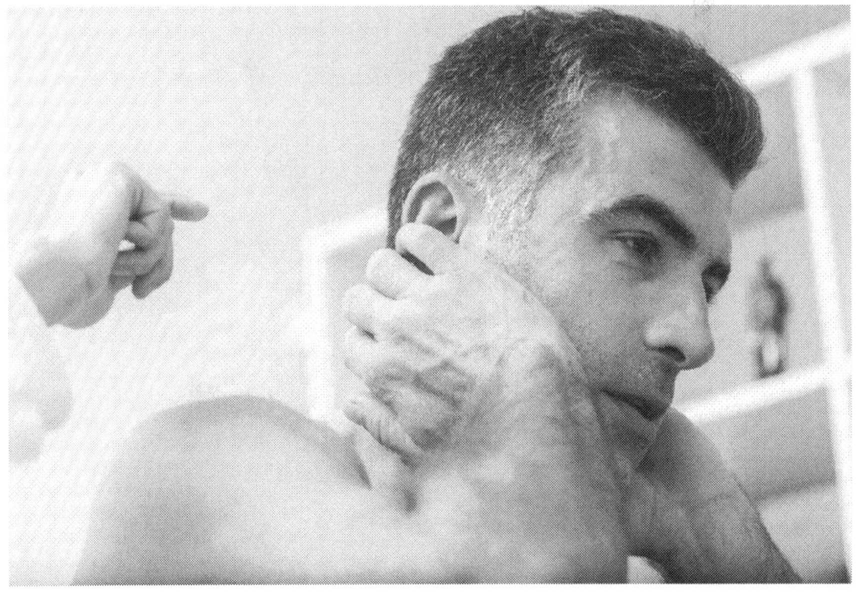

A Man Suffering from Tinnitus Does Massaging of the Muscles at the Base of the Head (Photo Credit: Shutterstock)

My Tinnitus Journey: Does This Exercise Really Work?

Yes, they can work. They worked for me, and maybe they can work for you, too, if you do exercises religiously several times a day.

Yes, finally I did i! For many years, I had been experiencing tinnitus symptoms, ever since I was in my 70s; I now in my 90s, my ringing in the ear is gone. Before, my tinnitus would come and go, every minute or a few weeks occurrence.

But now, my ringing in the ear is no more, and I think it's gone forever.

Before, for many years, in a few seconds, or a few minutes, hearing sounds or noises in my inner ear, was a continuing process, every day and night. It was frustrating, irritating, and depressing.

Wonder of all wonders! Gone are those days. Imagine, up to now, many doctors still consider tinnitus, as beyond cure, or reversion of the disorder is impossible.

Oh, my God! What a relief! Why didn't I discover this massage therapy many years ago, and why I knew about it only several months ago was regretting.

Chapter 24

Improving Your Balance to Prevent Falls

Brief Subject Summary

- Symptoms of Imbalance
- What Causes Falls?
- 2 Types of Balance
- Other Things That Cause Falls
- Stretching
- One-leg Standing Exercise (Left or Right Foot)
- Tai Chi Exercise
- Toe Gripping
- Toe Separators
- Do We Need to Undergo Physical Therapy to Improve Balance?

Bang!

That happened in the bathroom in the middle of March 2023.

I was shocked! My right leg gave way, my right knee just buckled, perhaps due to its weakness and instability.

Well, the accident was not rare. In fact, the Centers for Disease Control and Prevention (CDC) reports that in the United States, one in four adults (28%) age 65 and older, experience falls per year, although not all falls result in injuries.

These accidents result in about 36 million falls every year, making it the No. 1 cause of injury-related death.

According to the CDC, 20% of falls in adults lead to life-altering changes, primarily from broken bones or head injury. About 37% of those who fall reported an injury.

Thus, the accident that happened to me led me to do a thorough research on how to reduce the risk of falls among older adults, especially the oldest old, like me. Women are more likely to fall than men.

Symptoms of Imbalance

Signs of balance problems include:

- Confusion
- Feeling a floating sensation or dizziness
- Sense of motion or spinning (having tinnitus or vertigo)
- Loss of steadiness or balance
- Vision condition changes, like blurry vision

What Causes Falls?

The three main physical conditions that contribute to falls include:

- Weak stabilizer muscles
- Poor core strength
- Balance issues

Weak Stabilizer muscles. The stabilizer muscles are the ones that act to stabilize one joint so the intended movement can be done in another joint. Thus, these muscles are the ones that make you steady or balance, so that the primary muscles can perform their job.

If the stabilizer muscles are weak, then you can have a fall.

Poor core strength: Core means the central part of your body, including the pelvis, hips, stomach, and lower back.

To strengthen the core, you have to do some core exercises. There are four systems that work together to give you balance, while standing still, walking, jogging, or running.

The four systems are:

- Central nervous system
- Vestibular system of inner ear
- Vision
- Position-sensing nerves

Central nervous system: The central nervous system (brain and spinal cord) coordinates movements by sending motor signals to the eyes and muscles.

Vestibular system: The vestibular system (brain and inner ear) acts as the messenger to the brain about your head's position and movements, in relation to the ground or floor of your home, whether you are in the bathroom, in the kitchen or in the living room.

The vestibular system is divided into a central and peripheral system. It has a sensory and motor component to help you sense and perceive motion. It also provides messages regarding the movement of your head. It also gives information to stabilize the eyes in maintaining your gaze, with or without head movement.

To put it simply, your vestibular system aids the brain to coordinate numerous jobs, while you're walking, standing up, or reaching for something.

Visual system (brain and eyes): Your vision helps your balance because it shows where you are in relation to other objects, inside or outside the house.

Position-sensing nerves: These nerves, called proprioceptors, located in peripheral areas of the body, such as the legs, help you balance your body. They are embedded in your muscles, tendons, and joints to help you move around the house or outside, without stumbling or bumping into certain objects.

3 Things to Remember

Stability exercises should be based on these moves:

Exercising while seated: When you are sitting on a chair, your lower body has enough support, so you will be safe in your workout, doing your foot and hand movements.

Standing while exercising: When you stand to exercise, you will move your whole body that has no support. So let the body balance itself to avoid a fall, like your toes grip the floor or sole of your shoes or slippers, to have a steadier standing or walking. How can you this move? Curl and strengthen the toes to have a strong grip.

Standing in a wide stance: That is, let the two feet be wide apart to have the proper positioning of both feet towards a safe and effective exercise while standing.

In this way, you can increase your base of support for your body's balancing and stability.

Where Is the Sense of Balance?

"Your sense of balance is based in the brain. The brain integrates information from your inner ear organs, vision, and nerve endings and feelings in the feet, muscles, and joints, all the way up the spine," says Dr. Steven Rauch, medical director of the Balance and Vestibular Center at Harvard-affiliated Massachusetts Eye and Ear.

Rauch was quoted by Heidi Godman, Executive Editor, *Harvard Health Newslette*r, in an article published in the newsletter.

2 Types of Balance

The two types of balance are *static balance,* referring to the balance while you're standing still, and the *dynamic balance,* that you do while you are in motion or moving.

Clearly, the answers to balance problems is doing different proper exercises, and eating a balanced semi-plant-based diet (more plant foods than animal foods) to be healthy.

As Albert Einstein said: "Life is like riding a bicycle. To keep your balance, keep moving."

Other Things That Cause Falls

Many things can cause falls, including:

- Certain conditions such as diabetes, heart disease, or problems with your thyroid and diseased blood vessels
- Mild cognitive impairment or certain types of dementia in older adults
- Taking many medications. some of which cause side effects, like dizziness or confusion
- Safety hazards at home or community living environments
- Too much blood pressure drops when you suddenly get up from bed or from sitting (called postural hypotension)
- Rushing to the toilet, if you have overactive bladder or incontinence issue
- Painful or injured feet

Different Type of Balance Exercises

The simple but good exercises that you can do, are usually done after you wake up in the morning include the following:

- Stretching
- Tai chi (Chinese exercise)
- Toe gripping
- Balance Exercises

Before you embark on an exercise regimen, consult with your doctor on what types of exercise you can do, based on your physical fitness. You do this for safety concerns.

1. Stretching

Stretching, like any other simple and easy exercises can help you improve your balance and reduce your risk of falls, due to weak legs and buckling knees.

The beauty of it is, you can do your stretching anytime and anywhere, whether at home, in your office or outdoors. It's good to have better flexibility, in letting the joints move freely in whatever directions.

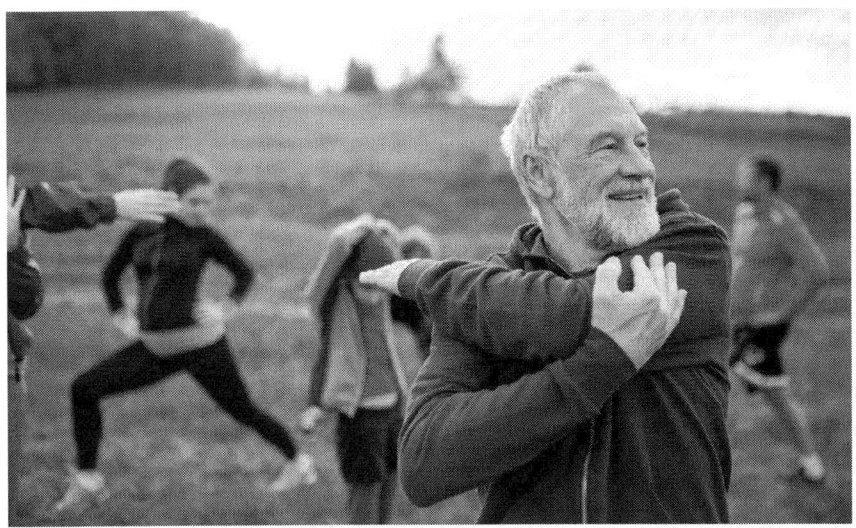

An Old Man Doing Stretching (Photo Credit: Shutterstock)

Benefits of Stretching

- Enable your muscles to work most efficiently
- Reduce your risk of falling that may result in injuries, broken bones, or even death
- Raise your blood flow in legs, hands, and the whole body

Before you do stretching, you must consult with your doctor on what kind of stretching you can do based on your physical condition, particularly if you have any chronic diseases. And you must do it in a safe way. The important thing is, to maintain your mobility and independence as you age.

2. Tai Chi Exercise

Tai chi, originally a Chinese exercise, and sometimes called "shadowboxing," is now practiced world-wide, from Asia to the Americas.

Tai Chi is a low-impact moving medications, involving slow movements of hands and feet, resulting in good blood flow, flexibility, and strength.

The low-impact moving meditation involves standing and balancing. The postures flow together without pause, doing slow, graceful dances that keep your whole body in action.

Since it's very low-impact exercise, it puts minimal stress on joints and muscles.

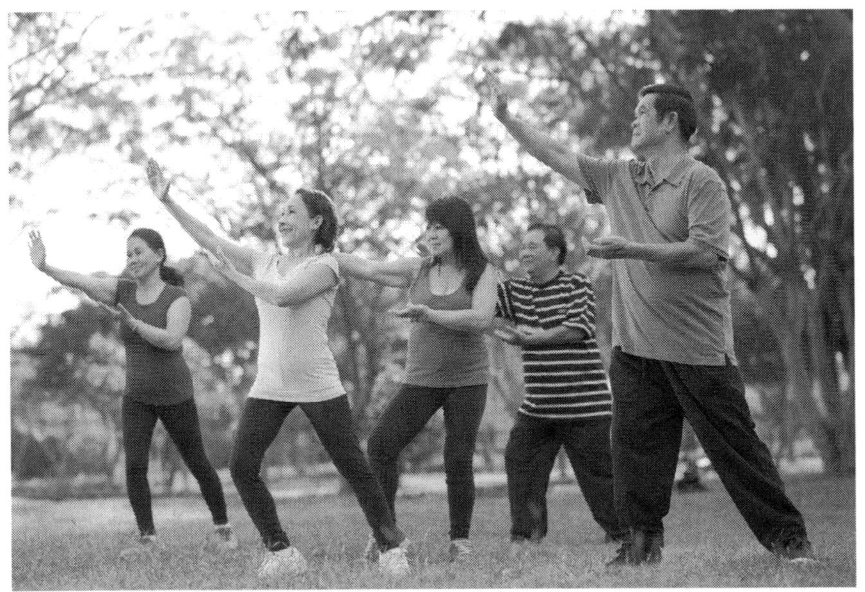

A Group of People Practicing Tai Chi

Photo Credit: Shutterstock

Components of Tai Chi

- Mindful Movements, a gentle exercise that moves, relaxes and stretches the body.
- Correct breathing that triggers de-stressing effects
- Increases circulation and energy, and enhances the body's natural healing process.
- Self-applied massage, stimulating energy and circulating blood flow throughout the whole body
- Meditation that relaxes the body and calms the emotions.

Benefits of Tai Chi

- Strengthens the muscles and bones to minimize risk of falls
- Increases blood circulation and energy
- Reduces high blood pressure

- Makes the glute muscles and pelvic floor stronger and flexible. (Glute muscles are located in your buttocks, with the *gluteus maximus*, giving shape in this body's area. The pelvic floor is a group of muscles that form a sling or hammock across the pelvic floor.

Names of Toes

The different names of toes include:

- Big toe (first finger or "hallux")
- Second toe or "digitus secundus peis"
- Third toe
- Fourth toe
- Fifth toe (or little finger)

The best well-known toes are the big toe and the little toe. The big toe, in any activity requiring balance, is the most important, among the toes, in playing its role in the foot's arch stabilization in times of joint mobility.

5. Toe Gripping

Toe gripping plays an important role in balancing of the body while standing, walking, or running. It is because the toes provide good posture, and balance and support your body weight

As Leonardo da Vinci once said, "The human foot is a masterpiece of engineering and a work of art."

Yes, that's true. For example, when your feet hit the floor (if you're barefooted) you'll notice that when each foot hits the house floor or ground outdoor, the feet distort and widen.

Why? Because they adapt to the unknown surface condition. Particularly, the toes grip, claw or clench the surface of anything, curling and strengthening themselves to have a better hold of the things, such as the floor or soles of slippers and shoes. This happens whether you are underweight or overweight, or you have a healthy weight.

To describe toe gripping, the process involves several muscles, including the parts that are called *flexor pollicis brevis, brevis, flexor pollicis longus,* and other muscles.

It may be considered that the toes are the best parts of the body in coordination with the whole lower body, that you can use to balance yourself, for stability and prevention of the occurrence of any falls.

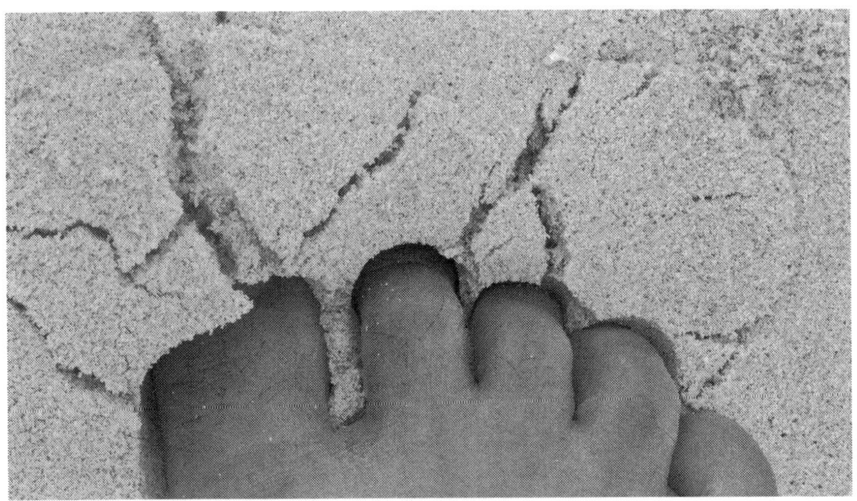

Photo Shows Toes Gripping the Sand

Photo Credit: Shutterstock

6. Toe Separators

What is a toe separator or spacer? A toe separator serves the purpose of keeping the different toes from rubbing each other, giving too much pressure to each other. The separator, also called spacer, goes between all of the toes. Needless to stay, its purpose is to make it sure that it won't move or shift when you use it. The spacer, by wearing it, provides balance. Not only that, it can prevent pain from corns, calluses, bunions, and blisters. In this way, there won't be any friction between each toe.

One other important thing. when the toes are slightly separated, you'll have a wider base to have a steadier balance and mobility, while standing still, walking, or running.

Usually, silicon is used for making toe separators. Silicon is a plastic that is considered as a member of rubber family, a hybrid between a synthetic rubber and a synthetic plastic polymer.

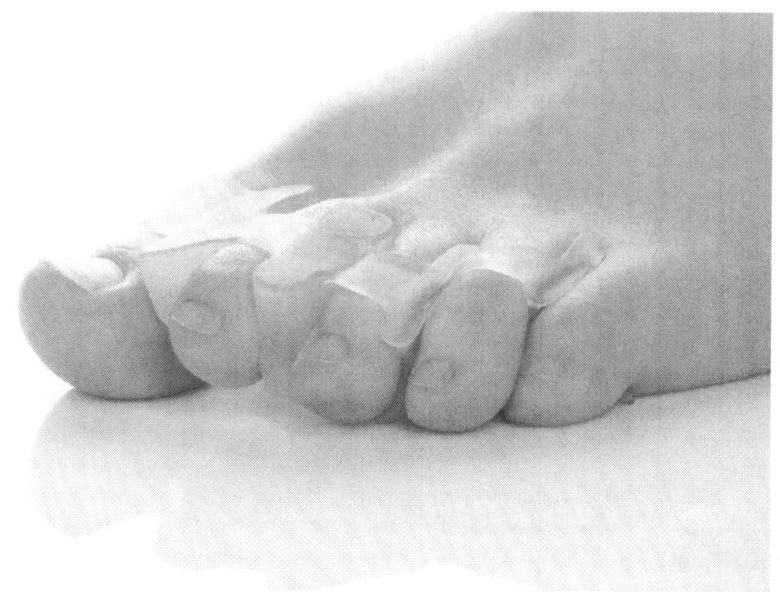

A Sample of a Toe Separator

Photo Credit: Shutterstock

First Line of Defense Against Falls

Actually there are at least two factors that can be used as the first and best defense against falls.

- Elimination of fall hazards
- Hand bars in the shower room or along the hallways or walking spaces for patient rehabilitation in hospitals.
- Toe gripping

Elimination of fall hazards: Fall hazards mean the things like pieces of rugs, crowded halls, unorganized furniture, not well-lighted rooms and hallways that can make residents trip and stumble.

So the best way is to organized your home, eliminating these fall hards.

Hand bars: Hand bars provide safety for the elderly in the shower area and proper spaces at home and in hospitals.

Toe gripping: In many or most nursing homes (if not all,) they offer toe gripping training in their facility for their residents.

My Journey: Imbalance

Yes, I had a fall in the bathroom several months ago. And it happened again for the second time, while I was turning to go to the kitchen. It was a frightening thing! That was really a wake up call for me: Improve my balance or else I will end up as a disabled person tied to my bed, forever.

So I did a research on how I could improve my balance. And what an amazing thing to discover the steps that I should do. That is, I must strengthen my legs, knees, and feet to have a steadier standing still, sitting, or walking.

Do We Need to Undergo Physical Therapy to Improve Balance?

And you know what? I requested my primary doctor to issue an order for therapy sessions at a local physical therapy clinic. Up to now, I'm doing balance-improving exercises at the Premiere Care Physical Therapy clinic in Sterling Heights, Michigan.

Dr. Andrew Afante, DPT, a Doctor of Physical Therapy and the owner and chief physical therapist of the clinic, has been teaching and training me the most effective exercises to make my feet and legs, hands, and the whole body stronger. All types of muscles must work. Yes, I enjoy all the balance exercises, although it was hard for me in the beginning. And I have noticed that I have been continuously improving my imbalance.

If you are an elderly and have balance problems, you may go to a local physical therapy clinic in your area and inquire if you are eligible to undergo the therapy for imbalance to be approved by your insurance. Just google "physical therapy clinic near me." I think that's easy to do. I did it, too. Before enrolling in a physical therapy program, you should verify if your insurance will pay for it. If not, you should be willing to pay for these imbalance exercises.

Yes, you can do many things at home or in a physical therapy clinic, to solve balance problems, through the means of doing proper exercises for that purpose. It's because the more we grow older, the more we will experience unsteadiness of our body while doing everyday activities. Remember, any falls can result in catastrophic events: with broken hips and bones, leading to your total disability. It's scary!

My Journey: Good News!

I must confess that since I started doing balance exercises at home and later at the physical therapy clinic mentioned above, I have not had any falls since I had two falls months ago in the toilet and outside the toilet. I think physical therapy works for me, and possibly it can work for you, too! Why don't you try to know if it's the right step for you if you are an elderly with imbalance problem?

Nowadays, before I go to the clinic (two or three times a week only), as soon as I wake up at 5.00 a.m., at home, I do exercises that Ive been doing at the physical therapy clinic. The whole workouts last for about 30 minutes every day, week after week. Daily, I also do my 3-session moderate-intensity walking outside, or on the treadmill at home to lower my blood sugar (yes, no diabetes medicine) and raise my heart rate for a stronger and efficient heart. What a joy to do this walking. I feel great!

Warning to Old People and Athletes!

For the past several years, many people do high-intensity exercises to be healthy by losing weight to be fit. Too much such exercises, for instance, like heavy lifting, can damage the different body muscles, leading to what is called rhabdomyolysis. This disease or condition, breaks down muscle cells, causing the release of a substance into the bloodstream, which may lead to kidney failure.

Dr. Chad Asplund, a Mayo Clinic sports medicine physician, points out that athletes at any level should know about rhabdomyolysis.

My reader, good luck to you in your exercise journey.

Have a nice day! And, enjoy life!

Final Thoughts

This new book, *Reversing Type 2 Diabetes, Kidney Disease, and Heart Disease: Exposing Old Age Secrets to Living in Your 90s, by Veltisezar Bautista by* Veltisezar Bautista, took the author almost five years to research, write, and publish the book. Now, this newly updated and expanded edition, 2 books in 1, is in your hands

I thought I could not have it published. But I did. I based the book on my disease journey and extensive research.

Why?

Because I desired that I would publish the original edition, only after I could have stopped, reversed, and put my diabetes into prolonged remission. I have also reversed and put my kidney disease into remission. Not only that, I reversed the severity of my heart failure and stabilized it into a better shape after several years. I would not dare to have this book published if I failed in managing my three diseases: type 2 diabetes, kidney disease, and heart disease. What will readers say if I didn't do it?

Not only that! I had an heart attack and survived it, when I was 63; now I'm in my 90s, the dream of my life. So also I have now I have accomplished my other dream: to live into my 90s.

All my secrets to reversing my three major diseases and being able to reach my 90s have been realized. You can use my secrets, so that you can do the same things that I did.

Yes, I did it! I based my disease reversal strategies on science and what modern technologies and other practical methods that can treat my unhealthy body. Against all odds, I have realized my dream of having a long life, at least, in my 90s.

I have revealed to you my success story. I've told you about my mistakes and accomplishments in life, dreams, and hopes, not to brag but to share the practical steps I formulated to reverse and put my type 2 diabetes and kidney disease into remission and to continue stabilizing my heart disease into a better condition.

I have given you all the tools you need to know my secrets to reaching the 90s and reversing your prediabetes, type 2 diabetes, kidney disease, heart disease, or whatever illnesses you may have resulted from major diabetes complications.

I also reached the 90s, in spite of the fact, that I have been afflicted with so many diseases and conditions.

The question is: When will you use the ideas, steps, and principles contained in this book?

What do you think of this book? Is it informative? Does it contain all the information you should know? Did the author provide you with clear explanations of complex things?

You may post on Amazon.com an honest review of the book if you want. In that way, other people with these diseases will know that a book like this exists. I hope that many people worldwide can benefit from this guide's tips, strategies, and other valuable information.

Thank you for reading this book. Enjoy life and be happy!

Statement of Declaration and Affirmation

December 16, 2023

State of Michigan

U.S.A.

To Whom It May Concern:

I, Veltisezar B. Bautista, in my 90s, solemnly and sincerely declare and affirm that the signature on this page is my signature and that every statement in the book about my longevity, type 2 diabetes, kidney disease, and heart disease is the truth and nothing but the truth.

Veltisezar B. Bautista

References & Recommended Reading

(Note: If you find any wrong links because of moving or deletion, type the article title and the institution's name to see the subject matter you are looking for.)

Chapter 1: The Secrets to My Living and Kicking at Age 88

Chapter 2: The Enigma of Insulin Resistance

MedicalNewsToday
http:/www.medicalnewstoday.com/articles/305567
What to Know About Insulin Resistance

Chapter 3: Prediabetes: If You Can't Stop It, You're Bound for Trouble!

Centers for Disease Control and Prevention (CD0
https://www.cdc.gov/diabetes/basics/prediabetes.html
Prediabetes – Your Chance to Prevent Type 2 Diabetes

EndocrineWeb
https://www.endocrineweb.com/conditions/pre-diabetes/pre-diabetes
What is Prediabetes? Here's What You Need to Know

DiabetesInControl.com
https://www.diabetesincontrol.com/simple-cure-for-remission-of-prediabetes/
Simple Cure for Remission of Prediabetes

Chapter 4: Type 2 Diabetes and Its Complications

EndocrineWeb
https://www.endocrineweb.com/conditions/type-2-diabetes/type-2-diabetes-complications
Type 2 Diabetes Complications

Diabetes Care of the American Diabetes Association
https://floridachest.com/pulmonary-blog/how-diabetes-impacts-your-lung-health
How Diabetes Impacts Your Lung Health

PAR
Pulmonary Associates of Richmond, Virginia
https://paraccess.com/diabetes-and-your-lungs/
Diabetes and Your Lungs

Healthline
https://www.healthline.com/health/type-2-diabetes/long-term-effects-prevention#short-term-complications
Type 2 Diabetes Complications and How to Prevent Them

MedicineNet.Com
https://www.medicinenet.com/blood_pressure_chart_reading_by_age/article.htm
Normal Blood Pressure by Age

Mayo Clinic
https://www.mayoclinic.org/healthy-lifestyle/nutrition-and-healthy-eating/in-depth/water/art-20044256
Water: How Much Should You Drink Every Day?

Chapter 5: Can Prediabetes and Type 2 Diabetes Be Reversed and Put into Remission?

Diabetes.co.UK
https://www.diabetes.co.uk/reversing-diabetes.html
Reversing Type 2 Diabetes

Diabetes.org.UK
http://www.diabetes.org.uk/guide-to-diabetes/managing-your-diabetes/treating-your-diabetes/type2-diabetes-remission
Diabetes Remission

Healthline
https://www.google.com/search?client=firefox-b-1-d&q=Emergency+Highs%3A+How+to+Lower+Blood+Sugar+Quickly
Emergency Highs: How to Lower Blood Sugar Quickly

Diabetes.co.UK
https://www.diabetes.co.uk/reversing-diabetes.html
Reversing Type 2 Diabetes

PMC
U.S. National Institute of Health
https://www.ncbi.nlm.nih.gov/pmc/articles/PMC6520897/
Reversing Type 2 Diabetes

Chapter 6: Pancreas Islets Transplant for Type 1 Diabetes; Next, Pig Islets?

Centers for Disease Control and Prevention (CDC)
https://www.cdc.gov/diabetes/basics/type1.html
Type 1 Diabetes

Medpage Today
https://www.medpagetoday.com/endocrinology/type1diabetes/92126
FDA Panel: Pancreatic Islet Transplant Should Be Option for T1D

Verywell Health
https://www.verywellhealth.com/islet-cell-transplant-type-1-diabetes-5094749
Islet Cell Transplant Helps One Woman Become Insulin Independent

Diabetes Research Connection
https://diabetesresearchconnection.org/pancreatic-islet-cells/
Advances in Pancreatic Islet Cell Transplantation

Medical University of South Carolina
https://muschealth.org/medical-services/ddc/patients/gi-surgery/chronic-pancreatitis-surgery/islet-cell-transplant-surgery
Islet Cell Transplant Surgery

StateNews.com
https://www.statnews.com/2019/08/27/islet-cells-transplant-type1-diabetes/
Transplanting Islet Cells Can Fix Brittle Diabetes, Why Isn't It Available in the U.S.?

WebMD
https://www.webmd.com/diabetes/islet-cell-transplantation
Islet Cell Transplantation for the Treatment of Diabetes

Islet Cell Research & Transplant Centers in the US
UCSF (University of California San Francisco)
https://transplantsurgery.ucsf.edu/conditions--procedures/islet-transplant-for-type-1-diabetes.aspx
Islet Transplant for Type 1 Diabetes

PMC
U.S. Institute of Health
https://www.ncbi.nlm.nih.gov/pmc/articles/PMC6345654/
Current State and Future Evolution of Pancreatic Islet Transplantation

Chapter 7: How to Reverse and Put Kidney Disease into Remission

Mayo Clinic
https://www.mayoclinic.org/diseases-conditions/chronic-kidney-disease/symptoms-causes/syc-20354521

PMC

U.S. National Library of Medicine

National Institute of Health

http://www.ncbi.nlm.nih.gov/pmc/articles/PMC5029805

Chronic Kidney Disease in Primary Care: Outcomes after Five Years in a Prospective Cohort Study

National Kidney Foundation
https://www.kidney.org/professionals/CKDGuideline
What's New About the New CKD Guideline?

National Kidney Foundation
https://www.kidney.org/content/10-common-habits-that-may-harm-your-kidneys
10 Common Habits That May Harm Your Kidneys

National Kidney Foundation
http://www.kidney.org/newsletter/what-difference-between-scr-egfr-acr-and-bun
What Is the Difference Between sCr, eGFR, ACR, and BUN?

National Kidney Foundation

https:/www.kidney.org/atoz/content/ckd-diet-how-much-protein-right-amount
CKD: How Much Protein Is the Right Amount?

National Kidney Foundation
https://www.kidney.org/news/ekidney/october11/top5
Top 5 Most Important Kidney Health Numbers

References and Recommended Reading

Kidney Cars
https://www.davita.com/education/ckd-life/lifestyle-changes/walking-an-ideal-exercise-for-people-with-kidney-disease
Walking Your Way to Healthier Kidneys

Healthline
https://www.healthline.com/nutrition/foods-to-avoid-with-kidney-disease#L-Dark-colored-soda
The 20 Best Foods for People With Kidney Disease

Medscape
https://www.medscape.com/viewarticle/864043
Remission Common in British Kidney Disease Patients

Durham Nephrology Associates, PA
https://www.durhamnephrology.com/can-you-reverse-kidney-damage/
Can You Reverse Kidney Damage?

American Kidney Fund
https://www.kidneyfund.org/kidney-disease/chronic-kidney-disease-ckd/stages-of-chronic-kidney-disease/
Stages of Chronic Kidney Disease (CKD)

Heart in Health Care
https://www.heartsinhealthcare.com/kidney-disease/is-remission-of-kidney-failure-possible.html
Is Remission of Kidney Failure Possible

National Kidney Foundation
https://www.kidney.org/professionals/CKDGuideline
What's New About the New CKD Guideline?

National Kidney Foundation
https://www.kidney.org/content/10-common-habits-that-may-harm-your-kidneys
10 Common Habits That May Harm Your Kidneys

National Kidney Foundation
https:/www.kidney.org/atoz/content/ckd-diet-how-much-protein-right-amount
CKD: How Much Protein Is the Right Amount?

(Note: If you find any wrong links because of moving or deletion, google the article title and the institution's name to see the subject matter you are looking for.)

Science Daily
https://www.sciencedaily.com/releases/2014/05/140515173331.htm
Walking May Have Profound Benefits for Patients with Kidney Disease

Chapter 8: Can You Reverse Your Heart Disease Severity and Put It into Better Condition?

Centers for Disease Control and Prevention
https://www.cdc.gov/heartdisease/prevention.htm
Heart Disease

Mayo Clinic
https://www.mayoclinic.org/disease-conditions/heart-failure/diagnosis-treatment/c dc-20373148
Treatment of Heart Failure

Medical News Today
https://www.medicalnewstoday.com/articles/326514#how-to-lower-blood-pressure
What to Know About Blood Pressure Rates After Exercising

Australian Eggs.org
https://www.australianeggs.org.au/healthcare-professionals/topics/cholesterol-and-heart-health
Eggs, Choleserol & Heart Health

American Heart Association
https://www.heart.org/en/health-topics/consumer-healthcare/what-is-cardiovascular-disease
What Is Cardiovascular Disease?

CNN
http://edition.cnn.com/2008/HEALTH/conditions/11/11/sleep.blood.pressure/index.html
Less sleep in older adults linked to heart attack, stroke risk

References and Recommended Reading

John Hopkins Medicine
https://www.hopkinsmedicine.org/health/conditions-and-diseases/congestive-heart-failure-prevention-treatment-and-research
Congestive Heart Failure: Prevention, Treatment, and Research

Verywell Health

https://baptisthealth.net/baptist-health-news/diabetes-drug-can-treat-or-reverse-heart-failure-promising-study-finds/
Diabetes Drug Can Treat and Reverse Heart Failure, Study Finds

Centers for Disease Control (CDC)
https://www.cdc.gov/heartdisease/heart_attack.htm
Heart Attack Symptoms, Risk, and Recovery

PMC
U.S. National Institute of Health
https://www.ncbi.nlm.nih.gov/pmc/articles/PMC5324874/
CRT-D or CRT-P in CRT-indicated patients?

(Note: If you find any wrong links because of moving or deletion, google the article title and the institution's name to see the subject matter you are looking for.)

MedicineNet.Com
https://www.medicinenet.com/blood_pressure_chart_reading_by_age/article.htm
Normal Blood Pressure by Age

Johns Hopkins Medicine
https://www.hopkinsmedicine.org/health/conditions-and-diseases/congestive-heart-failure-prevention-treatment-and-research
Treatment for Congestive Heart Failure

American Heart Association
https://www.heart.org/en/health-topics/heart-failure/warning-signs-of-heart-failure
Symptoms of Heart Failure

Healthline
https://www.healthline.com/nutrition/heart-healthy-foods
15 Incredibly Heart-Healthy Foods

Mayo Clinic
https://www.mayoclinic.org/diseases-conditions/heartburn/in-depth/heartburn-gerd/art-20046483
Heart Burn or Heart Attack: When to Worry

Verywell Health
https://www.verywellhealth.com/left-bundle-branch-block-lbbb-1745784
An Overview of Left Bundle Branch Block

Cleveland Clinic
https://my.clevelandclinic.org/health/treatments/16938-left-ventricular-reconstructive-surgery-modified-dor-procedure
Left Ventricular Reconstructive Surgery (Modified Dor Procedure)

National Institute of Health
https://www.researchgate.net/publication/271139559
Cardiac_Resynchronization_Therapy_History_Present_Status_and_Future_Directions
Cardiac Resynchronization Therapy

Healthline
https://www.healthline.com/health/heart-disease/exercise
Can Exercise Reverse or Prevent Heart Diseases?

(Note: If you find any wrong links because of moving or deletion, google the article title and the institution's name to see the subject matter you are looking for.)

Eat This, Not That!

https://www.eatthis.com/foods-that-cause-heart-disease/

The Most Common Foods That Raise Your Heart Attack Risk

CDC Centers for Disease Control and Prevention

https://www.cdc.gov/diabetes/library/features/diabetes-and-heart.html

Diabetes and Your Heart

Mayo Clinic

https://www.mayoclinic.org/ejection-fraction/expert-answers/faq-20058286

What Does the Term Ejection Fraction' Mean? What Does It Measure?

References and Recommended Reading

MedicalNewsToday

https://www.medicalnewstoday.com/articles/319649

Severe Heart Failure May Be Reversible

John Hopkins Medicine

https://www.hopkinsmedicine.org/health/conditions-and-diseases/congestive-heart-failure-prevention-treatment-and-research

Congestive Heart Failure: Prevention, Treatment, and Research

Cleveland Clinic

https://health.clevelandclinic.org/what-does-a-heart-attack-really-feel-like/

What Does a Heart Attack Really Feel Like?
National Instute of Health

National Institute of Aging
https://www.nia.nih.gov/health/high-blood-pressure-and-older-adults
High Blood Pressure and Older Adults

WebMD

https://www.webmd.com/heart-disease/news/20110427/heart-attacks-in-the-morning-are-more-severe

Heart Attacks in the Morning Are More Severe

Chapter 9: Walking System: Why It Works for Diabetes, Kidney Disease, and Heart Disease

Healthline
https://www.healthline.com/health-news/seniors-advised-to-walk-more-briskly

Older Adults Advised to Walk More Briskly
Just Walkers
https://justwalkers.com/pages/using-a-cane
Using a Can – Walking Cane User Guide

Centers for Disease Control and Prevention (CDC)
https://www.cdc.gov/physicalactivity/basics/measuring/heartrate.htm
Target Heart Rate and Estimated Maximum Heart Rate

Science Daily
https://www.sciencedaily.com/releases/2014/05/140515173331.htm
Walking May Have Profound Benefits for Patients with Kidney Disease

Healthline
https://www.healthline.com/health-news/seniors-advised-to-walk-more-briskly
Older Adults Advised to Walk More Briskly

Centers for Disease Control and Prevention (CDC)
https://www.cdc.gov/physicalactivity/basics/measuring/heartrate.htm
Target Hear Rate and Estimated Maximum Heart Rate

Chapter 10: 6 Nutrients That Make Your Body Alive

Healthline
https://www.healthline.com/health/food-nutrition/simple-carbohydrates-complex-carbohydrates
Simple Carbohydrates vs. complex carbohydrates

American Heart Association
https://www.heart.org/en/healthy-living/healthy-eating/eat-smart/fats/dietary-fats
Dietary Fats

Chapter 11: Best Diets for 2022 for Diabetes, Heart Disease, and Good Health

U.S. News & World Report
https://health.usnews.com/best-diet/dash-diet
What Is a DASH Diet?

Healthline
https://www.healthline.com/nutrition/flexitarian-diet-guide
The Flexitarian Diet: A Detailed Beginner's Guide

U.S. Institute of Health
MedlinePlus
https://medlineplus.gov/ency/patientinstructions/000110.htm
Mediterranean Diet

References and Recommended Reading

(Note: If you find any wrong links because of moving or deletion, google the article title and the institution's name to see the subject matter you are looking for.)

Chapter 12: Semi-Plant-Based Diet: Best for Meat Eaters with T2D, CKD, and Heart Disease

Popular Science
https://www.popsci.com/plant-protein-healthier/
Here's Even More Evidence That Plant Protein Is Better for You Than Animal protein

Everyday Health
https://www.everydayhealth.com/diet-nutrition/scientific-benefits-following-plant-based-diet/
9 Scientific Benefits of Following a Plant-Based Diet

Healthline
https://www.healthline.com/nutrition/plant-based-diet-guide
What Is a Whole-Foods, Plant-Based Diet

MedicalNewsToday
https://www.medicalnewstoday.com/articles/322827
What Is the Difference Between Animal and Plant Proteins?

U.S. Institute of Health
https://www.ncbi.nlm.nih.gov/pmc/articles/PMC5503680/
Diet and Diabetic Disease: Plant vs Animal Protein

Healthline
https://www.healthline.com/nutrition/7-nutrients-you-cant-get-from-plants
7 Nutrients That You Can't Get from Plants

Healthline
https://www.healthline.com/nutrition/animal-vs-plant-protein#TOC_TITLE_HDR_3
Animal vs. Plant Protein—What's the Difference?

Healthline
https://www.healthline.com/nutrition/10-foods-almost-pure-protein
10 Foods That Are Almost Pure Protein

(Note: If you find any wrong links because of moving or deletion, google the article title and the institution's name to see the subject matter you are looking for.)

Chapter 13: Foods: Eat These, Not Those!

Every Day Health
https://www.everydayhealth.com/type-2-diabetes/best-fruits-for-diabetes/
8 Best Fruits for a Diabetes-Friendly Diet

American Diabetes Association
https://www.diabetes.org/healthy-living/recipes-nutrition/eating-well/non-starchy-vegetables
Non-Starchy Vegetables

Nestle Health Science
https://www.nestlehealthscience.com/understanding-glycemic-index-and-glycemic-load
Understanding Glycemic Index (GI) and Glycemic Load (GL)

Mayo Clinic
https://www.mayoclinic.org/fructose-intolerance/expert-answers/faq-20058097
Fructose Intolerance: Which Fruits to Avoid

Healthline
https://www.healthline.com/nutrition/low-carb-diet-for-diabetes
A Guide to Healthy Low-Carb Eating With Diabetes

Everyday Health
https://www.everydayhealth.com/type-2-diabetes/best-oatmeal-type-2-diabetes/
The Best Oatmeal for Type 2 Diabetes

Chapter 14: Rice and Whole Grains Feed the World

Grains & Legumes Nutrition Council
https://wholegrainscouncil.org/whole-grains-101/whole-grains-z
Types of Grains
Oldways Whole Grain Council
https://wholegrainscouncil.org/whole-grains-101/whole-grains-z
List of Whole Grain

healthline
https://www.healthline.com/nutrition/9-benefits-of-whole-grains
9 Health Benefits of Eating Whole Grains

Healthline
https://www.healthline.com/nutrition/ezekiel-bread
Why Ezekiel Bread Is Healthiest Bread You Can Eat

Very Well Fit
https://www.verywellfit.com/are-sprouted-grains-gluten-free-562843
Are Sprouted Grains Gluten-Free?

Chapter 15: Fatty Fish: Are They Good for You or Not?

News Medical Life Sciences
https://www.news-medical.net/health/Fatty-Fish-and-Type-II-Diabetes.aspx
Fatty Fish and Diabetes

American Heart Association
https://www.heart.org/en/healthy-living/healthy-eating/eat-smart/fats/fish-and-omega-3-fatty-acids
Fatty Fish and Omega 3 Acids

Men's Health
https://www.menshealth.com/nutrition/a27150227/protein-in-fish
These Are the 14 Fish That are Highest in Protein

Men's Journal
https://www.mensjournal.com/food-drink/top-10-fish-proteins-ranked/
Top 10 Fish Protein: The Top Fish Proteins, Ranked

SF Gate
https://healthyeating.sfgate.com/much-protein-fish-have-6418.html
How Much Protein Does Fish Have?

Chapter 16. Which Bread Is Good for You?

Real Simple.com
https://www.realsimple.com/food-recipes/cooking-tips-techniques/whole-wheat-whole-grain-breads-0
What's the Difference Between Whole Wheat, Whole Grain, and Multigrain Bread?

Oola.com
https://www.oola.com/life-in-flavor/2390731/the-different-types-of-bread-from-around-the-world/
The Different Types of Bread From Around the World

Chapter 17: Drinking Water, Coffee, and Tea: Their Benefits and Risks

MedicalNewsToday
https://www.medicalnewstoday.com/articles/318619
What Happens If You Drink Too Much Water?

Healthline
https://www.healthline.com/health/ph-of-drinking-water
What pH Should My Drinking Water Be?

Centers for Disease Control and Prevention (CDC)
https://www.cdc.gov/healthywater/drinking/home-water-treatment/water-filters.html
Choosing Home Water Filters & Other Treatment Systems

Healthline
https://www.healthline.com/nutrition/carbonated-water-good-or-bad
Carbonated (Sparkling) Water: Good or Bad?

MedicalNewsToday
https://www.medicalnewstoday.com/articles/313681
Is Alkaline Water Good for You?

Consumer Report
https://consumerreportsguide.com/water-ionizer/
Best Ionized Water Filter Machines

References and Recommended Reading

Healthline
https://www.healthline.com/health/food-nutrition/alkaline-water-benefits-risks
Alkaline Water: Benefits and Risks

WebMD
https://www.webmd.com/diabetes/daily-control-19/diet/slideshow-diabetes-friendly-drinks
What You Can Drink, Besides Water, When You Have Diabetes

Water Research Center
https://water-research.net/index.php/ph
The ph of Water

Good Housekeeping
https://www.goodhousekeeping.com/health/diet-nutrition/a46956/how-much-water-should-i-drink/
How Much Water Should You Drink Every Day, According to Experts

Healthline

https://www.healthline.com/health/food-nutrition/alkaline-water-benefits-risks
Alkaline Water: Benefits and Risks

CaffeineInformer.com

https://www.google.com/search?client=firefox-b-1-d&q=Dunkin%27+Donuts+Coffee+Caffeine+Content+Guide
Dunkin' Donuts Coffee Caffeine Content Guide

Mayo Clinic
https://www.mayoclinic.org/healthy-lifestyle/nutrition-and-healthy-eating/in-depth/caffeine/art-20049372
Caffeine Content for Coffee, Tea, Soda, and More

McCafe Coffee
https://www.caffeineinformer.com/mccafe-coffee-caffeine-content
McCafe Coffee Caffeine Content

American Heart Association
https://www.heart.org/en/news/2018/09/28/is-coffee-good-for-you-or-not
Is Coffee Good for You or Not?

Caffeine Informer
https://www.caffeineinformer.com/coffee-and-diabetes
Coffee, Caffeine and Type 2 Diabetes

Mayo Clinic
https://www.mayoclinic.org/diseases-conditions/type-2-diabetes/expert-answers/blood-sugar/faq-20057941
Caffeine: Does It Affect Blood Sugar?

CaffeineInformer
https://www.caffeineinformer.com/coffee-and-diabetes
Coffee, Caffeine and Type 2 Diabetes

WebMD
https://www.webmd.com/diabetes/diabetes-and-caffeine
How Does Caffeine Affect Your Blood Sugar?

Caffeine Informer
https://www.caffeineinformer.com/coffee-and-diabetes
Coffee, Caffeine, and Type 2 Diabetes

MedicalNewsToday
https://www.medicalnewstoday.com/articles/311180
How Does Coffee Affect Diabetes?

Chapter 18: Sweeteners: Are They Good for Diabetes?

Healhline
https://www.healthline.com/nutrition/common-food-additives
12 Common Food Additives – Should You Avoid Them?

Ornish Living
http://www.ornish.com/zine/consume-stevia-small-quantities-negative-health-effects/
Why Should We Consume Stevia in Small Quantities? Are there Negative Health Effects?

International Food Information Council Foundation
https://www.google.com/search?client=firefox-b-1-d&q=has+sevia+been+approved+by+FDA+to+be+used+as+a+sweetener%3F
Re: SweetLeaf Stevia

International Food Information Council Foundation
https://www.google.com/search?client=firefox-b-1-d&q=has+sevia+been+approved+by+FDA+to+be+used+as+a+sweetener%3F
Re: SweetLeaf Stevia

(Note: If you find any wrong links because of moving or deletion, google the article title and the institution's name to see the subject matter you are looking for.)

Chapter 19: The Quest for Healthy Aging & Longevity

PRB
https://www.prb.org/resources/fact-sheet-aging-in-the-united-states/
Fact Sheet on Aging in the United States

MedlinePlus
https://medlineplus.gov/genetics/understanding/traits/longevity/
Is Longevity Determined by Genetics?

NIH News in Health
National Institute of Health
https://newsinhealth.nih.gov/2016/06/can-you-lengthen-your-life
Can You Lengthen Your Life?

Active for Life
https://activeforlife.com/tips-for-long-healthy-life/
10 Tips for a Long and Healthy Life from 90-yea-old Grandmothe

MedlinePlus
https://medlineplus.gov/genetics/understanding/traits/longevity/
Is Longevity Determined by Genetics?

Chapter 20: How to Live into Your 90s and Beyond

MedlinePlus
https://medlineplus.gov/genetics/understanding/traits/longevity/
Life Span Has Little to Do with Genes, Analysis of Large Ancestry Database Shows

Sixty&Me
https://sixtyandme.com/7-habits-to-help-you-live-long-and-prosper-into-your-80s-and-90s/
7 Habits to Help You Live Long and Prospr into Your 80s and 90s

Mcgregor
https://mcgregoramasa.org/2022/04/25/living-90-years-and-beyond/
Living 90 Years and Beyond

The Disabled World
https://www.disabled-world.com/fitness/longevity/#:~:text=Significant%20factors%20in%20life%20expectancy,%2C%20genetics%2C%20and%20lifestyle%20choices.
Longevit:y Extending Life Span Expectancy

MedlinePlus
https://medlineplus.gov/genetics/understanding/traits/longevity/
Life Span Has Little to Do with Genes, Analysis of Large Ancestry Database Shows

Trickle
https://trickle.app/drip/14897-its-important-to-differentiate-between-longevity-life-expectancy-lifespan-and-healthspan/
It's Important to Differentiate Between Longevity, Life Expectancy, Lifespan and Healthspan

Lifestyle
http://longevity.technology/lifestyle/how-to-live-longer-what-is-longevity-and-how-can-you-improve-it/
How to Live Longer: What IS Longevity and How Can You Improve it?

NIH National Library of Medicidne
PMC Pubmed Central
https://www.ncbi.nlm.nih.gov/pmc/articles/PMC3373258/
The Oldest Old and the 90+ Study

NIH in Health
National Institute of Health
https://newsinhealth.nih.gov/2016/06/can-you-lengthen-your-life
Can You Lengthen Your Life?

Chapter 21: Overcoming 8 Grand Challenges of Aging

Centers for Disease Control and Prevention
dc.gov/aging/pdf/perceptions_of_cog_hlth_factsheet.pdf
What Is a Healthy Brain? Research Explores Perceptions of Cognitive Health Among Diverse Older Adult

References and Recommended Reading

Chapter 22: Aging in Place or Elsewhere

TopTenReviews
https://www.toptenreviews.com/10-dangers-of-seniors-living-alone
5 Challenges of Seniors Living Alone, and How to Solve Them

A Place for Mom
https://www.aplaceformom.com/caregiver-resources/articles/senior-isolation-facts
Understanding the Shocking Facts About Senior Isolation

TopTenReviews
https://www.toptenreviews.com/10-dangers-of-seniors-living-alone
5 Challenges of Seniors Living Alone, and How to Solve Them

TopTenReviews
https://www.toptenreviews.com/10-dangers-of-seniors-living-alone
5 Challenges of Seniors Living Alone, and How to Solve Them

Senior Housing
https://www.helpguide.org/articles/senior-housing/independent-living-for-seniors.htm
Independent Living for Seniorsd

Aegis Living
https://www.aegisliving.com/where-to-begin/how-to-choose-a-community/what-is-skilled-nursing-care/
Five Types of Senior Care Communities

Centers for Disease Control and Prevention
dc.gov/aging/pdf/perceptions_of_cog_hlth_factsheet.pdf
What Is a Healthy Brain? Research Explores Perceptions of Cognitive Health Among Diverse Older Adults

NIH National Institute of Aging
https://www.nia.nih.gov/health/aging-place-growing-older-home
Aging in Place: Growing Older at home

Merck Manual
https://www.merckmanuals.com/professional/geriatrics/social-issues-in-older-adults/older-adults-living-alone
Older Adults Living Alone

NIH National Institute of Aging
https://www.nia.nih.gov/health/aging-place-growing-older-home
Aging in Place: Growing Older at home

NIH National Institute of Aging
https://www.nia.nih.gov/health/aging-place-growing-older-home
Aging in Place: Growing Older at home

PASSi
https://passi.us/2021/03/how-to-stay-in-your-home-as-long-as-possible/?gclid=EAIaIQobChMInJn8kNOF_AIVQ4NbCh2JNgwoEAAYAiAAEgKabvD_BwE
How to Stay in Your Home as Long as Possible

Retirement Living
https://www.retirementliving.com/arcd-community-typesDefinitions of Community Types of Community Living Types
Definitions of Community Types

Senior Living Blog
https://www.leisurecare.com/resources/what-are-independent-living-communities/
What Are Independent Living Communities?

Reach
https://www.reachcils.org/what-independent-living/
What Is Independent Living?

Helpguide.org
https://www.helpguide.org/articles/senior-housing/independent-living-for-seniors.htm
Independent Living for Seniors

Consumer Affairs
https://www.consumeraffairs.com/health/senior-living-options.html
10 Types of Senior Living Options

References and Recommended Reading

Aegis Living
https://www.aegisliving.com/where-to-begin/how-to-choose-a-community/what-is-skilled-nursing-care/
Five Types of Senior Care Communities

NIH National Institute of Aging
https://www.nia.nih.gov/health/aging-place-growing-older-home
Aging in Place: Growing Older at home

Chapter 23: 11 Senior Common Diseases & Disorders

Centers Disease Control and Prevention
https://www.cdc.gov/aging/publications/features/lonely-older-adults.html
Alzheimer's Disease and Healthy Aging

Centers for Disease Control and Prevention
dc.gov/aging/pdf/perceptions_of_cog_hlth_factsheet.pdf
What Is a Healthy Brain? Research Explores Perceptions of Cognitive Health Among Diverse Older Adults

World Health Organization
https://www.who.int/news-room/fact-sheets/detail/mental-health-of-older-adults
Mental Health of Older Adults

Mayo Clinic
https://www.mayoclinic.org/diseases-conditions/dementia/symptoms-causes/syc-20352013
Demantia

National Kidney Foundation
https://www.kidney.org/news/monthly/wkd_aging
Aging and Kidney Disease
Cleveland Clinic
https://my.clevelandclinic.org/health/diseases/9170-dementia
Dementia

PMC
National Library of Medicine
National Institute of Health
https://www.ncbi.nlm.nih.gov/pmc/articles/PMC5175057/#:~:text=As%20is%20seen%2C%20the%20most,and%20colorectal%20cancers%20in%20women.
Cancer in the Elderly

Download Wellness
https://www.downloadwellness.com/post/get-rid-of-tinnitus-with-massage-therapy#:~:text=Experts%20say%20that%20muscle%20and,%2C%20head%2C%20and%20jaw%20appropriately.
Get Rid of Tinnitus With Message Therapy

Chapter 24: Improving You Balance to Prevent Falls

Life Energy Foundation
https://www.thelifeenergyfoundation.org/components-of-a-fall-what-you-need-to-know?gclid=EAIaIQobChMIsYCN69TW_AIVo45bCh0m_wp3EAAYAiAAEgK5APD_BwE
Components of a Fall: What You Need to Know

John Hopkins Medicine

https://www.hopkinsmedicine.org/health/wellness-and-peventio/fall-prevention/fall-prevention-exercises

Fall Prevention: Balance Strength Exercises for Older Adults

MedicalNewsToday
https://www.medicalnewstoday.com/articles/balance-problems
Balance Problems: Causes, Prevention, and More

Mayo Clinic
https://www.mayoclinic.org/diseases-conditions/balance-problems/symptoms-causes/syc-20350474
Balance Problems

References and Recommended Reading

PMC
National Library of Medicine
U.S. Institute of Health
https://www.ncbi.nlm.nih.gov/pmc/articles/PMC8752848/
The Effect of Toe-grasping Exercises on Balance Ability in Home-based Rehabilitation: A Randomized Controlled Trial by Block Randomization

National Institute on Aging
National Institute of Health
https://www.nia.nih.gov/health/falls-and-fractures-older-adults-causes-and-prevention#:~:text=Age%2Drelated%20loss%20of%20muscle,all%20risk%20factors%20for%20falling.
Falls and Fractures in Older Adults: Causes and Prevention

PubMed
NIH National Library of Medicine
National Center for Biotechnology Information
National Institute of Health
The Effects of Toe Grip Training on Physical Performance and Cognitive Function of Nursing Home Residents

Index

Made in the USA
Las Vegas, NV
24 February 2024